W9-BKZ-387

STRANGER THAN FICTION

When Our Minds Betray Us

Also by Marc D. Feldman, M.D.—

Patient or Pretender: Inside the Strange World of Factitious Disorders
(authored with Charles V. Ford, M.D., and Toni Reinhold)

The Spectrum of Factitious Disorders (edited with Stuart J. Eisendrath, M.D.)

About the Authors

Marc D. Feldman, M.D., is Vice Chair for Clinical Services in the Department of Psychiatry and Behavioral Neurobiology of the University of Alabama at Birmingham (UAB). He is also Medical Director of the UAB Center for Psychiatric Medicine and is a recipient of an Exemplary Psychiatrist Award from the National Alliance for the Mentally Ill.

Jacqueline M. Feldman, M.D., is Associate Professor and Director of the Division of Public Psychiatry in the Department of Psychiatry and Behavioral Neurobiology at the University of Alabama at Birmingham. She is also Executive Director of the UAB Comprehensive Community Mental Health Center and Medical Director of the UAB Community Psychiatry Program. She has been awarded the Exemplary Psychiatrist Award of the National Alliance for the Mentally Ill.

Roxenne Smith, M.A., is a professional writer and gerontologist. A former research assistant at the University of South Florida, she has published articles in the areas of aging and mental health.

STRANGER THAN FICTION

When Our Minds Betray Us

Marc D. Feldman, M.D.,

and

Jacqueline M. Feldman, M.D.

With Roxenne Smith

Washington, DC
London, England

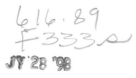

616.89
F333ρ
JY 28 '98

Note: The essential psychological issues in each case in this book reflect real-life events. The authors have, however, made ample changes to disguise the patients' identities, except when names and descriptions were already provided elsewhere in the scientific or general media.

The authors have exerted every effort to ensure that drug selection and dosage set forth in this text are in accord with current recommendations and practice at the time of publication. However, in view of ongoing research, changes in government regulations, and the constant flow of information relating to drug therapy and drug reactions, and because human and mechanical errors sometimes occur, the authors recommend that readers follow the advice of a physician directly involved in their care or that of a member of their family. The reader is also urged to check the package insert for each drug for any change in indications and dosage and for added warnings and precautions.

Books published by the American Psychiatric Press, Inc., represent the views and opinions of the individual authors and do not necessarily represent the policies and opinions of the Press or the American Psychiatric Association.

Copyright © 1998 Marc D. Feldman, M.D., and Jacqueline M. Feldman, M.D.
ALL RIGHTS RESERVED
Manufactured in the United States of America on acid-free paper
First Edition   01   00   99   98   4   3   2   1

American Psychiatric Press, Inc.
1400 K Street, N.W., Washington, DC   20005
www.appi.org

Library of Congress Cataloging-in-Publication Data

Feldman, Marc D., 1958–
    Stranger than fiction : when our minds betray us / Marc D. Feldman
and Jacqueline M. Feldman ; with Roxenne Smith.
        p.   cm.
    Includes bibliographical references and index.
    ISBN 0-88048-930-8
    1. Mental illness.   I. Feldman, Jacqueline M., 1953–
II. Smith, Roxenne, 1948–   .   III. Title.
    [DNLM: 1. Mental Disorders.   WM 140 F312s 1998]
RC454.F45   1998
616.89—dc21
DNLM/DLC
for Library of Congress   97-5481
                                                                              CIP

British Library Cataloguing in Publication Data
A CIP record is available from the British Library.

John Dewey Library
Johnson State College
Johnson, Vermont 0565(

*To Lee and Sara,
who bless us daily and doubly.*

*To Brian and Mim Anne,
whose love makes all the difference.*

CONTENTS

INTRODUCTION

What Is a Lie of the Mind?

The human head is bigger than the globe.
It conceives itself as containing more.
It can think and rethink itself and ourselves
from any desired point outside the gravitational
pull of the earth.
It starts by writing one thing and later reads
itself as something else.
The human head is monstrous.

—Günter Grass (1927–),
"Racing with the Utopias," *Die Zeit*

MARIA PLUCKED EVERY *other* flower petal when daydreaming about her love: "He loves me . . . he loves me . . . he loves me" was her mantra. No possibility ever of "he loves me . . . *not.*"

The object of her obsessive love was a regular customer at her bank. Something about his manner, his smile, his hand grazing hers as he exchanged deposit envelopes for receipts and cash at her window—*something* had convinced her that he was secretly mad about her.

In reality, nothing remotely personal characterized their transactions during more than two years of regular contact. But in Maria's "reality," their relationship was a smoldering romance that had to be hidden because of his marriage to the woman whose name appeared with his on his personal checks. Maria *knew* that the customer didn't love his wife the way he loved her—she could see it in his tender gazes—but she reasoned that he simply hadn't found the right time yet to confess his passion and divorce his wife.

Maria's preoccupation with their unspoken relationship led her to quit her job. Her work suffered from the constant longing, which in turn was heightened by her own husband's lack of affection. This would-be object of a secret admirer was actually suffering from a psychiatric syndrome—*erotomania*—that turned romantic daydreams into uncontrollable desires reflecting deep, unexpressed needs.

▌ The Mind Under Siege

Although mental illness rarely results in acts of senseless violence, it is precisely such swift and merciless actions that cause us to ask, *Why does thinking become so extreme? How does a person begin to accept these distorted beliefs as reality?* Such questions have become especially pressing in the wake of the April 1995 bombing of the Alfred P. Murrah Federal Building in Oklahoma City. Many have grappled with how a belief many of us share ("Government has too much influence") could snowball into the behavior of Timothy McVeigh, who was convicted of the bombing. News accounts have confirmed that his thinking went far beyond alternative political beliefs. Though he did not belong to a cult, his fanaticism became just as potent. Consumed with rage, he networked with others who reinforced his contorted thinking and his infatuation with firearms. Among the beliefs McVeigh and individuals like him share: that through an evil conspiracy Americans will soon be enslaved, computer chips implanted in their hands or buttocks to control them via orbiting satellites; that the markings on the backs of certain traffic signs are coded messages to help the conspirators' tanks invade; and that salt mines beneath Detroit hold Russian troops waiting to force a catastrophic United Nations takeover of the United States. Far from a simple curiosity or a reified phenomenon of interest only to psychiatrists, it appears to have been precisely this type of thinking that claimed 168 lives.

And the distorted thinking continues on, with new twists and inventions. Members of the radical right, for instance, quickly regrouped after the bombing to claim publicly that the federal government bombed its own building in a scurrilous, clandestine effort to justify its coming imposition of martial law. Thus, they believe, the stockpiling of weapons and the paramilitary training must proceed with even greater zeal.

As with erotomania, such paranoid thinking and many other psychiatric phenomena are explored in *Stranger Than Fiction: When Our Minds Betray Us*, our first joint writing project. Organized by types of symptoms and disorders, *Stranger Than*

Fiction invites you into a fascinating world where reality temporarily goes awry. With us as your guides, you will see and feel the world from a decidedly new vantage point. As we embark upon this educational mission, we will also show you that many of the lies of the mind resist clear-cut categories, for just as individuals are messy sums of their parts, so are the mental conditions that afflict them.

▌ Understanding the Lie of the Mind

Throughout this book, we will use the term *lies of the mind* as a metaphor for how our minds betray us. We define a lie of the mind as *a condition in which a person's thinking unintentionally becomes distorted.* Sometimes these "lies" arise from deep within us (e.g., delusions); at other times, they are induced by others unwittingly (e.g., mass hysteria) or more actively, though still not deliberately (e.g., false memory syndrome). Some lies of the mind harbor little consequence. Fans of Powerball and Lotto lottery games, for example, momentarily ignore the astronomical odds against winning the pot as they fork over their dollar bills. Other, more substantive lies of the mind critically distort and even come to dominate our lives. With the lottery, some individuals create a self-imposed financial ruin when they come to believe that their winning is preordained. Acting upon this delusional belief, they spend hand over fist in anticipation of a windfall that never comes.

The chapters that follow illustrate the range of behaviors and beliefs that qualify as lies of the mind. Here, to better demarcate the lie of the mind, we present three phenomena that do *not* qualify, along with the reasons.

Lies of the Mind

. . . versus *lying.* In a way, it is an acquired skill to be able to "tell the truth and nothing but the truth." Preschoolers, for instance, often invent far-fetched stories—such as the mysterious elephant that broke the table lamp—and are totally unable to recognize the transparency of the falsehood. The difference between wish and reality is taught as parents gently confront the child about outlandish claims and point out the difference between make-believe and real life. But a child's vivid imagination is not a lie.

We are much less tolerant of those who are supposed to know better. Most of us find lying to be repugnant. We concur with Ralph Waldo Emerson that "[e]very violation of truth is not only a sort of suicide in the liar, but is a stab at the health of human society."

But even the self-evident statement "Lying is undesirable" has been contested. As Clare Boothe Luce wrote,

> Lying increases the creative faculties, expands the ego, lessens the friction of social contacts. . . . It is only in lies, wholeheartedly and bravely told, that human nature attains through words and speech the forbearance, the nobility, the romance, the idealism, that—being what it is—it falls so short of in fact and in deed.

Yet, even in this glorified reframing of the behavior, the gains of the lie remain fleeting. A person who lies is what he or she is, regardless of the thrilling house of cards that has been erected. And Luce failed to add that, even to achieve this momentary gain, the lie must be told not only "wholeheartedly and bravely" . . . but *convincingly.*

Another requirement that dooms most lies is that they must go *undiscovered.* A notorious example of lying that captured the spotlight involved *Washington Post* reporter Janet Cooke. In 1981, Cooke won the Pulitzer prize for her sensational article "Jimmy's World," about an eight-year-old heroin addict. Admiration for Cooke turned to skepticism and finally disgust when it emerged—after 11 hours of grilling by several editors—that she had fabricated the main elements of the story . . . as well as much of her resume. Amidst publicity greater than her original article had ever captured, Cooke was disgraced and fired, and the *Post* returned the tarnished award.

Another case of faux journalism—this time involving the smaller scale of a college newspaper—occurred in 1995. Like Cooke, student journalist Mary Leigh Summerton lied to garner admiration for her work and, in doing so, overlooked the divisiveness her work inevitably would have provoked had she not been discovered.

Summerton wrote a gut-wrenching column for the Arizona State University newspaper, *State Press,* in which she claimed that, during a U.N.-sponsored trip to Israel, she witnessed Orthodox Jews murder a quadriplegic man confined to an electric wheelchair. The college senior claimed that the Jews brutally stoned the man for violating the Sabbath, the day of rest, by operating the motorized equipment.

But members of the local Jewish community noted inconsistencies in the story. And, checking records, they discovered that the student tour group to which Summerton alluded had not visited the site of the alleged assault on the Sabbath.

Her credibility questioned, Summerton's protests became burlesque as lie was built upon lie. She feebly countered, for example, that *she* had not written the column—that unnamed "Israeli feminists" had. But a professor pointed out that she had previously submitted the very same column as a class assignment. Was she now admitting that she had violated academic rules by presenting the "feminists' " discredited work as her own?

Summoned to a meeting with the director of the school of journalism, Summerton finally confessed that her column had been pure fiction. With ongoing revelations in the media that she had chronically falsified her work and educational background to make them appear much more impressive than they really were, the press she had courted for so long had now become her enemy.

Such cases stagger the imagination with their audacity while reflecting their protagonists' deep-seated insecurities. Although deliberate lying can involve a host of wishes and motives, it is nevertheless a behavior in which the tale teller ultimately *chooses* to engage. Based on the pivotal elements of *choice* and *control*, then, we do not consider it to be a lie of the mind. Although it is outside the purview of the chapters that follow, interested readers can learn more about the psychology of willful deceit in materials in the References and Suggested Readings section at the end of this book.

. . . versus *cultural differences*.   As we will repeatedly illustrate, we need to take culture into account whenever we seek to determine whether a behavior or belief is a lie of the mind. Just as our culture both determines and reflects the values we hold, it also shapes our conceptions of illness—whether physical or mental.

In the tradition of the Native American Navajo tribe, "negative information" about health is to be rejected. Are Native Americans afflicted with lies of the mind if they refuse to listen to the surgeon's instructions about the potential risks of an upcoming operation?

The dialectic between mainstream and subcultural beliefs arises conspicuously in this case. In Western medicine, a discussion of such negative information—often including the risk, albeit minuscule, of death—is the standard of care. But in traditional Navajo culture, it is maintained that thought and language have the power to control events. Discussing potential risks of a medical diagnosis or procedure, in this internally consistent view, can be tantamount to *causing* these untoward outcomes to befall the patient. Instead, Navajo tradition advises *"hózhoojí nitsihakees"* (thinking and speaking in a positive way).

The term *cultural relativism* refers to the cross-cultural differences that affect one's self-concept, relationships with others, and worldview. It is our contention that one cannot dismiss the Navajo perspective on health and sickness based solely on a Western perspective.[1] A community of people does not suffer from a lie of the mind simply because it disagrees with the dominant culture—one that demands that practices and beliefs be based only on objective evidence. Rather, our emphasis on full disclosure as part of the process of informed consent must be balanced with a respect for culture.

History reinforces the need to evaluate the authenticity of apparent "psychopathology" within its multidimensional context; after all, the dominant culture in antebellum America described a disease in slaves called "drapetomania: the disease causing negroes to run away." The symptoms of this "illness" included a "sulky and dissatisfied attitude," and the recommended treatment was "whipping the devil out of them." We must resist the temptation to base definitions of illness on our preferences and prejudices, no matter how much in vogue.

. . . versus *"brainwashing."* The third phenomenon that we exclude from the rubric "lies of the mind" is *"brainwashing"* as practiced, for example, by leaders of cults. Cult members adopt misguided thinking, but, as for the unsuspecting recipient of any lie, these distortions have been deliberately induced by another person. In the case of cults, the lies are promulgated by a single charismatic "prophet" with whom these people have affiliated. Unlike the mental conditions we consider in this book, these sometimes overtly irrational beliefs have typically been created through extensive planning supplemented by increasingly bizarre tests of obedience and loyalty.

Still, a cult, like a plant, can grow only where the soil is fertile. The current generation of Japanese citizens, for example, has achieved unparalleled income, and many of them have desperately sought a corresponding spiritual wealth. One of the many cults eager to count them among their ranks is Aum Shinri Kyo—now believed to have been behind the 1995 poison gas attack on Tokyo's subway that killed 12 and left thousands injured. Among his outrageous teachings, Aum Shinri Kyo's leader, Shoko Asahara, asserts that, once they truly "believe," adherents will be able to fly and to meditate under water for hours without taking a breath.

Although they drew their membership base—as opposed to Aum Shinri Kyo—from the poor and disenfranchised, Charles Manson and Jim Jones led followers down similarly destructive paths. And, frighteningly, experts predict that these cult movements will become even more pronounced as the year 2000 approaches.

---

[1] Indeed, the ongoing Framingham (Massachusetts) Health Study revealed that middle-aged female study participants who believed they were going to suffer a heart attack were 3.7 times more likely to die from coronary conditions than those who didn't consider themselves susceptible.

Imbuing the dawn of a new millennium with mystical significance, many cult leaders are teaching followers that God will reward them with a place in paradise if they precipitate mass death through biological or chemical weapons.

▌ Social Change and Lies of the Mind

Despite the perverse and sometimes destructive plans of cults, most of us will be fortunate enough never to have any personal involvement with them. Instead, they will remain the stuff of newspaper and magazine articles we casually skim and cast aside. Even if efforts *are* made to recruit us, we will find the solicitation extremely easy to rebuff.

Nonetheless, the societal factors that help propel some into cult affiliation are relevant to the mental conditions we discuss throughout this book. Our own community and culture are constantly evolving, bringing pronounced shifts in family structure and fundamental values. Along with the unique biological and psychosocial influences that predispose some individuals to unusual beliefs and behavior, these societal factors may constitute part of the substrate from which lies of the mind arise. We comment here on a salient few.

Society in Flux

The United States is in an era of tumultuous social change, leaving us befuddled. As one example, the envelope of art is being jostled in ways confusing and discomfiting to many. A central part of Ron Athey's performance art, for instance, involves piercing himself with needles, slicing designs into the flesh of his assistant, and hanging bloody towels over the audience. He claims that his work fuses Hindu and African rituals with the immediacy of the issue of AIDS.

In considering Athey's work, we find ourselves wrestling with a question that would have been unimaginable in decades past: Is such elaborate, staged body mutilation truly *art*, or is it the grotesque expression of one man's mental illness? In short, is it *creativity* or *psychopathology*? As we debate the issue, we find ourselves unable to reach even a hazy consensus on the "legitimate" boundaries of artistic expression.

And we have lost our bearings in other, more serious ways. In the past 25 years, the United States has experienced a dramatic increase in homicides, resulting in the highest homicide rate in the industrialized world. The phenomenon is especially pronounced among males ages 15 to 34; in this group, homicide has emerged as the second leading cause of death. Part of the reason for this increase is that violent street gangs have multiplied as changes in society have left teens feeling adrift. Gangs provide status and purpose; they also confer an instant sense of belonging through their own style of dress, speech, music, and, paradoxically, their particular funeral rituals.

In dizzying numbers of cases across the country, irrational violence arises from unthinkably minor disputes. In Pennsylvania, an argument over a gerbil culminated in the slayings of four people. In New York, a deli owner shot and killed a teenager for complaining that the service was too slow. In Alabama, the despondent loser of an impromptu Bible-quoting contest savagely murdered the winner. And, although still a relatively small piece of the trade in death, contract killings used to be the repellent phenomenon only of organized crime. Yet sociologists now tell us that the notion of hiring a killer to rub out a relentless business competitor or an inconvenient spouse is one that increasingly has been embraced by the middle class. Even murder has become a negotiable concept for some, a matter of prioritizing competing expediencies.

Thus, traditional maxims and assumptions about how we and others should behave are continually being shattered just as blatant problems, such as illegitimacy, illiteracy, and poverty, loom larger than ever before. These continual assaults on our values and confidence in the future have left our emotional safety nets frayed—and for some, ready to collapse.

A Creeping "Pastlessness"

At the same time that long-standing are under attack, our society has developed an ever-expanding collective amnesia, a "pastlessness." We chew up news and spit it out, ever hungry for more. Pixels cascade across our TV sets and vanish, flickering images that vaporize as fast as they have been formed. In calling the O. J. Simpson murder case the "Trial of the Century," for example, we overlook the many other trials of the century, such as the 1906 trial of Harry Thaw, the 1935 trial of Lindbergh baby kidnapper Bruno Hauptmann, and the 1971 Charles Manson murder trial. Yet we also manage to remember the past as it never was. The "good old days" baby boomers wistfully recall were also the days of Jim Crow laws and of Lee Harvey Oswald, James Earl Ray, and Sirhan Sirhan—painful realities we seem eager to strike.

Other vanishing images come from our computer screens. Although it brings indisputable benefits, the expansion of electronic media has not only engendered further pastlessness but also shaken our very sense of social solidarity. People spend more time alone and don't even realize it. Riveted by the monitor, they become estranged from their own bodies, replaced by pseudonymous avatars. Human-to-human contact takes a backseat when we meet and chat not over coffee but via terminals and modems, our visits mediated by computer network gurus and enhanced by interactivists.

Is there a chance that our emotional lives will be reduced to "emoticons" (:-o)? Will spirituality be replaced by worship of the machine? And will "real life" be derided, as it already has in some silicon circles, as little more than the keyboard shorthand "RL"?

As presaged by Aldous Huxley's 1932 novel *Brave New World*, many now see this depersonalization of our society advancing to a disturbing degree. A survey of scientists, researchers, business experts, and scholars in the journal the *Futurist* predicted that "humans will one day become composite beings—part biological, part mechanical, and part electronic—as they continue to incorporate nonhuman elements into their bodies." The same group anticipates that people "may begin to forgo their 'real' identities . . . in the world of virtual reality."

Nelson Thall, research director for Toronto's McLuhan Center for Media Sciences, placed us under the shadow of these outcomes in an interview with the *Hartford Courant*. As he put it,

> Electric technology is an extension of the central nervous system. It makes our old heads fluid. You don't have a container anymore because your mind floats out to the data bank. Computer banks and networks dissolve the human image. When you're on the phone or on the air and moving at the speed of light, your identity gets lost.

Although Thall is enthusiastic and hopeful, others wonder whether, in a twist the makers of the film *Invasion of the Body Snatchers* presumably never anticipated, we will be inexorably transformed into "cyber" pod people. This possibility, like the shifting values and pastlessness we have just described, surely does not cause lies of the mind. But all of these fundamental concerns do fuel the ambiguity and unease that, for the predisposed individual, make the world a frightening place; they further loosen the grip on reason and reality that, for some of us, is already weak.

■ Defense Mechanisms and Insight

What is it about a person that predisposes him or her to lies of the mind? How do clinicians tease apart the threads of personality, biological makeup, and experience to find out why a patient has moved so far beyond the range of normal thinking and behaving?

One of the crucial determinants of susceptibility to lies of the mind is our unconscious *defense mechanisms*. Observation of the particular defenses a patient uses can alert the psychiatrist to his or her likely problem areas even before these conflicts have been discussed. Similarly, our level of *insight* has critical implications for our capacity to recognize and modify the working of our own minds.

The Double-Edged Sword of Defense

All of us rely on a range of defense mechanisms to cope with stress and anxiety. Our ability to deal with tense work situations and charged emotional encounters is directly related to defense mechanisms that range from the mature and healthy (e.g., *anticipation*, in which an individual prepares for future events that might involve emotional conflict) to the primitive and unhealthy (e.g., *denial*, in which an individual refuses to accept some painful aspect of reality).

For example, picture this cartoon depicting *sublimation*, a healthy defense mechanism. A man is sitting, slumped and exhausted, paintbrush still in hand, in front of a massive painting filled with violent images of fists, screaming faces, and lightning. His wife says to him, "Feeling better?"

He almost certainly is. The man has been able to transform *(sublimate)* his inner turmoil into an outpouring of creative energy—the work of art.

Humor is another mature defense we can use to distance ourselves from frightening or painful memories or experiences. In Pat Conroy's novel *The Prince of Tides*, the character Tom struggles with the demons of his childhood as he recounts the horrible experience in which he, his sister, and his mother were raped by escaped convicts. At the opening of the story, his sister, Savannah, who at first tries to sublimate the reality of the rapes by transforming the horror into a story about a child's nightmare, is finally unable to cope and attempts suicide. When Tom seeks out her psychiatrist in order to understand his sister's suicide attempt, he is confronted with his own defense mechanisms: when he uses sarcasm to deflect the psychiatrist's questions, the doctor asks him, "Do you always hide behind your humor?"

The use of unhealthy defenses can easily result in the distorted thinking at the root of lies of the mind. Like Maria, whose story opens this introduction, Conroy portrays Savannah as a person whose deeply sensitive nature finally contributed to an unconscious refusal to acknowledge realities that were too painful; indeed, Savannah's early attempts to integrate the pain proved overwhelming. But Tom, bestowed by Conroy with a more balanced life and personality, was able to confront the memories and begin to heal once he became aware of how he used humor as a defense.

Defense mechanisms can help us understand why some individuals fall prey to lies of the mind and others are able to ward off mental illness. Although factors such as heredity and environment come into play as well, patients who use more mature defenses generally have fewer problems needing clinical attention.

The Armor of Insight

Earlier, we alluded to members of survivalist and militant militia movements. Unlike cult members, their slanted thinking does not arise from planned indoctrination. Instead, their lies of the mind are kindled by what psychiatrist Robert Jay Lifton has called the "post-Cold War confusion"—the uncertainty about "whom to hate" now that the omnipresent threat of the former Soviet Union has evaporated.

We have seen that a lack of purpose sometimes drives desperate young men in inner cities to the illusory remedy of the gang. Among young and middle-aged rural white men and women, the same factor can turn them to the radical right. Less educated, and facing stiff competition for unskilled jobs, members find that militias give them an instant place to fit in. Guns and violence then become the language of their discontent. Preferring extremist literary fare and linked by a jerry-rigged network of faxes, shortwave radios, and the Internet, they isolate themselves from mainstream media. In doing so, they cut themselves off from any information that might disconfirm their paranoid theories of Zionist plots and U.N.-enforced slavery. Extreme, even apocalyptic beliefs predictably arise in this insular setting. Fantasy becomes fact and finally fanaticism. Unable or unwilling to confront their own cognitive distortions, adherents remain convinced that it is the rest of us, blithely trusting, who are gruesomely out of touch with reality.

The critical factor that could thwart the destructive paths of these people—insight into their own circumstances and thinking—is tragically missing.

Insight shapes how we understand the world around us, how we filter experience, and how we come to know ourselves. It is a jumble of features, including self-awareness, self-control, proper judgment, and the capacity to think beyond the exigencies of the moment. And limitations in insight are at the heart of many of the lies of the mind we consider in this book.

If people lack insight, they are not aware of their own deficits and distortions. We are all too familiar with the limitations in insight that are characteristic of teens, for instance. Adolescents casually disregard basic truths—such as their own mortality—when they engage in the characteristic risk taking that older people would find incomprehensible. Newspapers regularly provide appalling accounts of such risk taking gone awry: a carload of teens is killed when they try to beat a freight train across the tracks, or a high school boy dies from an impulsive game of Russian roulette. And even as we shake our heads, newly invented ways to defy the odds emerge. "Subway surfing," "car surfing," and "train surfing" are new sports among adolescents in the United States, Brazil, and Europe, for instance—but with the thrill of hanging off the speeding vehicles has come the utterly predictable limb loss and death.

Some young adults remain slow to develop the insight that would otherwise temper their actions. In one recent survey, more than a third of 20- to 22-year-olds admitted to having engaged in unprotected high-risk sexual behavior in the previous six months. Perhaps they have convinced themselves that AIDS is an affliction exclusive to older gay men. Perhaps they haven't buried enough of their friends yet. Or perhaps they have retained the adolescent fantasy that they are invincible.

Although multiple factors, such as intelligence and education, contribute to each individual's level of insight, strong evidence suggests that the foremost lobes of our brains—the *frontal* lobes—imbue us with the basic physiology to have insight.

Due to a combination of a birth defect and an accident at age four, for example, British research subject "JP" was left with essentially no frontal lobe functioning. His behavior was the worst-case scenario of the absence of insight. As early as elementary school, he bullied, stole, and lied outrageously; lacking insight, he necessarily lacked morality. He was forever incapable of learning from punishment and was in essence controlled by his own whims.

Remarkably, all of us function on a continuum with the extreme cases in which insight is grossly impaired. If we lose the capacity to evaluate ourselves and our situations realistically, or refuse to exercise the insight we *do* have, any of us can come to believe that which is not true and find ourselves unable to resist our own thoughts.

In clinical care, mental health professionals know that the gradations in insight from person to person can be massive and that poor insight tends to lead to poor prognosis. This single factor explains the observation that even patients with the same psychiatric malady can differ appreciably in the critical matter of acceptance of their illness—the very foundation of the treatment alliance.

▌ Why This Book—and Why Now?

The ubiquity and consequences of mental disorders are staggering. The National Comorbidity Survey has disclosed that 48% of us will develop a psychiatric disorder at some time in our lives, with depression, alcohol dependence, and the phobias being the top three problems. We know from the Medical Outcomes Study that the disability associated with mental disorders is startling: the level of disability resulting from major depression, for instance, significantly exceeds that associated with hypertension, diabetes, arthritis, or lung disease. And according to the Institute of Medicine, disability from mental and substance-related disorders translates into an estimated total cost of $249 billion per year in the United States, due to the direct costs of care as well as factors such as reduced productivity.

Yet, as "managed care" continues to expand, we wrestle with the dilemma of how to balance the high cost of treatment against individual human need. Managed care is a diverse set of strategies aimed at controlling health care costs by controlling the use of resources. Generally, managed care systems limit the amount of treatment patients receive and negotiate for discounted services from clinicians and hospitals. We mental health professionals are therefore being challenged to resolve our patients' problems in less time and with fewer dollars, but—in spite of restrictive insurance plans—our patients continue to come to us in pain that often defies easy categorization and prompt cure.

The media have begun to acknowledge the importance of mental disorders, including their social, economic, and personal impact. They are starting to recognize the *continuum* of mental and emotional experience, no longer so uniformly relegating people with mental disorders to pariah status. Films such as 1996's *Shine*, although depicting the very real consequences of serious mental illness, approach their subjects (in this case, Australian pianist David Helfgott) with empathy and even love. Another film considers an even better-known victim of mental illness: Brian Wilson of the Beach Boys. The documentary *I Just Wasn't Made for These Times* takes an unsentimental look at the bipolar disorder (manic depression)—compounded by drug use—that derailed his career.

But the battle for understanding still wages. In 1994, for instance, NBC's stolid *Nightly News* characterized psychiatry's official diagnostic manual, the *Diagnostic and Statistical Manual of Mental Disorders* (DSM), as "a handbook of sorts for those looking for a way to say 'It's not my fault.'" The segment went on to ask, "[I]n a society where many people want to be victims, is psychiatry treating them or helping to create more?" Such statements from an esteemed news organization are disappointingly akin to those of antipsychiatry zealots (such as Thomas Szasz) and movements (such as Scientology) that attempt to dismiss mental illness as the misguided invention of authoritarian Western doctors.

In reality, the evidence suggests just the opposite. Across developed and developing countries, there is generally a remarkable consistency in the character of the psychopathology from which patients suffer, and their levels of disability are profound worldwide. Psychological illness thus has global public health significance, and it always has: in Eber's Papyrus, an Egyptian medical tract from 1600 B.C., conversion and dissociation—both described in subsequent chapters—are among the many psychiatric ailments discussed.

Our task is to help close the gap between the general population and those who suffer from the lies of the mind by demystifying symptoms that to some may seem inexplicable. In doing so, we will demonstrate that most mental disorders are caused by a combination of factors, both internal (psychological, biological, emotional) and external (societal, cultural, contextual).

We also will illustrate how mental health care professionals can help guide patients through the process of liberation from mental conditions—taking them from prisoners to escapees . . . and even on to achievers. Many public figures have helped show the way. William Styron and Rod Steiger, for example, have emerged from severe depression to share their experiences with others. Ted Turner, Patty Duke, Margot Kidder, and Mike Wallace have gone public with their struggles with bipolar disorder. Writer Kaye Gibbons, author of acclaimed novels such as *Ellen Foster*, has spoken poignantly of her own bipolar disorder; with medication, support from her family, and the "therapy" of her writing career, she has managed not simply to keep her life in control but to excel. And Lori Schiller describes her own battle with serious mental illness in her book *The Quiet Room*. Finally liberated at age 41 from the tormenting hallucinations, delusions, and mood swings she first experienced at age 17, Schiller writes,

> I have been to a place where all too many people are forced to live. . . . I want to tell others about my journey so that those who have never experienced it will know what life . . . has been like, and so that those who are still left behind will have hopes that they too will find a path out.

From our perspectives as clinicians, we will take you on an engaging journey through the human psyche and its many pathways. We will share case studies that best dramatize the symptoms and reveal the causes, effects, and ultimate consequences for individuals suffering from lies of the mind. *Stranger Than Fiction*, as our title promises, is a collection of characters and stories that could have been lifted from the pages of a fanciful novel. But they are even more compelling precisely because they are real.

ONE

PHOBIAS

Fear Itself

I have three phobias which, could I mute them,
would make my life as slick as a sonnet, but
as dull as ditch water. I hate to go to bed,
I hate to get up, and I hate to be alone.

—Tallulah Bankhead (1903–1968),
Tallulah

THE POET ANNE SEXTON, whose work "The Other" opens our chapter on dissociative disorders, was a one-woman show when it came to phobic disorders. As author Diane Wood Middlebrook describes in *Anne Sexton: A Biography*, Sexton developed a morbid fear of being alone with her babies shortly after the birth of her second child. When job demands pulled her husband away overnight, leaving Sexton alone with the children, she would stop eating, wallowing in a fear so intense that it sometimes left her panting and sweating.

Throughout her life, Sexton experienced a variety of other phobias that took turns on center stage, sometimes taking the spotlight, sometimes moving into the wings, but never going away entirely. Sexton was chronically afraid of mingling with strangers. At many points, the sheer thought of leaving her house terrified her (this type of phobia is called *agoraphobia*). Opening a car door was itself a frightening act because it meant abandoning the privacy and insulation of the automobile for the world of interactions with others. As Middlebrook puts it,

> [Sexton] yearned to browse in bookstores and libraries, but couldn't go unless a friend accompanied her. Grocery stores, drugstores, and department stores terrified her, and she refused to enter them unless someone . . . coached her ahead of time and stayed with her while she shopped.

Ultimately, Sexton sidestepped her fear of grocery stores by placing exactly the same order every week by telephone. At first eager to expand her literary horizons by attending writing classes, and eventually called upon to travel to distant spots to give poetry readings, Sexton tapped myriad friends to accompany her. These familiar faces anchored her and helped counter the possible humiliation lurking on public transportation, in new cities, among unknown people.

Even after achieving remarkable success, Sexton remained a victim of her phobias. She considered passing up the numerous poetry awards that quickly came her way if it meant traveling. Airplanes were particularly frightening (a *specific phobia*). One prize carried with it a trip to Europe. Sexton elected to go by boat, not so much to enjoy the leisurely pace and the dazzling horizons as to avoid air travel.

Even then, Sexton's journey was marred by her continual worries about finding places to go to the bathroom in complete privacy. She also disliked eating in public; a meal with a peer interested in her work might mean frequent interruptions as Sexton, ravaged by nerves, escaped to the bathroom to throw up (examples of *social phobia*).

Like many patients with severe phobias, Anne Sexton sought to "medicate away" her fears through the use of alcohol and sleeping pills. A series of double martinis at a reception, for example, would help counter the shaky hands that might betray her terror. If she were to read her own work to an audience, shots of vodka were a necessity before the performance, and she was so swept up in her anxiety that it took several days to recover. Even attending a lecture *by someone else* would require a few anticipatory drinks.

■ Anxiety: A Universal Experience

Anxiety is a sensation each of us has at times. Although Anne Sexton might have disagreed, anxiety—at least when it is only mild— is not only normal but often desirable. It propels us out of complacency, stimulates us to action, and—as long as it's not severe—enhances the way we perform. The person who is a little anxious during a test, for instance, is more attentive and attuned, and so he or she is likely to score better. Anxiety makes us sharper as we surmount obstacles, such as a physical threat to ourselves or someone we love; it is the exact kind of booster we need at such times. Anxiety about the likely consequences also helps us get out of bed each morning; it creates an internal alarm clock that gets us to work on time (on most days, anyway).

Anxiety has effects on both the body *(soma)* and the mind *(psyche)*. The bodily component commonly includes some stomach discomfort ("butterflies" or "knots," depending on our interpretation), chest tightness, and restlessness; the psychological component includes a vague sense of anticipation or worry.

But, like any emotion, anxiety can get out of hand. Remember the character Aaron Altman, portrayed by Albert Brooks in the movie *Broadcast News*? Facing TV news anchor duties for the first time, this former back-scenes reporter finds the role more terrifying than he had ever imagined. As Altman trembles, stammers, and gulps, tributaries of sweat pour off his face to converge into a river gushing down his shirt. Because Altman knows that his panic is obvious to millions of viewers, the terror multiplies, ultimately destroying the very performance he had yearned for years to deliver. Nobelist Marie Curie's famous dictum—"Nothing in life is to be feared. It is only to be understood"—would have been of pathetically little solace even to this most intelligent of individuals.

While rarely so overwhelming as depicted in *Broadcast News*, anxiety is nonetheless a genuine problem for many of us. Over 12 million Americans experience such frequent or severe anxiety that they seek treatment. And across the world, anti-anxiety medications are the most commonly prescribed drugs, a fact certainly not lost on pharmaceutical companies, which market "new and improved" varieties each year.

Whenever a patient with problem anxiety appears at our doorsteps, a number of questions run through our minds. Is the anxiety related to a particular *situation*, such as a threatening, authoritarian boss? Is there a *physical* explanation, such as thyroid disease or cocaine use, which escalates the metabolic rate and with it the level of anxiety? Or does the person have a formal *anxiety disorder*?

Within the last category are the *phobic disorders*, among the most troublesome of all the conditions in which anxiety erupts. In this chapter, we'll discuss and illustrate the three phobic disorders recognized by psychiatrists: 1) *specific phobia*; 2) *social phobia*; and 3) *agoraphobia*. They share several common features: victims suddenly experience irrational horror when they are in situations that are actually harmless; they have insight into the fact that the fear is indeed excessive; and yet they either try to avoid the feared stimulus or else endure it with dread.

▌ Specific Phobia

The fear of flying *(aerophobia)* is one of the most common forms of specific phobia, afflicting 25 million Americans. Although they may know that more people die each day on the nation's highways than in a whole year of commercial aviation, many people who are otherwise dynamic and self-assured are reduced to near whimpering at the thought of boarding an airplane. Even celebrities whose careers depend on their public appearances have fallen prey; examples are singer Michael Jackson and football commentator John Madden. They sometimes choose to spend many hours traveling via the road (albeit in plush converted buses or RVs) instead of the skies.

Denise [as told by Marc][1]

I've never understood how airplanes work. How can tons of metal take flight when the meticulously folded paper airplanes I make for my children can manage only a few feet?

I also don't know how the TV works. Or the garage door opener. Or my computer. At the same time, I've never cared enough to check into it. I realize that there *are* people, more mechanically or electronically savvy than I, who understand these things. When I board a plane, I have no concerns about the paradox of airborne machinery. I trust the pilot to take care of me, and my only distractions come from the skinniness of the seats and the blandness of the songs on the airplane headsets.

At the same time, I know that if I *really* thought about it—that, housed in a tiny metal tube tens of thousands of feet above the earth, I'm being hurled at hundreds of miles an hour—I might just start to worry. Thus, I can empathize with the many patients I have seen for whom flight is less an intriguing mystery than a terrifying prospect.

Denise, a homemaker with two children, was such a patient. Raised on a farm, she had not flown until the age of 15. Her initial excitement on the airplane turned to anxiety when, as so often happens, there were several episodes of turbulence. The pilot's grandfatherly voice over the speaker, gently

---

[1]As we take turns presenting each case vignette, we will indicate for the sake of simplicity whether it is "as told by Jackie" Feldman or "as told by Marc" Feldman. In addition, recognizing that language reveals key elements of personality and culture significant to the therapeutic process, we have made every effort to preserve our patients' own voices in recounting their stories. Dialect is therefore incorporated into the narrative where appropriate. Similarly, the various forms of address we use with patients reflect our respect for different subcultural norms and our patients' individual preferences. Both devices are used in the interest of preserving the authenticity of our patients' stories.

suggesting that the passengers buckle their seat belts as if it were just for fun, only agitated her further. She recognized suddenly that there was nothing she could do to control what was happening to her, and a feeling of raw terror struck. White-knuckled for the rest of the trip, she resolved never to travel via air again.

Fortunately, she had little interest in traveling anyway, and her desire to focus on child rearing kept her rooted to home. But Denise did have an interest in entertaining her kids. She had begun to take them to a nearby fast-food restaurant, partly for the food but mostly for the playground, the best one in town. The kids loved crawling through the maze of colorful suspended cylinders, waving at her through the Plexiglas windows as they worked their way through.

One day at the playground, her younger child, Marni, got mad at her son Ryan, and Marni refused to budge from a tube high off the ground. Denise started up, intending to retrieve her, when a familiar, painful feeling hit: she recognized instantly that she was once again off the ground, closed in by curved walls. She was petrified. Breathless and perspiring heavily, she begged Ryan to help her out, and she needed 20 minutes to recover.

Denise sought treatment for her phobia. I shared her concern about its having spread in a way that made a return trip to the playground a frightening thought. Denise also said she hated to think that family vacations would forever have to be planned around her and her fear of air travel. Marni was already talking about "Mickey" and "Disneyland" in her imploring—and irresistible—way.

We discussed the treatment options and settled on one; though it would involve considerable inconvenience and a hefty drive, we agreed that Denise would take advantage of the "fear of flying" classes offered at a regional airport.

Denise attended the class weekly for two months, surrounded by other pupils with the same problem. The first few sessions were led by pilots and mechanics who provided a primer on the numerous layers of safety and maintenance always in place. After that, a psychologist took over. She taught the group deep breathing and relaxation exercises to allow them to combat the anxiety at the moment it appeared. At the same time, they learned cognitive therapy techniques to confront the negative and irrational thinking that would otherwise increase their anxiety. The class culminated in an actual flight.

I met with Denise one more time a few months later. The dreadful feelings of panic had not returned during a repeat performance of Marni's obstinacy in the tubular maze or even during the trial flight. Denise remarked that now her only anxiety about Disneyland was the one facing every parent: being able to afford the three-day pass.

Josh (as told by Jackie)

While air travel was optional for Denise, in other cases airplane phobia actively curtails a career. Josh, a 35-year-old physician, had flown occasionally and without incident until he became an Air Force doctor five years before I first saw him. During that period, air travel had been a continual event. Although Josh never actually *avoided* being around the military aircraft, he started to become anxious many days before a scheduled flight. Takeoffs and landings were no problem; as with Denise, his horror came from being suspended in midair in a cabin. When his military service ended, he thought his problems with airplane phobia had ended as well.

But since then, Josh had moved into medical research, and now his academic career was, metaphorically speaking, taking off. He was invited more and more frequently to give presentations on his work, and air travel was again a necessity. His advancement as a medical school faculty member also depended upon his accepting such invitations.

Like far too many physicians, Josh had attempted to treat the problem on his own. Prior to boarding one recent flight, he had taken a hefty dose of an antianxiety medication and then downed two drinks on top of it. What happened next was recreated from information Josh got from others: he had become wildly agitated and incoherent during the flight, and the pilot was forced to make an emergency landing so that Josh could be whisked off to the hospital. After a day on a medical unit, he was transferred to a psychiatric ward with the presumption that he had willfully abused drugs and alcohol. The mess got sorted out, but, as Josh put it, "It's definitely not something I'd care to do again" and not the type of event that helps an associate professor gain tenure.

Josh talked with me about his dilemma, and I referred him to a psychologist who specializes in the treatment of anxiety disorders. With the use of biofeedback, Josh learned how to relax his muscles when anxiety tightened them up. The psychologist also desensitized him to the feeling of dizziness by literally spinning him (gently) in a chair designed for that purpose; in this way, Josh became better able to tolerate the sense of disequilibrium, of "being suspended in midair," and to accept that nothing catastrophic would happen if he had a similar feeling aboard a plane. When they finally took a brief plane trip together, both Josh and the psychologist were satisfied that treatment had been effective.

As noted in Denise's case, specialized treatment is now widely available through the airline companies themselves—and they have a 95% success rate. They recognize that the fear of flying is widespread. They know too that it is in their best interest to avoid emergency landings and convert airplane phobics into paying customers.

A Discrete Fear

As the term *specific phobia* suggests, afflicted individuals fear *particular* stimuli or situations. Many of us have an undeniable distaste for things that creep or crawl, such as spiders *(arachnophobia)*. And we can easily identify with the young lad in an Emily Dickinson poem whose fondness for the Earth's creatures does not extend to the snake, the "narrow fellow in the grass":

> [I] never met this Fellow
> Attended, or alone
> Without a tighter breathing
> And Zero at the Bone—

If we consider our own fears cowardly, it may help us to know that even supermacho Iraqi President Saddam Hussein has been reported to have an extreme fear of cockroaches.

But extreme fears are not necessarily phobias. Only for truly phobic people do such fears cause disruption of their lifestyles. They may shop only on the ground level of a mall because of a fear of heights *(acrophobia)*, refuse to walk on the street because of the risk of encountering a wayward cat *(ailurophobia,* which afflicted Napoleon Bonaparte), or walk up 20 flights rather than get into an elevator *(claustrophobia)*. The most common phobias are "situational"—for example, traveling over bridges *(gephyrophobia)*—and they tend to begin either in childhood or early adulthood. Specific phobias also often occur in multiple members of the same family, although the precise reason is unknown. Over 10% of the population will experience a specific phobia—and sometimes several—during their lives. And, as illustrated by Freud's famous patient Little Hans, one phobia can breed more. Five-year-old Hans's fear of horses *(hippophobia)* had evolved into a fear of carts, furniture vans, and buses before treatment finally succeeded.

Fears for All Occasions

The complexity and occasional perversity of the human animal is richly illustrated by the specific phobias. Experts have catalogued examples ranging from the understandable (such as *rhabdophobia*, or the fear of being beaten), to the redundant (such as *phobophobia*, or the fear of fear), to the paradoxical (such as *hedonophobia*, the fear of pleasure), to the bizarre (such as *autophobia*, the literal fear of oneself).

Russian novelist Leo Tolstoy's profound *thanatophobia* (fear of death) vastly affected both his personal and professional life. At age 41, with a successful literary career well established, Tolstoy became paralyzed by the insurmountable fear that death was stalking him. One day, while on a carriage ride in the country, Tolstoy's phobia expressed itself in a classic panic attack. He was forced to stop at an inn to recover, but his anxiety only increased as he lay in his room, which became for him "a square red and white tomb." Over time, this immense fear became the focal point of his life, taking utter control. For years, Tolstoy was unable to write any fiction at all, but he reemerged at age 57: his work, *The Death of Ivan Ilych*, became a turning point in that Tolstoy had discovered—through the character he created—that love has a power far greater than death.

Although easy targets for humor or derision because of their odd and colorful qualities, phobias—as in Tolstoy's case—can actually be as disabling as any medical illness. Researchers from St. Louis University described a 35-year-old woman whose driving phobia rendered her unable to drive on highways, in the rain, in traffic, on long flat stretches, or alone or to ride as a passenger. How is such an individual to get about, let alone function as an adult? In this case, the installation of a mobile phone allowed the patient to expose herself to the feared stimulus (driving) while readily accessing the therapist or others for help or reassurance. Eventually, she experienced enough success during progressively longer trips that her confidence increased and the phone could even be removed.

In the case of an eight-year-old boy, a food phobia resulted in such pronounced weight loss and malnutrition that hospitalization became necessary. The child had been well until six months earlier, when he had choked on a hot dog. Subsequently, he avoided or spit out foods he had previously liked, eventually reaching the point where he had eliminated all solids from his diet. Subsisting on yogurt, ice cream, and instant breakfast drinks, he would tremble, cry, and try to escape when invited to taste other foods or liquids, and his health had obviously suffered. Ultimately, a combination of behavioral techniques—including teaching self-relaxation exercises, gradually reintroducing the forbidden foods, and ignoring his tantrums—cured the problem. He left the hospital at a normal body weight.

Perhaps more pertinent to many of us is dental phobia, described in one article as the "holy trinity of fear, pain and the dentist." A British survey, for example, revealed that the majority of adults refuse regular dental checkups, 26% giving their reason as "being scared." This avoidance takes a toll on teeth. Some phobic patients choose to face abscesses and tooth loss rather than endure the dentist's drill. Special goggles called "i-glasses!" may be a remedy for some. Plugged into a VCR or TV, i-glasses! allow anxious patients a measure of visual distraction while the dentist is drilling away. For the patients who actually *enjoy* dental work, however, the glasses can be rigged to allow them to view their own procedures as they unfold, up close and personal.

The Legitimacy of a Phobia

Occasionally, interesting legal and ethical questions emerge regarding the "legitimacy" of particular phobias. In 1993, for example, a white woman in Miami was awarded hefty disability compensation based on her phobia of African American males. According to the claims judge, she was entitled to the payments because this particular phobia prevented her from working at any company whose employees included men of that race. Seven years before, while on the job, she had been beaten and robbed by a young African American man, and this event was the apparent cause of her present phobia. As news of the disability claim reached the public, people everywhere were outraged both by the nature of the phobia and its validation by the courts. Nevertheless, with the woman's mental condition medically confirmed as "disabling," we are left to grapple with the issue of what constitutes a *legitimate* phobia, and, more to the point, what constitutes an appropriate use of scarce entitlement dollars.

In another Florida case fraught with similar implications, a paramedic claimed he was disabled based on his blood phobia, a fear that surfaced after he discovered that he had administered mouth-to-mouth resuscitation to an infant with AIDS. His newly acquired fear of blood made it impossible for him to work in emergency medical services. In view of the precedent established in the Miami case, this man might have been awarded workers' compensation benefits if not for his history of psychiatric problems. The pensions board ruled that his phobia stemmed from a personality disorder, not the resuscitation incident, and thus his claim was denied.

In both cases, the phobia curtailed the activities—and opportunities—of the claimants. Both individuals needed treatment and financial assistance to get past their fearsome obstacles. But regardless of how such claims are finally adjudicated, they always create a no-win situation because they appear to pit one group of victims of social prejudice (those with phobias) against another (such as those devalued because of race or disease). The successful pursuit of disability based on aversion to other types of people appears, on the surface, to endorse prejudice. In reality, however, patients with true phobias never "choose" to walk the life-limiting path of fearing others.

Fearing What We Do

Although many of us complain that at times we hate our jobs, this phrase takes a literal turn when an individual becomes phobic about some aspect of his or her vocation. Gas mask phobia has afflicted soldiers since World War I, when battle began to include the threat of biological and chemical weapons. Some soldiers have so feared and despised their masks that they have ripped them off even when there was the risk that deadly gas was still in the area.

In a similar way, paralyzing underground phobia has occurred in coal miners, particularly following near accidents (such traumas often elicit subsequent phobias). A laboratory technician in England developed phobic anxiety over his genetic inability to smell cyanide, which was manufactured in the chemical plant in which he worked. A male stockbroker had a career-stultifying phone phobia. And mothers have, fortunately rarely, experienced phobic reactions toward their own babies. A 1992 report from Australia described nine cases that parallel Anne Sexton's response to her children when she was left alone with them. One mother was so upset and frightened by her infant daughter's crying that she became entirely unable to care for her, enlisting her mother-in-law as a surrogate parent. Another described unwarranted but persistent and incapacitating fears of dropping the baby. Unlike most specific-phobia patients, however, these mothers also tended to have other serious emotional disorders such as depression. Maternal support, marital therapy where indicated, and a variety of behavioral techniques (described in the next section) played a role in restoring the ill-formed mother-child connection in these cases.

Inevitably, technological progress has bred new phobias—at times, actively curtailing people's vocations. The term *technophobia* has been proposed to describe those who view the term *user friendly* as a dreadful oxymoron—the person, for instance, who quits her job immediately after the boss unveils the new computer mainframe and proudly announces, "Put on your helmets! This office is about to go high tech!"

Addressing the Problem

As we've indicated, behavioral therapies (addressed in the Final Thoughts chapter as well) have a special role to play in all of the phobic disorders. *Systematic desensitization* in particular can be remarkably effective. In systematic desensitization, the therapist first teaches the patient muscle relaxation and deep breathing techniques, then aids the patient in imagining increasingly fearsome situations; the resulting anxiety is quelled by the new relaxation skills until the original stimulus is not nearly so frightening. For example, a patient with an airplane phobia might be asked to think first about waking up on the morning of a flight. When his anxiety about this thought subsides due to the relaxation exercises, he then sequentially imagines packing for the flight, driving to the airport, obtaining the boarding pass, and entering the plane, with takeoff the final target. With each step, relaxation is used to topple the anxiety.

In contrast, *graded exposure* presents the patient with the actual stimulus, but in small increments that he or she can tolerate. A patient with needle phobia who required daily medication injections, for instance, alternated relaxation with stepwise behaviors such as actually filling a syringe, preparing the injection site, and placing the needle against his skin. Ultimately, he succeeded in self-administering his injections on a regular basis with no anxiety whatsoever. One New Age Southern California therapist has employed such graded exposure to cure driving phobias—supplementing the technique, predictably enough, with music, astral projection, and an exploration of the budding driver's past lives.

Graded participant modeling is an indirect route that can be effective. Here, the patient observes a fearless person interact with the phobic stimulus (for example, by touching and holding a snake or dog) until he or she gains enough courage to try it firsthand. In contrast, *flooding* takes a monumentally more direct approach, with overtones some might see as sadistic: the patient is exposed at full intensity to the stimulus or situation he or she fears most; because one can sustain peak anxiety for only so long, the panic inevitably begins to wane and with it the phobia. Imagine having *pediophobia* (fear of dolls) and being locked in a room filled with Malibu Barbies!

The technique of flooding, this time for *phonophobia* (fear of noise), proved highly successful in the treatment of a 21-year-old college student named Bill. Ever since childhood, Bill had had a disabling fear of loud noises. The simple circumstance of a car backfiring could trigger a full-blown panic attack. By the time he sought help, Bill's social relationships were suffering greatly. His fear of noise had evolved more specifically into a fear of bursting balloons and ultimately of balloons themselves. A description of Bill's treatment was published by psychologist Daniel Houlihan and colleagues:

> In the first treatment session, Bill followed the therapists into a treatment room . . . with 100 large multicolored balloons. . . . It was immediately apparent that Bill was bothered a great deal by the balloons in that he huddled very near the door and was visibly shaking. . . . While one experimenter stayed close by Bill, the other began popping the balloons. At this point Bill was visi-

bly shaking. Tears were streaming down his face and he began to turn pale. Bill asked for a chair in that his legs were shaking so hard he was having difficulty standing. . . . After popping about 50 balloons with a pin, the second experimenter reverted to popping them by standing on them. . . . [Bill] cried and tried to look away.

Despite the magnitude of the anxiety evoked in flooding, investigators have reported few adverse effects. In fact, in Bill's case, the technique was credited with his recovery from a phobia that had tormented him almost all of his life. By surviving the high-water mark of his greatest fears, Bill's phobia was washed away and he felt that his life had been restored.

Most recently, *cybertherapy*—using computers as therapeutic tools—has joined the list of treatment options in specific phobia. The software Spider Phobia Control, for example, presents the arachnophobic person with computer images ranging from a genial cartoon spider to a video of an actual tarantula. And in a study performed by researchers from Atlanta's Emory and Georgia Tech universities, 10 college students who feared heights were exposed during weekly sessions to computer-generated scenes that culminated in depictions of their worst nightmares. Wearing headsets and body-tracking devices that allowed them to interact with virtual objects, the participants were whisked away to vivid computer-created environments: they found themselves riding a glass elevator up 49 stories, for instance, or walking across a narrow footbridge perched 260 feet over a canyon river. Within seven weeks, the use of "virtual reality" had sharply reduced their acrophobia.

▌ Social Phobia

Many people would rather die than have to give a speech—literally. In a survey asking the general public "What is your deepest fear?" the fear of death ranked sixth, but the fear of public speaking ranked at the very top. Even among business executives who regularly make presentations to large groups, 20% said they would rather figure their income taxes than give a speech; another 20% would rather try to lose 10 pounds in a month; and 15% would rather have a cavity filled.

Social phobia has been called the "mental disorder of the 1990s." Previously underdiagnosed and misunderstood, social phobia is now known to afflict one out of every seven Americans at some time in their lives. Going far beyond simple bashfulness, social phobia is defined as the marked and persistent fear of social or performance situations in which embarrassment might occur. In fact, any exposure to the dreaded situation almost invariably leads to immediate and intense anxiety. In contrast, the person feels fine when alone.

Although we all feel self-conscious at times, people with social phobia will go to great lengths to avoid speaking, eating, drinking, or writing when others are around. Some, like Anne Sexton, fear using a public rest room (dubbed *bashful kidney syndrome*). They are afraid that others will notice their frazzled appearance—their trembling and clammy hands, shaking voices, sweating foreheads—and that they will be thought of as weak, foolish, or ridiculous. In most cases, the fear of scrutiny spans more than one social situation. For instance, a person may simultaneously fear meeting new people, participating in conversations, using the phone, and eating in restaurants.

Remarkably enough, even some of our best-known celebrities have been victims of social phobia. Barbra Streisand's fear of forgetting song lyrics led to a self-imposed absence from the concert stage for 20 years. The recording successes of Carly Simon and Van Morrison might have been even greater had the singers not been so burdened by stage fright. Baseball legend Mickey Mantle's fear of making personal appearances led him to escalate his use of alcohol, which culminated in full-blown alcoholism and fatal liver cancer. And actress Lauren Bacall stated in an interview with *New York Magazine*,

> People think that I have no frailties at all, that I don't need anyone to help me do anything, and of course nothing could be further from the truth. . . . I've always been frightened going into parties, going into crowded rooms. I've never felt secure. I probably never will. I put on a big act. I'm by myself and I walk in . . . [and] say to myself, "You're gonna do this thing. Just walk in, goddamn it." But inside, I quake.

Andy (as told by Marc)

Andy is a psychiatric colleague whose recovery from a severe public speaking phobia has been the most dramatic I've ever heard of. Andy recalls enjoying performing in public as a child. In elementary school, he hammed it up as a member of the school choir and was always a central figure in school plays ("People still get misty-eyed at my soulful depiction of *Oliver*," he recalls).

The lure of the greasepaint dwindled as Andy grew older, however. For several reasons, the usual self-consciousness of early adolescence was heightened in his case, and center stage was not where he wished to be. But of more immediate impact was an episode of dizziness and sweating Andy suffered during a choir rehearsal in eighth grade. Andy abruptly quit the choir and never performed again ("I realize now," Andy says, "that the dizziness was due to low blood sugar. I had skipped breakfast and lunch that day and paid the price. But at the time it seemed inexplicable and I was terrified.")

Andy became a stellar student, but one whose life was clearly constrained by his phobia of being the focus of attention, especially if it meant speaking in public: "I noticed that I felt panicky even when I asked a question in class. My voice shook horribly. If I had to be in front of the class, my hands shook too. It was absolutely visible. Students teased me and teachers seemed embarrassed for me. Sometimes my knees knocked; up until then, I had thought that 'knocking knees' was just an expression. I pretended not to know the answer to a math problem if it meant having to write it out on the blackboard."

"I got into a top college," Andy continued, "but I completed those four years literally without asking a single question in class. I'd wait until after class when I could be one-on-one with the professor, or I'd cajole another student into asking the question for me. If it were a really good question, he'd get the kudos."

At times, public speaking was unavoidable. The choice was either to endure a classroom presentation or to guarantee a failing grade. Andy would become increasingly frantic three weeks before the performance; he would scarcely sleep or eat and would vomit every morning. On the day of the presentation, he gobbled down over-the-counter antihistamines for the sedating effects, though they had the serious drawback of further drying his mouth: "By the time I was through, it was as if my tongue had been attached to my palate with Krazy Glue," he said. "One time, I overdid the antihistamines, and the police stopped me on the way to school because my car was weaving. I made up the excuse that I had reached down for some Kleenex and briefly lost control. They bought it, but it was a tremendous warning sign for me. A couple of times, I had also bought Valium on the street, and I was scared for weeks later that it would be discovered and spell the end of my medical career. I decided that I would commit suicide if that ever happened."

After entering medical school, Andy talked informally to a faculty member in psychiatry, who referred him to a psychologist for behavior therapy: "The idea was that I would learn relaxation exercises, then expose myself through systematic desensitization or graded exposure to increasingly stressful situations, each time practicing the relaxation techniques until I calmed down. The psychologist meant well, setting up a video camera to 'watch' me, or bringing in colleagues to serve as a mini-audience," he recalled. "But it didn't work. I never really grasped the relaxation exercises in the first place—I was too 'Type A,' I guess, and that doomed the whole thing. I was still scared to death. I started skipping therapy sessions. Eventually, the psychologist did too."

Improvement came during Andy's medical residency through a treatment rarely associated these days with phobic disorders, and one that most people cannot access because of its cost and limited availability: psychoanalysis.

"I entered treatment with a Freudian psychoanalyst to help me generally in life, but it turned out that it made a huge difference in my public speaking phobia too." Andy attended a session every morning before work, lying on a couch with the therapist out of view: "She would gently guide me, but *I* really did the work. After we had turned to the matter of the phobia and how crippling it was for me, I developed a lot of insight into the problem. I shifted from being frightened to being angry. I realized that it stemmed from the criticism and unrelenting pressure to succeed I faced as I was growing up. I decided not to be dominated by the past anymore."

There was still a lot of work ahead. Within the context of the psychoanalytic treatment, medication and behavioral approaches were added: "As a resident, I had ample opportunities to speak to both small and large groups, and I stopped dodging them. Prior to a talk, I would take an antianxiety medication the therapist prescribed and this relaxed me a little without drying my mouth. I always had a can of Coke with me at the lectern just in case, but I stopped worrying that taking sips now and then would betray my anxiety to everyone in the audience. As I had more and more success, my confidence soared. When I felt ready, we reduced the amount of medication, and eventually stopped it altogether." Andy remained in analysis for several years, solidifying his gains in maturity and security.

As I mentioned at the start of Andy's story, the undoing of his phobia has been essentially complete. Now in his early 40s, Andy has become a frequent medical commentator on television and radio: "I've even been quizzed on the air by Geraldo Rivera and never got hit in the nose once. I still carry around a little pillbox with a couple of antianxiety pills in it, and sometimes I'll take one before an especially important interview," he acknowledges, "but usually the can of Coke is enough to anchor me. As long as it's caffeine free."

Staring Down the Problem

Until recently, social phobia had been overlooked by health care professionals for two basic reasons: first, people with the disorder have rarely sought help, embarrassed even by the thought of talking about their affliction; and second, those (including many doctors) who have never experienced the disorder have often dismissed it as a sign of immaturity or, like a child's distaste for vegetables, something the person would eventually outgrow.

But the consequences of social phobia can be massive. Persons with social phobia are less likely to marry or to have friends. School or work performance may suffer because of excessive anxiety in taking tests, interacting with others, or speaking to the teacher or boss; as a result, some patients drop out of school, remain dependent upon their parents, and either miss opportunities for job advancement or do not even seek work because of their fear of being interviewed. More than 20% of patients with true social phobia end up on welfare.

In severe cases, panic attacks, depression, and agoraphobia (discussed later in this chapter) complicate the diagnosis. As we saw in the case of Mickey Mantle, substance abuse can be another devastating sequela, especially when social phobia has generalized to a number of different situations. Perhaps it is not surprising that the prevalence of suicide attempts for people with social phobia is almost 16 times higher than for the general population.

One might predict that social phobia would be a phenomenon unique to Western societies because of their emphasis on personal achievement and almost militant individualism. But even Japanese culture, which focuses on the group, not the individual, has its correlate. In fact, *taijin kyofusho* is a common Japanese psychiatric disorder characterized by the fear of offending others—in essence, losing the very inconspicuousness that Japanese society so values.

Who Is at Risk?

There is one period in a person's life when he or she is at particular risk for the onset of social phobia. As in Andy's case, this critical time is around puberty, when school performance and physical appearance are major concerns. Although "stranger anxiety" is universal among toddlers and preschool children, people who continue to seem inhibited or oversensitive beyond that time are at heightened risk as well. For some, a humiliating experience serves as the final trigger: for example, a shy teen publicly scolded in school may become extremely anxious about talking to the teacher at all, or an unfortunate slip of the tongue at a party may spawn shame in an already insecure individual. There are no racial differences in the frequency of the disorder, but a sex difference has been noted, with women affected twice as often as men.

In the case of social phobia, biology is not destiny, but it appears to play a role. Harvard researcher Jerrold Rosenbaum and his colleagues have suggested that human beings may be "wired" to fear scrutiny by others. Just as dogs become agitated when they are the recipients of fixed stares, humans too may perceive staring eye contact as a threat. Although this lurking evolutionary fear helped our ancestors escape imminent attacks from glaring predators, its persistence may set off false alarms even in the absence of true danger, taking the form of social phobia.

Driving the biological hypothesis is the fact that social phobia is familial, occurring much more often among first-degree relatives of those with the disorder than in the general population. But although a specific genetic factor may account for part of this familial trend, the quality of the environment in which the individual is reared seems to be involved as well.

Preliminary research using *magnetic resonance spectroscopy*, a way to get a glimpse of the biochemistry of the brain, appears promising. In a study conducted at Duke University, levels of some natural substances were decreased in specific parts of the brains of patients with severe social phobia. This finding suggests that a disturbance in brain chemistry may be a piece of the puzzle—though, if it is, we still don't know whether the altered levels cause or result from the phobia.

The Treatment Armamentarium

The good news: social phobia is eminently treatable. The bad news: all too often, the disorder is bathed in so much humiliation and secrecy that help is never even sought. Organizations such as the Anxiety Disorders Association of America (ADAA),[2] based in Rockville, Maryland, have been working to reverse the stigma of social phobia and to promote public and professional awareness of the many treatment approaches that are available to those with the disorder.

For example, professional actors, comedians, and others whose livelihoods depend on the excellence of their performances have long known that a single dose of a "beta-blocking" medication (propranolol, or Inderal, is an example) can alleviate troublesome sweating, trembling, and palpitations if taken shortly before a scheduled appearance. In one study, 27% of musicians acknowledged using beta-blockers to quell their tremor and anxiety prior to performances (lest a singer's sultry voice be transmuted into Tiny Tim's). If the frightening social situation is encountered often or unpredictably, consistent dosing may be needed. In addition to the beta-blockers, benzodiazepines such as clonazepam (Klonopin), antidepressants such as phenelzine (Nardil) or fluoxetine (Prozac), and other classes of medication may be extremely useful options.

Techniques that can be used alone or in combination with medications include systematic desensitization or graded exposure (both described earlier), social skills

---

[2] The address is ADAA, 11900 Parklawn Drive, Suite 100, Rockville, MD 20852; telephone: (301) 231-8369; URL: http://www.adaa.org/.

training, cognitive restructuring, and role playing. In *social skills training*, the therapist models appropriate social behaviors and the patient then rehearses them. This approach is best for those with deep-seated deficits in the social skills most of us naturally acquire as we grow up. *Cognitive restructuring* involves detecting and modifying the self-castigating, catastrophic thinking that perpetuates social phobia (such as the internal statements "Everyone finds me abhorrent" and "People find me odd and they don't like me"). *Role playing* helps therapists teach their patients how to handle the symptoms that develop in situations typically fraught with anxiety; through such activities, patients expand their self-confidence.

In 1993, during her presidency of the ADAA, Jerilyn Ross published an article in which she provided excerpts from a few of the thousands of letters the organization had received since its founding. One letter came from Heidi, a 21-year-old receptionist who experienced her first symptoms of social phobia at age 16. She wrote,

> I first learned that something was wrong when I couldn't do things that everyone else was doing. Sometimes I wouldn't be able to go to parties. Just the thought of having to talk to someone made me so anxious I had trouble breathing. I would avoid parties or school plays or football games, things like that. . . . I felt that everyone thought I was strange and that they would see me blush or tremble. . . . I felt like I was falling apart and that it showed and that I was embarrassing my friends as well as myself. . . .
>
> I didn't know it was a sickness or a problem. I thought it was something just happening with me and no one else. Since part of my problem included talking to doctors, I avoided that. . . . I never got any help.

Ultimately, Heidi was able to access treatment and regain control over her life. She described the impact of receiving appropriate care:

> When I found out I could get help for this, it was an incredible feeling. I didn't know that I could ever get over this. . . . I work as a front desk receptionist and have been for the past 3½ years, so I deal with people on a regular basis all the time, but I've never enjoyed it. . . . But now I'm starting to enjoy it. I like talking to people, I like carrying on conversations. And I like dealing with people . . . which I never thought I would do.

▋ Agoraphobia

Despite the colossal impact specific or social phobias can have on an individual's life, agoraphobia can still be the most disabling of all the phobic disorders. *Agoraphobia* is derived from the Greek words for "fear of the marketplace," and, at its core, it involves anxiety about public, crowded, closed-in, or wide-open spaces. More broadly, the agoraphobic person is fearful of being in situations in which embarrassing—if not incapacitating—feelings of panic might suddenly strike and escape or rescue would be difficult. As with specific and social phobias, the individual with agoraphobia avoids getting into these perceived predicaments in the first place, though they may be as seemingly benign as traveling in a bus, attending a concert, or standing in line.

In Alice Hoffman's modern novel *Illumination Night*, the raw terror of agoraphobia, and its confinement of an individual to an ever-smaller space, is presented through the eyes of its protagonist:

> You have read about force fields in science fiction novels, and now this force you thought existed only in fantasy has sprung up around you. If you come close to the force field, say walk out on the porch, a knot the size of a walnut forms in your throat. If you break through the force field by placing one foot on the porch steps, you are jolted back. You can feel the force field enter your body. If there were a string of electrons that shocked you each time you tried to leave the house you could not be any more trapped. . . . More than anything, you fear that the circle will continue to close in on you. Can anyone exist on a couch? Can anyone be broken down and then stored in a wineglass, a teaspoon, a thimble?

Agoraphobia, in contrast to specific phobia, strikes in a large number of situations. And unlike social phobia, the fear can develop even when the person is alone (for example, being alone outside the home is intolerable for some people with agoraphobia). Patients may refuse to go out without a trusted friend or family member, and—in the most extreme cases—an agoraphobic person will refuse to leave home at all. Imprisoned by the force field of their own minds, these people evolve into hermits confined to their only safe haven.

When Fear Strikes

Most often, agoraphobic patients experience panic attacks as well. During a panic attack, mind and body seem to conspire in a ruthless assault: the individual suffers an overwhelming sense of terror combined with imposing physical symptoms such as palpitations, hyperventilation, hot and cold spells, and hand and finger numbness. Panic attacks, which hit "out of the blue" and dissipate just as spontaneously, are routinely described by patients as the worst experience of their lives. In clinical settings, over 95% of patients who present with agoraphobia have a history of such frequent and severe panic attacks that they carry the additional diagnosis of panic disorder.

The dreadful combination of panic disorder and agoraphobia was poignantly described in an issue of the magazine *Cosmopolitan*. There, Katherine Weissman writes about her own battle:

> I'm walking along a familiar street in New York City, where I've lived for almost twenty years. I ought to feel safe. Endangered is more like it. My heart starts beating very fast, very loud. The thin clothes I am wearing might as well be wool. My mouth is dry. My eyes won't focus. . . . I seem to have forgotten how to walk. My legs are stiff and clumsy, as if they'd been clapped into metal braces; I have to swing them from the hip in order to take a step. People avert their eyes. Possibly they think I had polio or a bad accident. I lurch my way through the crowds, sweat pouring, praying I'll get the eight blocks to my destination. . . .
>
> Certainly, I didn't fit the popular perception of an agoraphobe—a housewife literally trapped in domesticity, a thin and suspicious recluse who never lived much in the world anyway. I worked in an office, earned a good living, had a grip on reality, dressed well, spoke clearly, and moved fast. Now, all that had changed. Twice I'd been disgraced and disabled in a public place [due to panic attacks], and twice was no accident. Those two episodes became the foundation of my phobia, the cornerstone of hard fear that brought an entire prison into being.

As in the celebrity cases of social phobia we mentioned earlier, agoraphobia has become paradoxically public. Some people who are now highly visible had battled agoraphobia earlier in their lives. For example, Howard Stern's spirited sidekick, Robin Quivers, revealed her own history of agoraphobia in her autobiography *Quivers* (a title that is appropriate on at least two counts). Panic attacks and agoraphobia have emerged in film; they burdened the sheriff's wife, Mary Peterson, in the film *Nell*, and they plagued Elliott Gould's character, Jimmy Morgan, in *Inside Out*. Agoraphobia has even insinuated itself into the literary fodder of today's youth. In a 1995 issue of *'Teen* magazine, a young woman's moving account of her personal struggle with agoraphobia ("When Fear Takes Control") is embedded within more traditional adolescent fare such as "Diet Resolutions" and "Female Bonding: Stronger Than Ever!" The article on female bonding may not be entirely beside the point, however: agoraphobia is yet another mental disorder that affects women more commonly than men.

Reading One's Way to Relief

A curious spin on agoraphobia comes from the case of Minnesota resident Gerald La-Pre. Dubbed a "biblio-kleptomaniac," LaPre, according to police reports, stole 30,248 books from Minneapolis-St. Paul public libraries over a period of years. Craving science fiction and fantasy novels, LaPre had stuffed two apartments, his car, and a storage room so full of books that it took a couple of pickups, a minivan, a 27-foot moving van, and two dozen police officers and firefighters to remove them all. The reason for this purloined collection? As LaPre put it during his interrogation, "[Books] are the only things in the world that keep me safe. . . . [They] are the only things that do not make demands on me, that do not hurt me, that do not frighten me." Under long-term psychiatric care and on disability, LaPre had been diagnosed with agoraphobia, and ultimately books had come to provide his main solace, his company. Barred from public libraries for two years as a result of his crime, LaPre nonetheless found a way to continue to surround himself with worlds safer than the real one: he joined six book clubs.

Determining the Cause

In many cases, agoraphobia descends after a stressful event. The young woman who published her account in *Teen* magazine traced the onset of her panic attacks to a bout of food poisoning that sapped her strength and triggered shortness of breath. She gradually felt well enough to work as a restaurant hostess, but the panic in public settings reintensified after her ranting boss swore at her in front of customers. Despite these two undeniable and influential stressors, however, she added that both heredity and emotional trauma in childhood may have played a role as well: "The potential to become agoraphobic had been inside of me for years; I had been verbally abused by my former stepmother and my natural mother had once suffered from both depression and agoraphobia." Studies do suggest that the disorder is more common in families in which other members suffer from an anxiety disorder or from alcohol abuse. Reinforcing this concept is the case of bookaholic LaPre. In a magazine interview, LaPre related his suspicion that his parents' alcoholism and the resulting childhood neglect played a role in his developing crippling anxiety (though he believes that a bizarre accident resulting in a head injury was also involved).

Some researchers suspect that agoraphobic patients process information differently from others. This quality makes them overattentive to potential threats in the environment, and so they anticipate being fearful even in relatively benign situations. Perhaps the unpredictability of the panic attacks they have had in the past—and their interpretation of these as calamitous experiences—"trains" them to be chronically fearful. If so, this finding would help explain why 40% of patients cannot identify any specific events or situations that contributed to their agoraphobia. These patients, like many with social phobia, may have had basic personality characteristics such as avoidance, timidity, and overdependence that predisposed them. Agoraphobia, then, may be a *forme fruste* of these faulty underlying personality traits.

In 1990, President Bush and the Congress officially designated the nineties as the "Decade of the Brain," and so it should not be surprising that explanations involving brain function have been advanced by those who prefer to study synapses rather than psyche and neurons rather than neuroses. Although this preliminary work may hold some promise, one initially compelling theory has been laid to rest: recent research has extinguished the notion that panic and agoraphobia are related to the cardiac rage of the 1980s, mitral valve prolapse. As research proceeds, other specious assertions—such as that made by a social security disability claimant who contended that her agoraphobia was due to "birth control pills, junk food, and large amounts of Tab"—will be more quickly and irrefutably debunked.

Containing the Fear

In the movie *Nell*, the title character—an unsocialized but knowing "wild child" played by Jodie Foster—is herself the unlikely, idealized cure for Mary Peterson's apparent agoraphobia. Fortunately, treatment approaches available to health care professionals are much less idiosyncratic than Hollywood would have us believe, and psychiatric care usually dramatically reduces the symptoms of agoraphobia.

The particular approach taken depends initially on whether panic attacks complicate the agoraphobia. If so, a large majority of patients will have their panic attacks remedied with medications, especially antidepressants. Antianxiety medications such as benzodiazepines appear to be effective as well, and they may make it possible for the patient just to get to the doctor's office in the first place—literally to take fledgling steps toward independence. Psychologist Alvin Pam and his team from Bronx, New York, for instance, reported on a man who had spent four years in self-imposed isolation in his room. His mother had even had to pass food, linen, and clean clothes through the door. He was finally hospitalized but was too fearful ever to leave the ward. How did he eventually accomplish the impossible and brave the imposing barrier of the unit doorway? By taking benzodiazepines to briefly tranquilize him. Once surmounted with a little pharmacologic help, the obstacle was no longer quite so towering.

A number of nonmedication interventions can be used too—alone or in combination with one another. With all of these techniques, patients who access treatment soon after their symptoms begin—that is, before their symptoms are entrenched—are more likely to improve. For example, Katherine Weissman, whose personal account was discussed earlier in this chapter, overcame her agoraphobia, in part, through behavior therapy. First enlisting her mother as a constant companion, she began to reacquaint herself with public transportation, such as the city buses she had dreaded. With time, she relied less and less on her mother's presence to make travel possible. Finally, she was able to take the bus to work on her own. This achievement led to others. She writes,

> Over the next year, I marked my recovery with milestones of a private kind: first subway ride, first movie by myself, first walk through the park, first cab, first train to the suburbs, and first plane to Paris. Small risks that got bigger month by month as I learned to trust myself again.

Behavior therapy for panic and agoraphobia, as in the case of Jackie's tenure-minded patient Josh and the twirling-chair technique, can sometimes involve actually evoking the troubling symptoms, albeit in a careful and controlled way. The therapist can then directly observe and help the patient to learn techniques to combat the symptoms.

Most often, though, behavior therapy incorporates the measures described in other sections in this chapter, such as graded exposure, breathing exercises, and systematic desensitization. Supplemented by cognitive therapy to block the "automatic thoughts" that lead the patient first to misinterpret any strong emotion as "anxiety" and then to equate "anxiety" with "doom," the agoraphobic person discovers that feelings of panic, though unpleasant to be sure, are not a death sentence.

Traditional psychotherapy has its place in some cases. A German team was certainly optimistic about the results with individual psychotherapy: they claimed that psychotherapy alone helped 6 out of 10 patients with agoraphobia. Psychotherapy can be employed to help the motivated patient identify the unconscious conflicts that display themselves through horrific anxiety. The childhood unavailability of a parent, for instance, might have triggered fears of abandonment that are revived with blistering urgency when the patient is alone in public places. Alternatively, overprotective parenting may have suggested to the impressionable youngster that the world is an erratic and menacing place. Supplementing the individual psychotherapy with a support group can compound the benefits by providing a social network that alleviates patients' isolation. Similarly, family therapy may be important:

families of patients with agoraphobia may have had to suspend their own lives to accommodate their loved one's disorder. Relatives and friends may also have functioned as "enablers" or "codependents." One well-meaning husband, for example, quit his job to be able to stay with his wife full-time . . . and therefore became every bit as entrapped by agoraphobia as she. In cases such as this, support and education for family members and significant others are indispensable.

A patient named Jacqueline wrote about her agoraphobia—a particularly severe case—in a professional journal. For months, Jacqueline had confined herself to her room, terrified even to venture to the bathroom. At the time she wrote her account, she was no longer so completely incapacitated, but group therapy remained the only "social" event she attended—and still she missed at least half the sessions because she never knew until the last minute whether she could manage to go. Nevertheless, her gradual improvement made her eager for more and hungry to help others. She stated, "I wish for myself and I wish for all agoraphobics: freedom, peace of mind—panic free—and a joyful life. If I ever succeed in becoming free, I will always dedicate my life to helping other people with agoraphobia."

We can only hope that her dream, which has seemed so far away, becomes a fulfilling reality.

■ Is There Life (Before and) After Phobic Disorders?

As we have seen in each of the cases in this chapter, the pain of phobic disorders and the sufferer's desperation for relief are inextricably bound. It is not surprising, then, that "alternative" remedies have been sought with such eagerness by beleaguered patients that they have created a $30 billion-per-year business. Writer Sara Davis recounted just such a trek in a recent article:

> I tried crisis counseling, est. . . . I talked to anyone who could give advice. I climbed narrow flights to the East Village apartment of an alternative healer who taught me meditation and tried to bring my cranium into alignment with my sacrum. I whooshed up silent elevators to the Fifth Avenue apartment of a noted hypnotherapist who elicited images of abandonment and loss. I consulted with a bioenergetics therapist on the East Side and an integrative therapist on the West Side. I swallowed homeopathic pills and drops of Bach Rescue Remedy.

Davis's relief finally came after she attended a workshop based on Dr. Brian Weiss's 1988 book *Many Lives, Many Masters*. The book is founded on an enormously provocative notion: that events from our "past lives" influence us today and that reexperiencing these prior-life events can furnish an understanding of the origins of our irrational anxieties. In the book, for example, Weiss describes his patient Catherine, whose phobias and anxieties vanished only when he took her back, via hypnosis, to her life as a 25-year-old woman named Aronda . . . in the year 1863 B.C. Over the next three years, Catherine's phobias faded as she recalled the nerve-racking events of dozens of past lives. Another patient, one who had presented with the curious problem of being unable to button her top shirt button, "recalled" that she had been guillotined in a previous life, making the neck an understandably sensitive region. Yet another attributed her acrophobia to having been thrown from a tower in the 16th century. These patients and many others are fans of Weiss's theories, though "past life therapy" may well be just about as "alternative" as it gets.

The theory of past lives is an undeniably enticing and reassuring construct, for it postulates that we never die. It is a self-aggrandizing concept as well, in its holding that each of us has extraordinary depth and complexity at which our humdrum exteriors only hint. Weiss maintains that we are continually recycled into new human forms (unlike reincarcation in the Hindu religion, past life therapy assures its believers that they need not fear coming back as cows). He has also stated, with notable imprecision, "We're probably all ageless and have been around from the beginning."

Despite its surface appeal, Weiss's work has not been subjected to scientific scrutiny; in fact, he claims that past life therapy is beyond such practicalities. But we note that it relies on the very same methods for memory retrieval—such as hypnosis, dreamwork, and regression—that have fallen into disrepute with the recognition of false memory syndrome (FMS), discussed in Chapter 4 of this book. As in FMS, the memories that most commonly emerge, according to Weiss, are those involving sexual abuse (that occurred not just during the past, but during a past life). He also believes that the total inability to recall a past life, even under hypnosis, by no means suggests that it did not occur. This contorted logic is simply a new spin on a theme now well recognized in FMS. Both past life and recovery movement therapists offer circular arguments to explain away data that do not support their preconceptions.

All that said, the past life theory may nevertheless have some value. It gives patients a face-saving way to move beyond their difficulties, and, unlike FMS, it brings no harm to family members, friends, and others: after all, how can you sue your 15th-century abuser? In allowing patients to cushion their distressing symptoms with layers of mysticism, intuition, and the paranormal, their problems are now somehow richer and more meaningful: they have been reframed as exciting spiritual signposts to the past.

Sara Davis does indeed say that she is happy and well. And one of our acquaintances found relief after retrieving memories of having been burned alive at the stake during the Salem witch trials—however, it is a common misconception that the presumed witches were burned; as described in Chapter 7 of this book, they were not. For some of us, the illusion is far more sumptuous, and perhaps even more liberating, than the reality.

TWO

SOMATOFORM DISORDERS

What Does My Mind Have to Do With It?

Imaginary pains are by far the most real we
suffer, since we feel a constant need for them and
invent them because there is no way of
doing without them.

—E. M. Cioran (1911–   ),
The Trouble With Being Born

Marc

At times, all of us seek to be coddled like newborn babies. Returning home
from a particularly trying day, I'll let Jackie know, "I'm spent. I have nothing
left. Every single person in the world wanted something from me today. My
head's splitting and I *have* to lie down and rest. Can you take care of the kids?
And let me know when dinner's ready?"

"Not so fast," she'll answer before I can escape. "You think *your* day was
bad? *You* sit in an office. Try seeing 30 patients at two different clinics—
across town from each other. Add to that a presentation to the city ....'
'headache boy.' "

"But I really *do* have a headache. You know about my neck problems."

"Save it for 'Oprah.' Lee's waiting for you to play on the computer with him. And if you want to eat, you'll have to help."

The couch, a glimmering mirage, suddenly vanishes. My "somatization" is rebuffed again.

▌ Mind and Body: Which Shall Reign?

Whether we do it consciously or unconsciously, all of us at times stoke our physical symptoms like embers on a cold day. Falling prey to the defense mechanism called *somatization*, we convert our psychological strain into physical symptoms that can range from mild nausea and dizziness to intense chest pain.

During any given week, 60% to 80% of the normal population experiences some sort of physical complaint. Even if we become concerned enough to consult a doctor, only infrequently will a straightforward medical cause be found. More often, it appears that—even as we're clutching our chests or grabbing the banister for support—we're actually just fine medically; at least, none of the conditions we might have, such as high blood pressure, is any worse than it has been.

Arising from a confluence of our emotions and the level of stress to which we're being exposed, our infirmities become the "language" of our distress. Typically, after mobilizing TLC from our families or gaining respite from the stress, we move on, our pacified psyches ready—for the time being—to relinquish the symptoms.

Psychiatrists reserve the term *somatoform disorder* for people whose ailments begin to loom like shadows on the wall of a dim room. So troubled are they by their self-perceived maladies that they are unable to handle their usual duties at home, school, or work. Perhaps no psychological phenomena better illustrate the meshing of mind and body than the somatoform disorders. They reveal to us not only that the mind can make it harder for us to cope with the authentic medical problems we do have but that psychological factors can cause the illusion of serious physical illness. In the somatoform disorders, what is at best a physical molehill becomes a portentous medical mountain.

It should not be surprising that primary care physicians (PCPs) see patients with somatoform disorders far more often than psychiatrists or other mental health clinicians. These patients minimize or are genuinely unaware of the psychological component to their symptoms. *Why*, they would ask, *would anyone go to a psychiatrist if the problem is so obviously physical?* Exasperated PCPs may find, negative exams and tests notwithstanding, that these patients tenaciously refuse to consider the possibility that the symptoms have a psychological explanation. They may also find that the reporting of vague, unexplained symptoms is increasing among their patients as the public grows increasingly intolerant of any kind of discomfort, seeking care for even minor or time-limited symptoms. Physicians must adroitly juggle the qualities of persistence and tact if they are even to broach the subject of a psychological overlay, let alone make a mental health referral.

In this chapter, we illustrate three somatoform disorders that, although very disparate, are characterized by a common core: troublesome medical complaints that lack a physical basis. The three are 1) *conversion disorder;* 2) *hypochondriasis;* and 3) *body dysmorphic disorder.*

■ Conversion Disorder

Mrs. Jasper (as told by Jackie)

As a second-year resident on my emergency room rotation, I served as the "front-line" psychiatrist each day in the ER. Business came unpredictably, from long dry periods to sudden gushers. During lulls, my medical student Tabitha and I would hang out in the back office we shared with the pediatric resident. In an effort to entice Tabitha into pediatrics, the pediatric resident routinely regaled her with quirky details that she apparently found fascinating—such as the differences among the various brands of infant formula. Although I thought Tabitha had no interest in psychiatry as a career, I countered with my own rendition—a scintillating laundry list of psychiatric side effects from different medicines.

Her eyes were glazing over when we received a consult request. The attending internist complained quietly as we walked to the patient's room.

"I can't get any information out of her. Literally. She won't even talk."

"Then why are you getting a psychiatry consult?" I asked, shaking my head. "We tend to emphasize the part where the patient talks."

"Well, I don't have the time to cajole her. That's what *psychiatrists* do." He pointed toward the exam room and started to walk away. "Let me know what you find out."

I turned to Tabitha as we approached the door. "Cute. You know, there are a million medical reasons why someone can't talk, and he assumes it's psychiatric. Typical."

As we entered the room, we were astonished by the number of people who had squeezed into the tiny space. A large woman occupied the gurney. She was lying on her back looking vacantly at the ceiling, her hands gently clasped on her chest. Modestly dressed, she had her wispy brown hair pulled neatly into a bun. No jewelry, really no adornments whatsoever, until I noticed that her hands were around something. Rosary beads.

I wondered about the assortment of people. I introduced myself to the patient, Mrs. Jasper, who looked at me pleasantly and smiled but said nothing back. I turned to the crowd.

"Now, who are y'all?"

One by one, they introduced themselves.

"Gary" identified himself as the patient's son. "Patricia" was her daughter, "Terri" her other daughter. "Sandra" and "Betty" were her sisters and "Martha" was her neighbor. I wondered where her husband was but quickly decided that the most pressing matter was to establish some breathing space.

"I'm sorry, but you can't all be in here," I said. I turned to Mrs. Jasper. "It's too tight. One person can stay in here with you if you'd like. Who should it be?"

She pointed to Martha. I asked the others to step out, which they did, exchanging glances among themselves and glaring ferociously at Martha. She ignored them as she stood by the gurney and patted Mrs. Jasper's shoulder.

I drew up a chair and Tabitha leaned against the wall.

"Okay, Mrs. Jasper, what brings you to see us today?"

She shrugged her shoulders and looked at the ceiling. Silence. More silence. I had told my medical student that sometimes if you wait long enough, the silent patient will get anxious and blurt something out, often something important. But there was no blurting this time, only a continuing quiet that made *me* uncomfortable. Martha said nothing either. I reached over to look at the patient's chart. The internist had examined her and found no physical reason for her lack of speech.

I finally gave in and broke the silence. "Look, Mrs. Jasper, we can't help you unless you talk to us. *Can* you talk?"

She shook her head no.

"Did this just start?"

She nodded.

"All of a sudden?"

Another nod.

"Doesn't it *worry* you that you can't talk?"

A subtle shrug.

"Are you feeling okay?"

Another shrug.

"Is there anything *bothering* you?"

A head shake indicating "no," although her grip on the rosary beads tightened somewhat.

"Are you depressed, or upset, or mad about something?"

Another no.

Then she finally opened her mouth. Aha, I thought, now it will all come out. She mouthed several words but there was no sound, not even a whisper.

"Try again," I urged.

She moved her lips, displaying emotion with her face and hands, but again, there was absolutely no voice.

I turned to Tabitha and asked her to go talk to the family. Had anything been happening? Had this happened before? In the meantime, I performed a quick neurologic exam myself and found it entirely normal. Through nods, shrugs, and mouthed words—a kind of impromptu pantomime—Mrs. Jasper denied any medical problems. She wasn't taking any medications and denied using any illicit substances. Martha seemed content to keep patting her shoulder, humming little songs in her ear, telling her that everything would be all right.

Tabitha finally called me out of the room.

"Something's strange," she said, "but I can't put my finger on it. Her family keeps hemming and hawing. I got nowhere."

This wouldn't do. I turned on my heel and went to the family.

"We can't figure out what's going on with your mom," I said. "It doesn't seem as if she's *refusing* to talk; she *can't* talk. And there also doesn't seem to be any medical reason for this. Has something traumatic happened? Sometimes when people are feeling overwhelmed, *really* overwhelmed, they temporarily lose function. Like they can't walk, or move some part of their body, or talk. If that's what's going on, then I can't help your mom unless I know what's been happening in her life."

They looked at each other as if they were trying to make a decision about whether to open up to us.

"Okay, if you won't tell me, maybe I should ask Mr. Jasper. By the way, where *is* Mr. Jasper?"

Bingo. The mention of his name set off the group.

Sister Betty: "That low-down sonuvabitch. If I ever see him, I'll kill him!" The other sister scowled fiercely and crossed her arms over her chest.

Son Gary: "Now, Aunt Betty, there's got to be some reason why he did what he did . . . ."

Daughter Patricia: "Of course you'd defend him. All you men stick together."

Daughter Terri: "I can't believe he would do this to us or to Momma. It's so embarrassing."

"What did he do that was so awful?" I asked.

Sandra exploded. "He's having an affair, that's what he did. A dirty, sneaking affair, and now he's took off with that 20-year-old thing last night and left his wife with nothing but a broken heart."

I wanted to get back to the patient, still sitting with Martha and Tabitha in the exam room. "Well, what was Mrs. Jasper's reaction?" I asked.

Patricia answered first. "There *wasn't* any reaction. Mom read the note after we got back from Mass last night. I don't even think she suspected anything. She read it and just got quiet and went to bed. This morning she got up and acted like nothing had happened. She hasn't talked since last night."

"What does your mom usually do when she gets angry or sad?"

"Do? *Do?*" exclaimed Betty. "She never *does* anything. She was always the calm one, the one we could turn to in any storm. And *now* look, she's falling apart."

I hardly considered not talking to be falling apart.

"Let me tell you what I'd like to do," I said. "I'd like to give Mrs. Jasper some medicine called Amytal to relax her. It might open her up, help her let the feelings out. It may not be easy for her to let the feelings go but it's got the best odds of helping her talk again, and quickly. Okay?"

Her family had no better ideas. They seemed willing to do whatever it would take to get her to speak.

I returned to Mrs. Jasper's room.

"Your family and I think there may be something bothering you that you don't want to think about, much less talk about. How about I give you some medicine that might help you talk?"

She simply closed her eyes. Martha turned from her and pulled me aside.

"What are you doing? If she doesn't want to talk, she doesn't want to talk."

"Martha, I think there's more to it than that. I think she *can't* talk right now, not that she's *choosing* not to talk."

After a little more discussion, Martha backed off. I then explained the procedure in detail to Mrs. Jasper, and Martha and I helped her sit up as she signed the consent form. We hooked up an IV and started to deliver the Amytal into a vein. Since Amytal is sedating, I wasn't too surprised when, after a few minutes, her eyes lost focus. She looked both a bit dazed and much more relaxed.

I asked simple, open-ended questions to allow *her* to guide the flow of the conversation. "Mrs. Jasper? Mrs. Jasper? Can you tell me how you're feeling?"

After a very long pause, and in a hushed voice, she said, "I'm so sad."

I pulled very close. "About what?"

"Lou left me." Her mouth turned down and a tear rolled down her cheek. "Lou left me. We had been together forever. I thought he loved me. I did everything for him. I did everything he wanted me to."

"Why do you think he left you?"

Her voice got louder, her brow suddenly scowling. She started to lift up from the gurney.

"I KNOW why he left me. His note told me. She's younger and prettier and thinner than me. Of course she's thinner; she's 30 years younger and has never had children. And *I* had his children and kept his house and took care of him and met his every whim, and NOW HE'S LEFT ME! I CAN'T BELIEVE HE'S LEFT ME! HOW COULD HE DO THIS TO ME AFTER EVERY-THING I'VE DONE FOR HIM? I HATE HIM I HATE HIM I HATE HIM! I HOPE HE ROTS IN HELL!"

Martha's eyes were huge. She pulled me close and whispered in my ear, "I have *never* heard her yell. She always told me her father would smack them good if they even raised their voices. But *he* screamed at *them*. It scared her."

We looked back at Mrs. Jasper. She seemed spent; the Amytal and the fervent emotions had taken their toll. She fell asleep within moments.

I spoke with her family as she slept. I recounted what had transpired and how they needed to encourage her to ventilate her feelings of rage and betrayal—even if they had never before heard her talk that way.

I went back to her room a few minutes later. She had roused herself and was starting to sit up. She said softly, a forlorn smile on her face, "I guess I'm angry."

"I guess you're angry, and probably sad and confused too."

"What can I do?"

"I don't know that you need to do anything right now. What's important for you to understand is that you have very strong feelings about Lou's leaving, and that's not surprising . . . or wrong. It's okay to have those feelings and to express them, even if it means yelling."

"But if I yell, I'll get into trouble."

It was my turn to take her hand. "Mrs. Jasper, that may have been true when you were little. But you're grown up now. It will cause you more problems if you don't recognize that you have *lots* of feelings about what's happened, and then *talk* about those feelings."

She nodded slowly, then got up and gathered her things together. She left with Martha and her family, an appointment card to see me—to talk things over—in her hand.

Abilities That Vanish

Mrs. Jasper suddenly lost an important ability—the capacity to speak—in a way that initially suggested a stroke or some other severe neurologic problem. This feature is at the core of conversion disorder, a problem diagnosed in 1% to 3% of patients seen in outpatient mental health clinics, and one that is even more frequent in hospitals. The conversion patient develops unexplained symptoms or losses in function that are judged to stem from psychological conflicts, not medical conditions. Described as early as 1900 B.C., the symptoms or deficits in conversion disorder tend to occur suddenly and involuntarily and to affect just a single body function.

Whereas some conversion patients, including Mrs. Jasper, experience motor deficits such as paralysis, incoordination, or an inability to swallow, others develop sensory problems that may include tunnel vision, deafness, or loss of the sense of touch. In one case, a woman temporarily developed conversion blindness when, on her wedding night, she saw something she had never seen before. . . .

Controversy About the Cause

We have been struck by the findings of researchers such as Watson and Buranen that around 25% of conversion disorder patients are later diagnosed with authentic medical ailments that account for their symptoms. Even a case of conversion disorder that appears classic can deceive us, and so we believe this diagnosis should be rendered only with exceeding care. Patients diagnosed with conversion must also be reassessed at regular intervals for underlying physical disease.

For example, a 15-year-old Chicago girl came to the emergency room complaining that she had precipitously developed a strikingly abnormal posture. Indeed, she was leaning markedly to the right and, when she tried to walk, her movements were hesitant and awkward.

Based on this sudden and bizarre change, the girl was diagnosed with conversion disorder. A psychiatrist was called in who endorsed the diagnosis, stating that the patient's anxiety over some recent surgery appeared to be the culprit—the stress had expressed itself in this disturbing physical way.

Several days later, the girl was correctly diagnosed with a medical problem—the graphically named "Pisa" (as in "leaning tower") syndrome. The cause was the side effects from medications she had been taking for a bout with nausea and vomiting. She was fine once these medications, which had interfered with proper muscular functioning, were out of her system.

In a case from Boston, a boy named "A.C.," only four years old, was also initially misdiagnosed with conversion. He had been hospitalized with right leg pain and an inability to walk. At the same time that the tests turned out to be negative, the staff learned that the boy's parents often fought and had recently separated; in addition, a cousin with an amputated right leg had just moved in and A.C. was preoccupied with the cousin's prosthesis. A.C. started to claim that he too needed a cane to walk. The diagnosis of conversion seemed self-evident.

The doctors shared their impressions with the family, and the boy was referred for both pediatric and psychiatric follow-up. But his symptoms worsened over the next few months, and serial medical exams started to uncover some clear-cut neurologic abnormalities. A.C. was readmitted to the hospital, where a computed tomography (CT) scan of his back showed a tumor in his spinal cord. Chemotherapy was started, and the focus of the psychiatric intervention switched to helping the youngster and his family cope with an illness that was all too real.

Mr. Davis (as told by Marc)

The complexity of conversion is magnified by the fact that genuine illness and conversion can coexist. Sometimes, for instance, patients with genuine epilepsy have conversion seizures as well. In a true *grand mal* seizure, a patient has massive electrical discharges from all the parts of his or her brain, leading to the body jerking and tongue biting with which most people are familiar. But patients with conversion seizures have normal brain activity even when they appear to be in the throes of a seizure.

For obvious reasons, some patients with genuine epilepsy are continually worried about having a sudden convulsion. As a result of their chronic anxiety, they develop an overlay of these conversion seizures, also called pseudoseizures (in a parallel way, some cancer patients receiving chemotherapy begin vomiting before their treatments). Separating out which seizures are real and which aren't is a task that can challenge even the most skillful neurologist.

Mr. Davis was one such patient. His neurologist had been surprised that Mr. Davis's convulsions still occurred frequently despite hefty doses of antiepileptic medications. The neurologist began to wonder whether Mr. Davis's lingering seizures represented conversion phenomena.

As the consulting psychiatrist on the case, I worked with the neurologist to carry out an experiment that we believed would ultimately benefit Mr. Davis. We asked him to relax on his bed and, after pasting more than a dozen surface electrodes to his scalp and placing an IV in his arm, we monitored his brainwave activity with an electroencephalograph (EEG). Normal. We then staged a ruse, telling Mr. Davis that, in order to test the intensity of his seizures, we needed to administer a medication that would precipitate one in a controlled environment. We also assured him that we had another medication handy, an antidote that would halt the seizure in its tracks. In reality, both "medications" were saline, or salt water, which would have no effects whatsoever.

As the saline started flowing into Mr. Davis's arm, the neurologist warned him, "Now in about five seconds, you've going to have a seizure." Moments later, Mr. Davis let out a small bark; his head tipped back and his eyelids fluttered. Seconds after that, he began to jerk violently on the bed.

I turned to look at the EEG printout: still normal.

Loudly proclaiming "Here comes the antidote," the neurologist inserted a syringe into the IV line and dispensed more saline. Mr. Davis rapidly settled down, looking spent and a bit dazed. "That was a bad one, docs," he said as he recovered.

The point of this little plan was not to deceive Mr. Davis. It was also not to "unmask" him; Mr. Davis experienced his persistent seizures as real, never suspecting the central role of the unconscious. Instead, the ruse was intended to assuage his fears about his epilepsy by showing him just how powerful the mind could be. Going over the EEG tracing with him later, we were able to point out that the antiepileptic medications were in fact doing their job—but that his mind was working overtime. He was tremendously reassured and grateful. Most importantly, the pseudoseizures came to a screeching halt—even without more of the "antidote."

Unlocking the Door and Keeping It Open

There are a number of clues to the diagnosis of conversion disorder. First are the characteristics of the patients themselves. As with the somatoform disorders in general, conversion disorder is more common among women because they seem to be more vigilant to their own bodies, and thus their bodies are more susceptible to psychological influences. There is also an increased incidence among people in rural settings and lower socioeconomic groups, those with anxious or dependent personalities, those who have had a somatoform disorder in the past, and those who have recently experienced extreme stress. In the last category are the World War I servicemen who fought in the trenches and were subsequently diagnosed with "shell shock," a type of conversion; after witnessing carnage of an unimaginable magnitude, for example, some soldiers simply erased it from their visual field by going "blind." In a similar way, over 100 survivors of Cambodia's "killing fields" developed conversion blindness after viewing unspeakably brutal beatings and murders at the hands of the Khmer Rouge.

Second, diagnosis is simplified when the conversion deficits defy the laws that govern the physiology of the human body. For example, a "paralyzed" arm may have intact reflexes and good muscle tone and function normally when the patient's attention is directed elsewhere. The distribution of "numbness" in a hand or foot may be incompatible with everything known about neurology. And, as we saw in the case of Mr. Davis, convulsions concurrent with a normal EEG are readily shown to be spurious. In other conversion states, lab tests that would be aberrant if the malady were authentic are perfectly fine.

Third, Mrs. Jasper's case illustrates the fact that the intravenous administration of the barbiturate Amytal or similar medications can help some conversion patients relax enough to become aware of the stressors that precipitated the loss of function. Hypnosis can also assist in unlocking the door, though, as we will illustrate in the chapter on false memory syndrome, both techniques must be applied in a way that avoids coercion.

Regardless of whether these procedures are used, ongoing psychotherapy is critical. It helps the patient feel understood and supported and also teaches him or her new ways to cope so that conversion disorder remains a thing of the past—even when difficult times hit again, as they inevitably will. The goal is for the patient to express through words and appropriate emotional responses, such as crying, what he or she had previously expressed through the body. Behavior therapy to reinforce efforts at normal function can be useful too. On the other hand, the clinician should always avoid vigorously confronting or trivializing the symptoms; these approaches will serve only to anger or embarrass a patient already in distress.

The prognosis for recovery from conversion disorder is generally good. A sudden onset of the conversion symptom or deficit, and the presence of a clear-cut stressor that precipitated it, are especially favorable prognostic factors. On the other hand, "rewards" accruing from the conversion (such as disability payments, or oversolicitous handling by family and friends that allows the patient to bask in the sympathy) are associated with a much more drawn-out course. The less prominent the gains, the better is the prognosis.

Mrs. Cox (as told by Marc)

One of the stranger examples of conversion disorder I've encountered involved a patient, Mrs. Cox, whom I met a few days before she was scheduled to undergo the amputation of her left arm. Mrs. Cox, a pleasant middle-aged woman, had suffered a severe nerve injury to the arm in a car accident. In an effort to preserve the limb, surgeons had performed a series of delicate operations. Initial hope was followed by devastating disappointment when Mrs. Cox slipped in the bathtub. She badly reinjured the arm, and all the progress—exacted at the heavy price of considerable pain and worry—was instantaneously reversed. She was left unable to move the arm at all. Repeated infections had then occurred in the limb, and her doctors, fearing that an infection might eventually spread into her bloodstream, reluctantly recommended amputation. She agreed, and the operation was scheduled for the next week.

Soon thereafter, Mrs. Cox's sister called the surgeon in a state of alarm.

Mrs. Cox had begun to act as if half of her body weren't even there. She would literally dress only her right side, the "good" side unencumbered by a paralyzed arm. She ate only from the right half of the plate. She combed only the hair on the right side of her head and was no longer presentable. It seemed that she had expunged her left side from awareness—"written it off," her sister said.

Her symptoms indicated *hemineglect*, a phenomenon in which patients blithely behave as if half their bodies don't exist. Individuals who have suffered strokes sometimes display hemineglect, and, realizing this fact, the surgeon ushered Mrs. Cox into the hospital. Extensive testing, such as an emergency magnetic resonance imaging scan of her brain, was both reassuring and befuddling: there had been no stroke or, for that matter, any other kind of brain injury. He asked me to take a look. Could her hemineglect be "psychiatric"?

When I met with Mrs. Cox and asked her about her recent behavior, she looked at me with a blend of perplexity and tolerance. I found her to be curiously detached, even bored, as I tried to learn more about this sudden change. At the same time, her sister battled her own anguish, pacing about the room, arranging toiletries, smoothing the towels; at times, she muttered "See? There it is!" when I performed a maneuver to test the tenacity of the hemineglect.

Retreating to the nurses' station, I looked over the mini-mountain of records that had accumulated since Mrs. Cox's initial injury. I could only imagine her feelings as she had undergone one operation after another in what ultimately proved to be a futile effort to save the limb: the succession of operations, the ever-climbing cost, the constant discomfort . . . and then the mishap at home that rendered it all for naught. Based upon the records, the negative medical tests, and my evaluation of Mrs. Cox, I surmised that her hemineglect was a variant of conversion disorder. It seemed that her unconscious had finally "banished" the "bad" side of her body—the side with the scarred, useless arm that even had the potential to threaten her life.

Despite this "psychiatric" finding, I saw no reason to delay the operation. Indeed, the risk of escalating medical problems from a paralyzed and infected limb remained as intense as ever, and the surgeon proceeded. The outcome helped reassure me that the diagnosis of conversion hemineglect had been correct: immediately after the amputation, the hemineglect disappeared. It seemed that when Mrs. Cox knew that she had undergone her last operation, and that the source of so many problems had been removed, her unconscious need for the hemineglect evaporated. Although obviously most people would experience an amputation as an unthinkably tragic event, for Mrs. Cox it was actually liberating. It allowed her finally to accept her body as it was.

Such an outcome, however, is in no way equivalent to the delusional patient's self-mutilation to get rid of a "bad" body part (see Chapter 5 of this book). In Mrs. Cox's case, the liberation that came with the amputation of her arm followed years of strife: limited mobility, pain, and invasive medical interventions.

▌ Hypochondriasis

"Hypochondriac" is one of those psychiatric terms that have insinuated themselves into everyday parlance. And we all know at least one person who qualifies for the title. Consider the following example, in which "Dear Esther" spoofs the "Dear Abby" and "Ann Landers" advice columns:

Dear Esther:

My aunt is a hopeless hypochondriac. She is flying down soon for her annual week-long visit. Last year she complained nonstop about her many ailments. My husband and children are threatening to go skiing in Aspen for the week unless I come up with a plan for dealing with "Auntie." Please help.
—Favorite Niece

Dear Fav:

These people have an appetite for attention that is not easily suppressed. Now my prescription is this: you must administer a megadose of attention to your aunt in hopes that it will knock the hypochondria into temporary remission. When Auntie arrives at the airport, have her picked up in style. Mind you, I'm not talking limos here. I'm talking about a big, shiny new ambulance. . . . After dinner, the family should go see Baryshnikov in his new play. Of course, tell your aunt that you wouldn't *dare* let her push herself, and not to worry because you were able to sell her ticket. . . . The next morning, make Belgian waffles for the family and Cream of Wheat (with white bread on the side) for your aunt. . . . I have a notion that by mid afternoon Auntie will be healthy as a horse.   —"Ask Esther," *The (North Carolina) Independent*, March 23, 1989

Hypochondriasis: Then and Now

In *hypochondriasis* (the formal term favored by psychiatrists), an individual is preoccupied not only with symptoms that lack a medical basis but with the conviction that the symptoms point to a serious disease lurking in the background. Each generation has witnessed the proliferation of "diseases du jour." In the early 20th century, Freud described patients with *neurasthenia*, a syndrome of weakness, vague aches and pains, and fatigue. More recently, reactive hypoglycemia, chronic fatigue syndrome, symptomatic mitral valve prolapse, fibromyalgia, myofascial pain syndrome, and total-body yeast syndrome have come into vogue. Some researchers maintain that these are all examples of "nouveau neurasthenia" and that efforts to treat them fall into the same dark category as astrology and channeling. They add that physicians aid and abet the process in their zeal to get to the bottom of the complaints, overtesting and overexamining patients at considerable expense. But others believe that most of these syndromes do have an authentic physical basis—though they'll usually admit that psychological factors influence the way the patient experiences the malady. The controversy is typified by our own beliefs: Marc doubts that these complaints reflect real physical illnesses, whereas Jackie accepts diagnoses such as chronic fatigue syndrome as true entities.

Most of us can accept a few fleeting pains as one of the vagaries of the human body. For others, however, symptoms such as these become ominous portents of serious medical illness. It is this belief that is at the core of hypochondriasis. Even illustrious figures such as Charles Darwin; Jiang Qing, the wife of Mao Tse-tung; biographer James Boswell; and piano virtuoso Glenn Gould have fallen prey to this mental disorder.

Hypochondriasis has also captured the attention of novelists. Molière wrote about it in his 17th-century play *The Imaginary Invalid*. In Edith Wharton's 1911 novel *Ethan Frome*, Zeena's obsession with her unfounded medical problems stripped Ethan of any hope for financial security and trapped him in a loveless marriage.

This mental malady has certainly continued to thrive into the present. Today, family doctors and internists encounter hypochondriasis in up to 9% of their patients, with its severity ranging from a relatively mild state of worry to an intense, nearly delusional belief that one is terminally ill. For the hard-core hypochondriacal patient, the *Physicians' Desk Reference* and *The Merck Manual* are just a little light reading. The most common fears hypochondriacal patients have are of cancer or heart disease; the most common symptoms are headaches, back pain, and dizziness. In their quest for reassurance about their physical condition, patients sometimes alienate family and friends. One woman, for instance, demanded reassurance of her good health from her husband more than 30 times a day.

Hypochondriasis tends to strike in early adulthood. The people at greatest risk are those who have had a serious illness in childhood, grew up in households dominated by parental "health hysteria," are facing high levels of stress, have coexisting depression and anxiety, or have recently experienced the death of a loved one.

Angie (as told by Marc)

As she left my office after her final visit, Angie handed me a copy of a letter she had sent to the hospital administrator. I've kept it to this day because it redoubles my enthusiasm for psychiatry whenever I read it. It has survived countless moves and it always will. The letter tells of "the worst year of my life," as she puts it:

"At my insistence, my doctor at home referred me to eight different specialists. Every doctor ruled out any major diseases, yet I became totally disabled. I had also become extremely depressed, but I didn't know it at the time.

"I'm happy to say I've come a long way. I am capable of enjoying my family, my home, my hobbies, and my job. I've learned to balance competing needs and to include *myself* on the list of people whose needs matter. I had an illness to be sure, but I hadn't realized that it was an *emotional* illness."

My relationship with Angie wasn't always so auspicious. Any physician will tell you that certain patients become unforgettable. Despite the thousands of faces and symptoms that pass by over the course of a career in medicine, a small percentage are etched indelibly. The reason may be a unique and perplexing pattern of symptoms, a rich friendship that builds over the years, or a particularly gratifying response to treatment. On the other hand, the cause may be rather ignominious, such as the patient's particularly overbearing or contentious personal manner. Sometimes a doctor-patient relationship, living thing that it is, becomes memorable as it evolves from detached and clinical to warm and nurturing.

My care of Angie began on the rockiest of roads. I groaned "Not again!" when my beeper went off. Angie, an inpatient on the neurology ward, had figured out how to page me directly using the phone in her room—no going through the nurse for her!

"I don't believe in going through channels," she said. "Channels aren't the kind of medicine I need."

But channels *did* work for me. Struggling as I was to juggle my clinical, administrative, and research loads, Angie's conviction—and her intuition into the intricacies of the paging system—meant that I could be interrupted at any time for any question or demand. And Angie had plenty of both. Still, I found myself grudgingly admiring her persistence; for example, I noted that she was housed on the opulent neurology floor despite having no diagnosable neurologic problem.

"Are my chemistries back yet? I feel worse. I'm too tired to move," she said. But you're not too tired to dial the phone, I thought. Yet I had to admit that her cheeks did look sunken, her color pale.

Angie's physical problems had eluded diagnosis, though they did seem truly to disable her at times. A stylish, articulate woman in her late 30s, she had functioned well as an executive secretary until the year before. Then her worries about her health began, multiplying and mutating until she felt entirely unable to work. She had been on leave, at partial salary, for four months, and for four months more she had received no salary at all.

"It started in August with the fatigue. It was bearable at first, but it only got worse and worse. It was so bad that just the stress of *trying* to function gave me headaches."

She whirled her finger around her head to show that the headaches were of the bandlike type that typically stems from chronic muscle tension.

"I had the headaches so much that it made me nauseated, and then the weight fluctuations started—up and down, up and down. The numbness in my fingers and the burning in my legs hit around that time. Also, it seemed like my temperature would never just stay put."

Angie had catalogued her symptoms, literally charting the development of each of them in a journal. She thus had documented with remarkable precision the time course over which the inexorable deterioration had occurred. The carefully recorded diary also served as her way of trying to master the symptoms that were so much out of control. The burning led to vertigo, she wrote, and then the bladder spasms hit. In a similar way, she had produced a staggering list of the physicians whom she had seen and the tests that had been conducted. Her growing facility with medical parlance, such as "Are 'my chemistries' back yet?" was perfectly understandable. She had acquired an education at the hands of specialists ranging from endocrinologists to otolaryngologists. I was impressed with her intelligence and eagerness to absorb whatever medical information she could; after all, I had been a novice medical student once. At the same time, I marveled at the likely cost of her medical care to date. I made a quick estimate of $200,000 to $300,000.

"Nothing and no one has helped," she informed me after she finally agreed to add "psychiatrist" to the list of specialists she had seen. "I *do* believe they've tried. And I believe the results of the tests they've done. But I also know that there are diseases yet to be discovered, so it only stands to reason that no one has designed a test for them. And I also know that medicine is as much an art as a science. So-called physicians used to believe in bloodletting and leeches, you know."

She had a point. I was embarrassed for my colleagues-in-antiquity. Would future doctors scoff at *me* and my primitive tools someday? Would they say

"*Psychotherapy*? He did *psychotherapy*? With the patient on a *couch*? Why didn't he just shake a gourd and deliver an incantation?"

Nonetheless, I knew that Angie had received excellent care even though all the efforts had had disappointing results. She had remained essentially bedridden, and her own theory was that she had an undetectable viral infection. Her husband had had hepatitis several months before she became ill, and though she tested negative for the hepatitis virus herself, she believed that "perhaps it's there but more in the *organs* than in the bloodstream, and so blood tests don't pick it up." She alternated this curious belief with the assurance of having "undetectable cancer."

As a psychiatrist, I had initially been consulted to help out with the growing conflicts within Angie's family. Her husband acknowledged over the phone that his compassion for Angie when her symptoms began had evolved into irritation as they worsened and the medical bills rose. He had had to assume increasing responsibility for caring for the children, cleaning up, and cooking the meals while holding a full-time job. In short, he was frustrated to find himself turning into a typical working mother.

"No, I've had it," he said when I broached the subject of our all meeting together for a marital session. "All we ever talk about is Angie and Angie's illness. I don't have time to travel up there anyway. Just send her back fixed."

I understood his resignation and negotiated simply to stay in touch with him over the phone. In the meantime, the focus of my work became a sort of one-on-one jousting with Angie. She was utterly direct: she let me know that she resented my daily meetings with her, feeling that the regular presence of a psychiatrist would delegitimize her symptoms in the eyes of the rest of the staff. "It's not all in my head, and by definition psychiatrists think it is," she stated. I refuted her, trying to match her directness, but some defensiveness crept in anyway. I felt compelled to point out to her that I had dual appointments in the departments of psychiatry and medicine: *I'm not just a shrink; I'm a real doctor.*

Over time, the jousting was transformed into supportive listening as I became better able to empathize with Angie. I understood just how disturbing her husband's bout with hepatitis had been. Though he had never been terribly ill, Angie nevertheless had been forced to confront his mortality, the likelihood that one day she would be without him—still intelligent, articulate, and forthright, but terribly alone. This realization was dramatically heightened when her father died unexpectedly of a heart attack. She submerged her feelings while handling all of the family matters as her husband recuperated. When he recovered, she fell apart.

I became convinced that a struggle with deep depression had fueled her feeling that she was "sick inside." I recommended an antidepressant medication to supplement our daily sessions and the dwindling testing and prescribing of her internist. We continued to talk about her background, the stresses of her life before her illness, her sources of support. We also talked about the "doctor shopping" she had been doing, the real risks of complications from the repeated testing, and the profound consequences to her family. Angie was able to admit that her job had been a reliable source of self-esteem for her and that she was frightened that she could never return to it. Her internist and I pointed out that months of near-total bed rest really had weakened her muscles and reduced her energy but that these were problems that could be solved. A physical therapist began to work with her on reconditioning exercises.

Somehow it all came together. In time, and with a focused determination, Angie began to show unmistakable signs of improvement. The hospitalization was long—just over five weeks—but nevertheless an important investment for her. It also provided an experience of growth and learning for me. By the time she left, Angie felt remarkably better, understanding the reasons for her preoccupation with illness and the bitter self-fulfilling prophecy it had become.

The last time I saw her in my clinic, Angie appeared marvelously fit and tanned, just back from a long weekend in the Bahamas. She admitted with a sly smile that she still scheduled appointments with her family physician fairly often, but she had decisively ended the doctor shopping. She was back at work, still a model of efficiency, but also willing to shut her office door and practice some physical therapy exercises when a twinge of a headache lurked. And she had abandoned her theory about the mysterious organ-dwelling virus.

As I said, Angie is etched indelibly in my mind indeed.

Why Me?

Traditional thinking has maintained that, as in conversion disorder, patients with hypochondriasis are expressing their inner conflicts via their illness obsessions. After all, it's more acceptable in our society to be sick than crazy. Other theories hold that genetics plays a role or that hypochondriacal patients have brains that are far too attuned to physical sensations (the so-called noisy body theory). We do know that the thresholds at which people experience pain and other noxious feelings vary considerably; for example, whereas some patients in the final stages of cancer rarely speak about their discomfort, we all have met physically fit individuals who feel compelled to highlight every ache in a rambling personal documentary.

But in some cases, the anxiety seems to be precipitated less by the symptoms patients are experiencing than by their intangible fears.

Alexander (as told by Marc)

Alexander ("not Alex and not Al" he told me up front) had scheduled his appointment with me only the day before. He had carefully explained to my secretary that he was in town visiting his family but that he would have to return to Vermont shortly: was there any way possible for me to fit him in?

Alexander was less than grateful when he appeared at my office, however. He had been misled by his family into thinking I was an infectious disease specialist. In reality, at that time my practice consisted primarily of patients whose problems had eluded medical diagnosis. The sign outside the clinic, "Psychosomatic Division," had startled and offended Alexander, as it had others. (I had wondered how many of my no-show patients had seen the sign and abruptly turned around. We later changed it to the markedly less provocative "Division of Behavioral Medicine.")

"I've been scammed, but I know why they did it," he acknowledged after asking me a series of questions about my practice and studying the diplomas on the wall. His initial antagonism began to fade, and I could tell that he was in considerable emotional distress.

"I only have part of a life these days," he said. "Maybe no life at all. I can't let go of it, of the anxiety that I have AIDS or that I'll get AIDS."

I saw this statement as an opportunity to identify any risk factors in Alexander's life and potentially to educate him about reducing the risk of HIV transmission. But there *were* no risk factors that I could detect, never had been in his case, and I didn't think Alexander was holding back any information. He was also well informed about HIV and AIDS; he knew, for example, that HIV couldn't be transmitted through casual contact. Still, this was an era when "AIDS hysteria" was everywhere and Ryan White was being barred from his Indiana school.

He astonished me with his next statement.

"In the past two years, I've been examined and HIV tested 26 times," he said. "All negative. I scheduled the appointment here to be tested again by a new lab."

"*The Guinness Book of World Records* needs a new category," I said. "You're in."

He chuckled. I had heard of cases of "AIDS delusions," in which people retain the conviction of being infected despite all evidence to the contrary. Delusions of rabies or syphilis had been reported too. I was also aware of "factitious AIDS," in which an individual knowingly makes false claims of being HIV-positive or having AIDS, typically in order to elicit attention and nurturance.[1]

In contrast, Alexander recognized that his preoccupation was excessive, and he could even tolerate some ribbing about it.

"I suppose my talking about this all the time hasn't exactly made me the life of the party," he admitted. "Sometimes I get bored with it myself. But it *is* awfully hard to let it go."

Did I know for sure that Alexander had never been exposed to HIV? That he was absolutely straightforward in all of his responses to me? Of course not. But I still felt confident in making a pronouncement, the very pronouncement that Angie, in the case above, would have been terrified to hear.

"I think it's all in your head," I said, the one and only time I've used that forbidden expression.

Alexander collapsed in the chair. "Oh, thank goodness," he sighed. "You have no idea how long I've been waiting to hear that. Every other doctor has hedged so much that I figured they just didn't want to be the one to break the bad news."

Alexander may eventually have gone on to HIV test number 62. I'll never know. But I do know that he left seeming genuinely at peace.

The Costs of Being "Sick"

My frank pronouncement to Alexander hinged on my belief (buttressed by 26 negative HIV tests) that his preoccupation with being infected was unfounded. Any time that hypochondriasis is diagnosed, the physician is implicitly stating that he or she has ruled out a genuine medical basis for the symptoms. But some diseases, such as multiple sclerosis and systemic lupus erythematosus ("lupus"), can be notoriously difficult to diagnose in the early stages. When has "enough" testing been performed? For the hypochondriacal patient, the answer is "Never." The dilemma is intensified by the ready availability of many thousands of lab tests, X rays, radionuclide scans,

---

[1] Factitious disorder, termed *Munchausen syndrome* in its most extreme form, can involve any ailment imaginable. Patients have falsified cancer by starving themselves and shaving their heads to mimic chemotherapy-induced hair loss. Others have injected themselves with bacteria to cause raging infections. In typical cases of a variant called *Munchausen syndrome by proxy*, a mother causes illness in her child in order to win the sympathy of family members, friends, and health care professionals. Those wishing to learn more about factitious disorder can consult the book *Patient or Pretender* in the References and Suggested Readings section of this book.

and the like. Why *not* get HIV test number 62, just to be really, *really* sure? And how about a biopsy and a liver-spleen scan?

We suspect that, paradoxically enough, the inexorable creep of managed health care will influence hypochondriacal patients more than any doctor ever could. Despite stalled plans for national health care reform, reductions in medical spending are being implemented *de facto* by businesses, insurance companies, managed care entities, and health care providers all over America. Not only will these initiatives further limit redundant testing for the purpose of reassuring the patient (or doctor), they will curtail the ready accessibility of the physician specialists on whom many hypochondriacal patients depend. *Fixed-benefit packages*, *medical gatekeepers*, and *precertification requirements* mean that the objective medical necessity of any desired care is being reviewed. Also, limits are being imposed on the amount of medical intervention any one patient can obtain, regardless of apparent need. Because the nonessential treatments administered to hypochondriacal patients cost the health care system $20 to $30 billion per year, the pains that patients with this disorder will increasingly feel will come from the pinch in their pocketbooks.

Although patients sometimes rev up the urgency and vociferousness of their symptom complaints to ensure their own continued access to physicians, it seems unlikely that a group effort—such as a "Hypochondriacs' Political Action Committee (Hypochondri-PAC)"—will be mobilized anytime soon to oppose these changes. Instead, and perhaps not coincidentally, home diagnostic instruments and blood tests have become a flourishing industry in the 1990s. At a reasonable cost, patients can buy their own automatic blood pressure cuffs; peak-flow monitors, to check how well they are breathing; blood-glucose sensors; ovulation and pregnancy tests; HIV tests; blood cholesterol kits; and stool occult blood tests. Home monitoring for nutritional deficiencies, strep throat, and venereal diseases is imminent. Although such devices have the potential to reduce overall medical costs by allowing patients to bypass the doctor at times, they may also serve as fodder for the hypochondriacal patient certain of having some kind of problem—if not today, then maybe tomorrow. Better check. And check again.

Treatment for What Ails You

Treatment for hypochondriasis is a puzzle. Part of the difficulty stems from the fact that these patients almost always lack motivation to lessen their medical vigilance. Thus, at the same time that they enlist help from medical professionals, they reject the conclusion that all is well; rarely is reassurance alone enough for them to let down their guard.

It's not surprising, then, that in their exasperation with patients' unremitting complaints, doctors may drop the loaded word *hypochondria*, with its implication of a sniveling, self-pitying doctor groupie. Even those who gently reframe the disorder—perhaps by telling the patient that he or she has a "pessimistic cognitive style" or a tendency to "worry too much"—may be viewed as insulting and infuriating. Doctor shopping—that is, transferring care to a new and "more understanding" physician, followed by another, and another—is the rule in these situations. Although they'd be loath to admit it, that tendency of patients to move on would delight a lot of their physicians. They feel badgered to join a game they can't possibly win.

Psychiatric medications can be helpful in some cases of hypochondriasis. In a report published in 1993, a 30-year-old man with fears of having a heart attack, AIDS, a brain tumor, and other serious illnesses centered his life around emergency room visits and doctors' appointments. All medical workups over a 10-year period had been negative, yet he was able to work only part-time and then just in a position that allowed for generous sick leave.

Although other medication trials had failed, the prescribing of a preparation called clomipramine (Anafranil is the brand name) led to a significant decline in his worries about illness. After several months, the man was looking for full-time work and, in his words, "trying to make up for 10 lost years." Up to the time of the report, this patient hadn't visited any emergency rooms or felt the need for any other types of medical services.

Psychotherapy sessions, when the patient is willing to commit to them, usually focus on careful explanations about the innocuousness of the physical complaints. At the same time, the patient's attention is redirected away from medical concerns, and his or her fears and beliefs about illness are gradually explored.

Behavior therapy can be helpful in some cases, taking a variety of forms. In a 1988 study reported in the *British Journal of Psychiatry*, the behavior-therapy techniques included *exposure* (e.g., having a patient frightened of a heart attack sit for long periods in a cardiology waiting room), *satiation* (e.g., having the patient repeatedly write down his or her fears in detail), *paradox* (e.g., having the patient strenuously exercise as if to try to "bring on" the baseless heart attack he or she fears so intensely), and the *banning of reassurance* (e.g., teaching relatives to withhold sympathy and forbidding the patient from undergoing further exams and tests). In this study, 6 of 13 patients responded well, experiencing no further anxieties about their health up to five years later. The remaining 7 went back to their old ways . . . and to their physicians.

Alternative techniques—such as self-hypnosis, yoga, aerobic exercise, and transcendental meditation—can increase some hypochondriacal patients' feelings of well-being. Distraction from physical sensations, perhaps through increased social activities or volunteer work, can help disrupt the focus on self-perceived ailments.

As in conversion disorder, patients who have had a sudden onset of their hypochondriasis—perhaps due to intense but short-lived stressors—have the best prognosis. Depressed hypochondriacal patients may also do well; treatment of the underlying depression—the factor propelling their so-called illness behavior—may remedy the problem. Still other patients seem to get over their hypochondriasis spontaneously. They get tired of the disruptive effect of continual doctors' visits, or of the expenditures on tests that are, in their eyes, relentlessly negative. Encountering undeniable illness, such as advanced cancer, in another person can also trigger the realization that the worries have been out of proportion, even shameful by comparison.

But certainly there is no sure-fire cure. For far too many patients with hypochondriasis, the preoccupation with illness becomes a way of life—a cuddly, warm blanket they refuse to give up.

▌Body Dysmorphic Disorder

First recognized in Europe over 100 years ago, *body dysmorphic disorder* (BDD) is also known as "the syndrome of imagined ugliness." Patients with BDD are convinced that something is, simply put, quite dreadful about the way they look.

Sometimes individuals with BDD are exaggerating a slight flaw of the face, the buttocks, or the hairline, perceiving themselves as grotesquely misproportioned and offensive—as if viewing themselves in a fun-house mirror invisible to anyone else. In other cases, the object of their self-perceived freakishness is another part of the body: an asymmetry in the eyes becomes a deformity; bulky arms and thighs become horrible and hideous. Some patients say that the maligned body parts feel abnormal as well.

Few of us are really satisfied with the way we look. A lucrative industry has arisen in malls throughout America: called "glamour photography," dramatic makeup, bold jewelry, and elaborate hairstyles allow women who feel plain to become fantasy supermodels. Liposuction, facial peels, permanent eyeliner and blush, hair implants, electrolysis, and a panoply of other procedures help the insecure feel a bit less self-conscious about the pockets of cellulite, the crow's-feet, the sallow complexion, the hair shafts that refuse to stay only where they belong.

But the two million Americans with BDD go beyond the so-called normal concerns about appearance. Instead, the preoccupation with ugliness dominates so much of their thinking that they may put their lives on hold. Lest they offend others with their appearance, they avoid work and social engagements. They worry that people will openly ridicule them or secretly joke about the way they look. Even though some patients retain enough insight to realize that their concerns are unrealistic, they may still continually examine their "defects" in mirrors, store windows, and even shiny car bumpers, as if to ensure that they're not getting any worse. Sigmund Freud's patient the Wolf-Man, for instance, compulsively checked out his nose in mirrors. Others assiduously avoid seeing their reflections, those cruel reminders of anatomy gone awry. As in hypochondriasis, many BDD patients constantly seek reassurance from family members ("Is my hairline receding?"; "What do *you* think of my eyes?").

The hair, nose, skin, buttocks, eyes, and thighs are the most frequent culprits in the minds of BDD patients. Yet, the average patient implicates three to four different body parts over the course of the disorder, failing to realize that their way of perceiving themselves—not the anatomy itself—is to blame. One patient named 13 different body parts that at various times he was convinced were aberrant.

David (as told by Marc)

Some people believe that psychiatrists are supposed to be immune to mental disorders. Others say that they must have been crazy to have gone into psychiatry in the first place. The reality is that many psychiatrists, like almost half the general population, will battle some form of mental disorder during their lifetimes.

A psychiatric colleague, David, shared with me his own bout with body dysmorphic disorder. This experience helped fuel his desire to pursue psychiatry as a career. I believe it has also made him a more empathic human being.

As he was negotiating the twists and turns of puberty, David became increasingly self-conscious about his appearance. "I could handle the zits and the gawkiness," he said, "but not the nose." His "button nose" had matured into a "honker, a snout, a facial Shamu," he said.

His parents never understood the problem or saw anything wrong. He rejected their efforts at reassurance and even the statements of other relatives that he looked darned handsome. "What else *could* they say?" he thought. " 'Sorry about the genes?' "

David admitted that his self-consciousness about his nose swamped all his other feelings in those days. "It was always on my mind. I still haven't broken the habit of holding my hand in front of my face when I talk. I figured my hand was better looking than my nose. I didn't want to offend anyone."

He underwent his first rhinoplasty (nose job) while still in high school. "My parents gave in," he said. "They accepted that I'd never date, never expand my horizons until I felt better about my appearance." As is so often the case with BDD patients, however, David wasn't satisfied with the results. "I really don't know what I wanted or expected, but that particular nose wasn't it." Additional plastic surgery consultations followed, leading to a total of six separate operations. "If one doctor assured me I looked great," he said, "I would find another willing to try to please me. The last two nose jobs were purely corrective to remove the scar tissue that had formed and made it hard to breathe. I can identify with Michael Jackson. I bet he's a mouth breather."

David showed me a photo of himself taken the day before surgery number one. His nose looked pretty much the same then as it does now. What allowed him finally to move on with his life?

"Two things," he said. "First, when I talked with my last surgeon about having another operation, he let me know that there was little viable tissue left. It was still mostly scar. Actually, he was more direct than that. He said the whole structure of my nose could collapse if we tampered with it anymore. I envisioned myself with nothing but two little holes in the middle of my face. That was a pretty arresting thought.

"But the most important factor," he said, "is that I fell in love. And my girl-friend particularly liked my nose. Who could argue with that? So I married her."

The Development of Body Dysmorphic Disorder

Adolescence and young adulthood are times when people are especially worried about fitting in. Self-esteem and body image, often based on the most superficial aspects of one's appearance, are particularly brittle during this period. BDD tends to evolve during this vulnerable time. And because, from infancy on, our culture stresses the importance of appearance for females more than males, we should not be surprised that in a 1996 report of 50 BDD patients, the diagnosis was more common among women.

Psychoanalytic theorists believe that BDD results from an effort at self-protection. Susceptible patients, they maintain, shield themselves from difficult emotional or sexual impulses by incriminating a particular body part as reprehensible and guilty instead of dealing directly with their conflicts. Biologically oriented psychiatrists invoke deficiencies of chemicals in the brain, such as serotonin. Sociologists note the influence of mass media depictions of beauty and the acceptance of plastic surgery in our society; in a similar way, anorexia nervosa and bulimia have been linked to unrealistic cultural physical standards. We suspect that all these factors are involved and that they act synergistically to create BDD.

In the most extreme cases of BDD, patients are utterly disabled. Convinced that they are ugly and unlovable, they try to conceal the body parts that torment them; failing that, they become shut-ins, perhaps venturing out only at night. Unable to work or to enjoy companionship, they often go on to develop severe anxiety and depression. Some try to "medicate away" these painful feelings by using alcohol or drugs. Others experience suicidal feelings that can progress to suicide attempts; indeed, a quarter of the BDD patients in two different studies had attempted suicide at some point during the course of the illness.

Joseph (as told by Jackie)

BDD is definitely not just a phenomenon of urban settings, where, compared to small towns, there is more likely to be a tremendous focus on appearance and style, and certainly greater access to plastic surgery as well. Following a brief TV appearance on an unrelated subject, I received a letter from a 40-year-old man living in a tiny North Carolina village. It spoke to his desperation that he confessed his deepest secrets to me.

Joseph, as I'll call him, was raised by a fundamentalist preacher and his wife. As he matured, Joseph felt deeply torn between his religious beliefs and his burgeoning sexuality. Though he was warned by his father and others in the church that masturbation is sinful, the urge got the best of him at times. Afterward, he felt profound guilt and shame. He repeatedly made vows never to repeat the behavior, but when he inevitably did so, it exacerbated his feelings of worthlessness.

He sheepishly confessed to the coach of the church softball team. The coach's condemnation was swift, and he also gave Joseph destructive misinformation about human sexuality. The coach indicated that masturbation, in his words, "destroyed the structure" of the penis and condemned the person to "a lifetime of premature ejaculation and inability to please any woman." Joseph believed every word and saw himself as doomed.

As his self-loathing over his own sexual desires increased, Joseph began to notice that his penis did indeed appear "different" in some way. He concluded that the damage had already occurred, and he was devastated by the thought that, still only in his teens, he had ruined any chance of a loving sexual relationship with a woman. It became a preoccupation, a burden on his shoulders that led him to avoid any women who seemed interested in dating him. Now, at age 40, he remained alone, imprisoned within walls of regret.

His reason for writing to me? In fact, it was not to share these grim secrets and perhaps avail himself of psychiatric care. Rather, he had noted during the TV show on which I had appeared that I was affiliated with a major medical center. Could I possibly arrange for a consultation with a urologist, he asked, so he could have surgery to correct the "destruction"? And could I explain to the consultant that he had rather limited insurance but was willing to work out a payment plan?

It was terribly sad to see how the quality of this man's life had been scuttled by blatant falsehoods. Whether the coach knew just how influential his statements would be, whether he honestly believed what he was saying, whether he thought that scaring Joseph would "straighten him out"—I don't know. All I could do in my return letter was to provide valid information about human sexuality. I tried to correct the distortions and encourage Joseph to understand that the intervention needed to be psychiatric, not surgical. And I asked him to update me on his progress. I later received a brief, nondescript note of thanks but, knowing how entrenched BDD can be, I am certain that my letter failed miserably in reversing over 20 years of mistaken ideas.

Facing Up to Body Dysmorphic Disorder

As the cases of David and Joseph illustrate, BDD patients often insist that the answer to this complex malady is in fact straightforward: corrective surgery by a plastic surgeon, a dermatologist, or a dentist. Yet, as David found out, cosmetic surgery generally provides only temporary relief. As one patient wrote in *New York Magazine* after liposuction, "Now I look better, not best. I've stopped assessing my stomach's hideousness every time I pass a mirror. . . . My arms still look a little chunky, though. I think I'd better have them done. And my back is disgusting." In cases in which one operation after another has been performed, the BDD patient's fears all too often become reality: the multiplicitous surgical interventions create a patently unnatural, if not grotesque, appearance. Such patients may have had more than 20 cosmetic operations.

We believe that surgery is rarely even part of the answer. Instead, we recognize that BDD is commonly entwined with other mental disorders—such as depression, social phobia, and obsessive-compulsive disorder—and that mainstays of treatment for these conditions apply to BDD as well: a judicious combination of medications (especially serotonin reuptake inhibitors such as fluoxetine [Prozac], fluvoxamine [Luvox], and clomipramine [Anafranil]) and psychotherapy. In some cases, behav-

ior or cognitive therapy improves the chance of success. Overall, treatment can reduce the intensity of the symptoms of BDD in at least 50% of patients—not bad odds
with such a potentially disabling condition.

Maintaining Perspective

Undeniably, ours is a culture that worships beauty. In *Autobiography of a Face*, Lucy
Grealy recounts the searing peer rejection she experienced as a result of the childhood cancer surgery that had disfigured her face. A veteran of more than 30 recon-
structive procedures, she writes,

> I spent 5 years of my life being treated for cancer, but since then I've spent 15
> years being treated for nothing other than looking different from everyone else.
> It was the pain from that, from feeling ugly, that I always viewed as the great
> tragedy in my life. The fact that I had cancer seemed minor in comparison.

As Grealy—and the friends that mattered—finally came to realize, beauty is
not only thoroughly subjective, but almost always incidental. She notes,

> It was easy for me to ascribe to physical beauty certain qualities that I thought
> I simply had to wait for. It was easier to think that I was still not beautiful
> enough or lovable enough than to admit that perhaps these qualities did not
> really belong to this thing I thought was called beauty after all.

In the same way, Alice Walker, author of acclaimed books such as *The Color Purple*, has spoken of the change in her own perceptions of other African Americans after
she lost an eye in an accident. She had been instilled with the common belief that
darker skin is less attractive than lighter skin and had tended to evaluate the beauty
of other African American women within that framework. After the accident, Walker
realized that, even though the appearance of her prosthetic eye was not quite "normal," her identity and personal strengths had been untouched. Just as she would not
have others judge her based upon their biases about appearance, she would never
again do the same to them.

    In certain segments of our culture, the emphasis on beauty is always at a fever
pitch. We know, for example, that actors and actresses, braving a business preoccupied with evanescent beauty, fixate on their physical flaws even more than the rest of
us. Indeed, winsome Demi Moore, the highest-paid actress in Hollywood history, despaired over her own looks in a 1995 interview with *Rolling Stone*. She compiled an
impressive list of faults: "You know . . . eyes too small, I don't have a good smile, I'm

square, I have no waist, and I'm never thin enough." In *Cosmopolitan*, singer Dolly Parton despaired over her having "short legs, little hands, and a tiny frame," whereas TV star Heather Locklear complained that "my legs are . . . too thin. And I'm knock-kneed." Many women would eagerly trade their features for the self-classified faults of these three celebrities.

The moral is that even the most comely of us may approach the mirror with a jaundiced view. We can regain our bearings by reminding ourselves of what poet Charles Baudelaire wrote 150 years ago: "[J]ust as we have our own particular emotions, so we have our own beauty."

■ Somatoform Disorders in Context: The Body Speaks Its Mind

In an interview for the PBS series *Healing and the Mind*, host Bill Moyers asks research biologist Candace Pert a question that betrays his Western mind-set: "Are you saying that the mind talks to the body . . . through these neuropeptides?" he asks. Pert ignores the question, instead spotlighting Moyers's assumption with a question of her own: "Why are you making the *mind* outside the *body*?" she wonders. This same assumption pervades Moyers's interview at every turn, and he finally attempts to exonerate himself by reminding Pert that the mind-body distinction has been "knocking around the West for a long time."

Indeed. Since the 17th century, René Descartes's enduring axiom, "I think, therefore I am," has capsulized the dualistic thinking of Western civilization—as if the body and mind were distant cousins. The somatoform disorders tell us otherwise, but now we also have proof at the molecular level that the distinction between mind and body is far hazier than we had ever imagined. Dr. Pert would tell us to speak not of "mind and body" but rather of "mind *in* body" and even "mind *is* body." Historically, this ethereal concept has been largely unacknowledged in Western medicine. Instead, the study and treatment of human beings has been compartmentalized. Because it has been more tenable scientifically to break us down into parts, we treat the mind on one hand and the body on the other. And we treat a cancer, for example, rather than the whole human being.

In recent years, however, influences from the East have been challenging our notions of where the body ends and the mind begins. Tai chi, yoga, meditation, and massage are gaining ground as adjunct therapies. The public's overwhelming reception of Deepak Chopra's books, including *Ageless Body, Timeless Mind*, is a clear indication that Americans are searching for more than what medical science has offered on its own. Chopra, a physician from India whose feet are planted firmly in both cultures, brings to Western medicine an Eastern approach to "total healing." Drawing from ancient Ayurvedic principles, Chopra soothes us with the notion that we are our own masters—that through "mind-body discipline" we can control our organic processes and bring our lives into "balanced harmony."

Although Chopra has not gained a massive following among American physicians, his influence has been felt in the medical community. Even within the ivy-covered buildings of academic institutions, investigators are beginning cautiously to measure the effects of nontraditional therapies on disease processes. If not in full agreement that patients are the sole masters of their own healing, medical science is recognizing that they are essential partners in the process and that thoughts and feelings can advance or forestall the progression of disease. In works such as 1986's *Love, Medicine, and Miracles*, Dr. Bernie Siegel regales us with convincing stories about the healing power of love. If there is an abiding connection between mind and body that influences the healing process, so claims Siegel, there is also a personal connection between physicians and patients that shapes the attitudes of each. The notion is not new, but our willingness to subject it to scrutiny is.

Thus, so-called complementary medicine is now being tested in austere laboratories. The National Institutes of Health opened an Office of Alternative Medicine to explore these very issues, and corresponding university-sponsored World Wide Web sites have been established.[2] The findings that have just started to emerge have been provocative: formal explorations into the mind-body connection seem to verify that mind and body truly are inseparable.

Nowhere is this connection more dramatically illustrated than in a 1989 report of 86 women with metastatic breast cancer. This study, led by Dr. David Spiegel of Stanford University, was designed to measure the effects of supportive group therapy on the women's quality of life. Spiegel expected to find that women receiving the group therapy enjoyed a higher quality of life. But the results went much further: not only was their quality of life much greater, but those who had participated in the therapy lived an average of twice as long as those who did not.

The specialty of psychiatry, as a field discrete from other areas of medical practice, has itself sometimes reflected the split perception we have historically had of mind and body. As sectors of the medical community become involved in examining the effects of mental processes on health and illness, our roles as physicians may

---

[2] Try http://www.gen.emory.edu/MEDWEB/keyword/Alternative_medicine.html.

become less rigidly circumscribed. We may see greater overlap and collaboration to the benefit of patients. Just as we must advocate for the advancement of science, we must also advocate for opening the door to new ways of looking at health and healing.

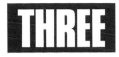

DISSOCIATIVE DISORDERS

Who Am I Today?

When someone kisses someone or flushes the toilet,
it is my other who sits in a ball and cries.
My other beats a tin drum in my heart.
My other hangs up laundry as I try to sleep.
My other cries and cries and cries
when I put on a cocktail dress.

—Anne Sexton (1928–1974),
Selection from "The Other"[1]

THE DISSOCIATIVE DISORDERS are controversial, and this controversy has turned them into media darlings. Over the past 10 years, the popular press has increasingly seized on dissociative phenomena such as multiple personality disorder, amnesia, and the

---

[1] From *The Book of Folly*: Copyright © 1972 & 1973 by Anne Sexton. Reprinted by permission of Houghton Mifflin Co. and Sterling Lord Literistic, Inc. All rights reserved.

John Dewey Library
Johnson State College
Johnson, Vermont 05656

"memories" that have apparently been liberated after years of repression. When the book *The Three Faces of Eve* appeared back in 1957 and Joanne Woodward went on to win an Oscar in the movie version, multiple personality disorder was viewed as an engrossing phenomenon, but one that was extraordinarily rare. Hardly something a therapist—or journalist—could build a career on.

Now, multiple personality disorder has itself multiplied, such that some psychiatrists claim that it afflicts one of every 20 patients on psychiatric wards, which translates roughly as one in 20,000 people in the general population. Other psychiatrists insist, with equal firmness, that the phenomenon is ridiculously overblown and that in 40 or 45 years of practice they've never seen a single valid case.

The burgeoning interest in dissociative disorders among medical professionals is reflected in the exponential increase in scientific articles on the subject. A journal devoted to nothing but dissociation has been launched. And professionals who have assumed the mantle of "multiple personality research" have been transmogrified into media fixtures.

▍Understanding Dissociation: A Shutoff Mechanism

Normally we have a solid grasp of who we are, where we are, and where we've been. And barring a bad night's sleep, we feel reasonably alert on most days. But when a person "dissociates," this natural integration among thoughts, feelings, and actions breaks down—sometimes to a limited extent, sometimes massively and disastrously. As a result, the person's memory and sense of self are undermined.

Most of us can recall having experienced dissociation in its mildest form at some point, especially in childhood or adolescence. We might suddenly have experienced a few moments during which we felt profoundly detached from the world, as if we were outside observers or characters in a dream. We had a sense of unreality, of strangeness. This brief sensation, called *depersonalization*, is a common, benign form of dissociation that we tend to outgrow. Marc remembers just such an experience when he was six:

> My brother, the kids from next door, and I were all immersed in a rowdy game of softball when the whole experience suddenly took on odd overtones. Inexplicably, I felt entirely removed, suddenly an impassive observer rather than a participant. The laughter of the other children became distant and artificial, as if I were hearing it through a tunnel; the air seemed thin and the sky unnatural. But within moments, this episode of depersonalization came to an end. The world became "real" and I was once again ready to join in.

Dissociation can also be an important defense mechanism that is mobilized in response to extreme stress, such as sudden violence. When overwhelming trauma strikes, people feel utterly helpless, actively manipulated by forces they cannot control. They recognize that their own wishes are, at least for a time, completely irrelevant. They know that they or the ones they love may well be severely injured physically or harmed in other ways, regardless of anything they do. A patient of Marc's vividly described such an experience:

> My Mom and I had been Christmas shopping and she was battling heavy traffic to get us safely home. I was in the passenger seat nursing my infant son. My two-year-old was buckled into the backseat. At some point we became aware of the urgent dissonance of many horns competing for attention. I turned around and saw that the back door was open. On a four-lane thoroughfare, cars were forming a safety shield behind my son, who was running for all his might down the busy highway. We stopped and I got out of the car, baby still at my breast. I saw my son running toward us in slow motion, black pavement burns marking his chubby legs. My mother responded quickly to her panic, running toward him into the lane of traffic, but I stood perfectly still, thinking it was all a dream.

In such intolerable situations, dissociation can become our way to "shut off" awareness. In a sense, it becomes an adaptive mechanism that helps us to be less cognizant of the possible damage and in that way to protect ourselves from the acute, devastating experience of the trauma itself. We "escape" from the constraints of reality as if these terrible events are not really happening.

This "protective" effect of dissociation has aided employees who have witnessed shootings in their office buildings, victims of assault and rape, survivors of combat, and witnesses to mass murders. For example, in the aftermath of the bombing of the Federal Building in Oklahoma City, hospital authorities were initially unable to identify a wounded teenager who had lost her capacity for intelligible speech. She had retreated to a childlike state, retaining only three words in her vocabulary: Mama, Daddy, and Dana. Victims of natural disasters, such as the Coconut Grove fire in Boston, the Oakland/Berkeley firestorm, and the Los Angeles and San Francisco earthquakes, have also used dissociation as an unconscious coping technique. They mentally flee the reality so they won't have to experience the raw anguish of the situation.

Although mild, infrequent dissociation is universal and even necessary, dissociation that occurs in response to relatively innocuous events or that persistently limits the person's ability to function is abnormal. It is in this situation that psychiatrists formally diagnose a dissociative disorder. In this chapter, we discuss three disorders involving dissociation: 1) the development of alternate identities *(multiple personality disorder)*; 2) estrangement from one's own identity, typically associated with unexpected travel to a new place *(dissociative fugue)*; and 3) the "pure" loss of memory *(dissociative amnesia)*.

Of all the lies of the mind, the dissociative disorders are perhaps the easiest to mimic, sometimes being employed as shams by people who are either consciously or unconsciously motivated. For this reason, we will also discuss the phenomenon of feigned dissociative disorders, how to recognize them, their prevalence in modern psychiatric practice, and the motivations that produce such extreme behaviors.

▌ Multiple Personality Disorder

Multiple personality disorder (MPD) is the coexistence of two or more distinct identities or personality states, often called *alters*. These different personalities or identities recurrently take or share control, causing changes in the individual's behavior for which he or she later has little or no memory.

As we've said, information about MPD (formally termed *dissociative identity disorder)* has become widespread in contemporary American society. Many people first encountered MPD through the book *Sybil*, published in 1972, which brought to life the riveting personal story of a young woman with 16 separate alters. Within its first year of publication, the book sold more than 170,000 copies, catapulting it onto the bestseller lists; today, more than six million copies are in print. The compelling portrayal of Sybil's suffering has profoundly affected those who have read the book or seen the movie. The sheer visibility of this case has been one of the central forces creating the public perception that MPD is not rare.

However, readers and moviegoers were not privy to the behind-the-scenes negotiations that brought Sybil's story to the printed page and screen. The author, Flora Reta Schreiber, was intimately connected with the publishing world, and she knew how to sell books. She also knew that Dr. Herbert Spiegel, one of Sybil's psychiatrists, had repudiated the diagnosis of MPD in this case. But when the book went to print, Spiegel's opinion was excluded. The controversy about Sybil persists to this day, and it reflects a problem inherent to MPD: even the most seasoned and experienced psychiatrists have extreme difficulty discerning true from false MPD.

Further, in more recent years it seems that all sorts of people are coming out of the closet claiming to have double-digit personalities. Part of the reason is that dramatic claims of MPD are virtually guaranteed to propel one into the news—if not the front page any longer, then at least the "Lifestyle" section. For instance, the comedienne Roseanne announced on a talk show that she had been diagnosed with 21 personalities. Predictably, national newspaper coverage mushroomed. But when Roseanne went on to say that MPD is "not a debilitating thing. It's a gift that allows you to be multiply gifted," she trivialized the very real pain of most MPD patients.

On the same talk show, Roseanne was upstaged by her friend, Truddi Chase, who claims no fewer than 92 personalities. Perhaps not surprisingly, Ms. Chase has written a book about her story. Marcia Cameron's *Broken Child* and Gene Stone's *Little Girl Fly Away* are also recent literary efforts, incorporating new, fantastical spins on the MPD theme (for example, in the latter, one personality stalks another). Even the real "Eve," Chris Costner Sizemore, points out in *A Mind of My Own* that she ultimately had 22 different personalities, not just the paltry three depicted in the original book and film. The subsequent alters, given nicknames such as "The Purple Lady" and "The Strawberry Girl," had remarkably different medical problems and talents; some needed glasses or had food allergies that the others didn't, and one was a seamstress even though Ms. Sizemore herself couldn't sew a stitch.

Attention to MPD has certainly increased in the professional community as well, with both positive and negative effects. Some solid research has been performed to develop a better understanding of MPD, increasing the likelihood that actual cases will be recognized and treated. But the professional proponents of MPD tend to overdiagnose it, and this overdiagnosis accounts for the phenomenal increase in cases during the past decade. We agree with authorities such as Dr. August Piper of Seattle that most of the recent scientific literature on MPD is one-sided because it has been written by acknowledged proponents of the diagnosis. By so overtly lobbying for the diagnosis, they sometimes overstate their position to the point of absurdity. For example, among the most visible MPD advocates is Dr. Colin Ross, former president of the International Society for Dissociative Disorders, who has argued that MPD afflicts as many as 5% of college students in Canada (and presumably elsewhere). He also has asserted that, through systematic abuse using "flotation tanks" and "enforced memorization," the CIA has implanted MPD into "thousands or tens of thousands" of children; in this way, the alters are able to carry more secret information than any one person. Ross claims that these "Manchurian candidates" are being used "for espionage and surveillance purposes and possibly for assassinations." MPD proponents lose credibility when they fail to counter such outlandish remarks.

We believe that hard-core MPD lobbyists do not distinguish between an alternate "personality state" and the behavior any of us would be expected to show when angry or happy. Should we all be labeled with MPD just because sometimes our thoughts and feelings markedly change? Although we have seen real cases of MPD, we conclude that the phenomenon is exceedingly rare, a raindrop that is being amplified into a pounding thunderstorm.

One MPD lobbyist insists that even the total absence of MPD symptoms in a given patient does not in any way disconfirm the diagnosis. But, we ask, if we ignore what patients tell us and show us about themselves, just how do we function as doctors? Shouldn't we prevent our personal feelings and preconvictions from governing the way we diagnose and care for our patients? In each case, we must remain responsive to all the data, whether they support or dispute the diagnosis.

Jason (as told by Jackie)

Take, for instance, the case of Jason. I first became aware of Jason's strong alterations in appearance and manner when, one day during a therapy session, I questioned him about his feelings concerning his mother's impending marriage. Suddenly, I became aware of another presence in the room, one so palpable that I remember glancing over my shoulder to see if someone had quietly entered the office. When I turned back to face Jason, I saw a different person. Jason's dark eyes, generally hesitant and fearful, were now focused on me with extraordinary rage. From his slouched posture on the couch, he had assumed a commanding position and was towering over me. His small, childlike voice had acquired a raspy tone. It was the first of many alters that I would meet during the course of Jason's therapy, alters so compelling—and consistent—that my initial skepticism vanished.

I recall one Friday in particular when Jason stumbled into my office and flung himself into a chair. Friday afternoon was a terrifying time for him. It meant a lonely weekend, typically without any outside contact at all. He was estranged from his family, and his erstwhile girlfriend had fought with him and left—again. The strain of his circumstance was evident in the drawn lines of his face and the wide, startled eyes that betrayed the cool exterior he tried to project. He told me that he had worked a full week and had come to the clinic directly from his job, but his appearance told me that this was unlikely. I was surprised at how different he looked. Typically neat, he was dressed far too casually for the middle management job to which he somehow managed to cling. His hair, usually worn in a ponytail, was shoved under a heavy knit cap despite the fact that it was 65 degrees outside.

Jason began to articulate his week's complaints in his usual fashion, starting with his arrival at work on Monday morning and continuing through five consecutive days of unrelenting snubs and outright rejections, interrupted only by his bouts of overeating, fatigue, and "the masses" (his term for his alters).

I couldn't help but think to myself that over the weekend Jason probably wasn't going to be alone after all—that without the distraction of his job, he was going to feel overwhelmed by the hordes inside him. He wept as he begged me to put him in the hospital to "keep me company. I'm so tired of fighting with all of them," he said. "And we can't watch *him* anymore. . . ." He curled up on the couch and seemed to drift off to sleep momentarily. I sat quietly in my chair, waiting.

He woke up abruptly, and immediately started speaking in a very soft voice.

"Timmy needs to stop," he said. "He's just so mad."

"Mad about what?"

"Mad at everyone. At the world. At us. And when he's mad he hurts himself and I'm afraid he doesn't know that he's with us, so he might hurt himself too bad and take us all."

"Has he hurt you all today?" I asked.

"Not today. Last night he got mad and took a razor blade."

"Show me."

Jason pulled off his hat. Huge chunks of hair were missing. I was horrified by this new development in Jason's behavior. He had sometimes threatened such actions, but never before had he gone so far. And this wasn't the worst of it. Jason replaced his cap, carefully concealing the damage he had done, and then pulled up his grubby shirt sleeves. His arms were crisscrossed with dozens of thin cuts, all sealed with dried blood, like a burgundy cobweb. None of the cuts was deep or infected, but it was his taking the step of cutting—so many times—that concerned me. The risk of self-mutilation would make an already-rocky therapy that much more treacherous.

My worry increased as Jason continued. "And someone else is coming," he whispered. "Jason can't stop him. He's new. He's scary. We don't know what he'll do. Timmy will hurt us, but I don't think he'd kill us. But this new one, I just don't know."

A new alter had entered the picture, one that threatened to dominate the others. Jason was appearing more and more agitated. I wanted to distract him by shifting the subject a bit.

"Who am I talking to now?" I asked.

"You know who I am. It's Tessie. I take care of everyone."

"And how many do you take care of?"

"Oh, at least 20 have come and gone. Some have died. I think nine are left."

This window into Jason's MPD had never been opened so far. I was being offered an opportunity to explore the questions that continued to plague me about Jason's past. I intuitively felt that proceeding with caution and intelligence might yield the long-sought key to personality integration. More than anything, I wanted to help Jason confront the masses who tormented him with their opposing needs and desires. Not sure of where it would lead, I began with an innocuous question.

"And how old are you all?" I wondered.

"Well, Jason is 52. Timmy is in his 40s but he's like Jason's dad. And I'm 7. I dunno," he said, suddenly seeming both fatigued and frustrated by the questions. He summarily ended his answer: "The others are all different ages."

Suddenly he closed his eyes for a moment, then shuddered. I could tell immediately from the change in his voice, his posture, even the look in his eyes that Jason was back. The window was again closed.

"You need to take care of me. Of us. We can't keep this new one under control much longer. And no one will be with me this weekend. I can't go to work until Monday and there won't be anything to occupy my mind."

These were always the most personally difficult points in my sessions with Jason. Jason was like a wounded rabbit caught in the jagged jaws of a hunter's trap and struggling desperately for freedom. I wanted just as desperately to spring him loose—to relieve him of his terror—but to spring the trap and leave him profoundly wounded was not the answer. I had watched my patient suffer these recurring bouts of anxiety long enough. The quick fix of hospitalization was a tempting alternative but no longer tenable.

We had discussed this many times before. Jason certainly knew we couldn't hospitalize him just to keep him "busy." We had also discussed his tendency to regress, to become even more dependent, in the hospital. We were aiming for independence and the long-term solution. He must have seen the look in my eye, and he laughed.

"Okay, okay, I know we've gone down this road before," he said. "You won't let me off the hook for a second, will you?"

Instead of grasping at a faulty quick fix, we spent the next hour planning an agenda for the weekend. We debated and compromised, trying to fill in many of the gaps but also allowing for some time for Jason to "practice" being alone. We agreed that he would call on some friends and church members when he needed it. As we brainstormed and finally developed a "recipe" for how he would handle his free time, he appeared encouraged. By the end of the hour, he was visibly relaxed, and I believed him when he said he felt comfortable leaving and driving himself home. I worried about Jason over the weekend but soon discovered what, as a therapist, I am continually relearning: that our patients, however troubled, have deep inner resources, surprising strength even in their vulnerability, and courage beyond measure. On Monday morning, I confirmed that Jason had handled the weekend with prideful self-reliance and a significant boost to his self-esteem.

It was a victory we celebrated together.

The Backdrop to MPD

MPD patients appear almost always to have been victims of severe physical and/or sexual abuse in childhood. The trauma—so overwhelming just as these children are forming concepts about the world and themselves—is often compounded by a lack of nurturance from parents and others who could otherwise have helped restore the child's brittle sense of security.

Interestingly, however, the disorder rarely manifests in childhood, although a few children have been diagnosed as early as three years of age. When diagnosing children, the psychiatrist must differentiate normal "fantasy" behaviors and the creation of imaginary friends from true MPD symptoms. Some clues to MPD in children are a demonstration of radically inconsistent knowledge, fluctuating abilities at various tasks, and other evidence of erratic access to information and skills.

The most common time for MPD to manifest is in the late teens and early 20s, when the feeling of devastation can no longer be sustained and is shut out through dissociation. This development is especially likely if the child has already been "wired" through experience or biology toward use of dissociation; this explains why most people who have suffered childhood trauma do not have MPD—they are not predisposed. Clearly, though, our understanding of all the forces propelling an individual toward MPD is still rudimentary. Much of the research to date has been sketchy. We deeply empathize with the patients still struggling to answer the question, *Why me?*

A Real Whodunit: MPD in the Courtroom

As MPD has hit the headlines, it has entered the courtroom as well. When a defendant claims more than one personality, the courts face imposing legal and ethical dilemmas. For example, which one should be put on trial after a crime is committed? Consider the 1993 case of *Commonwealth of Massachusetts v. Roman*.

Norma Roman was arrested in Lowell, Massachusetts, after police discovered a stash of heroin and cocaine in her home. She was charged with possession of heroin with intent to distribute. At her trial, Ms. Roman claimed not only that she suffered from MPD, but that "Vicky," one of her seven alter personalities, had brought the drugs into the house. She emphasized that, as Norma, she opposed drug abuse and discarded the drugs whenever Vicky brought them into her home.

On the stand, Vicky admitted that she had sold drugs and took responsibility for the police discovery. Another alter, "Alice Meijas," concurred that Vicky, not Norma, had done the buying and selling.

Ms. Roman sought to be judged "not guilty by reason of insanity." Instead, she was convicted. On appeal to the State Supreme Judicial Court, her attorney argued that Ms. Roman should not be punished for behavior over which she had no control. However, the court rejected that argument, pointing out that it could not possibly try to apportion criminal responsibility among a number of different personalities housed in the same body. Their decision presaged claims such as that of a 23-year-old defendant, who contended that one of her 3,817 personalities was responsible for the crime with which she was charged.

Although most judges have ruled in this way, the legal community has sometimes been divided. One legal scholar has argued that, unless all the personalities participated in the crime, it is unfair to convict the individual on trial. This line of thinking, however, would lead to a quicksand of impractical—if not impossible-scenarios. Whenever an MPD patient signed a contract, for example, each personality would have to sign independently for it to be valid. If an MPD patient were arrested, the police would have to read the Miranda warnings to every identity state. And, carrying the argument to the point of near absurdity, if the alter "in charge" at the time of a crime were a minor, the trial might have to take place in juvenile court. Such cases, entangling the criminal justice system in shifting culprits and alternating identity states, present judges and juries with tasks from which even Solomon would have recoiled. To date, no clear precedent has been set regarding how to try MPD cases.

Alter as Victim

The courts struggle not only when a person with MPD is the perpetrator of a crime, but when he or she is the apparent victim. In a 1990 case in Wisconsin, a 29-year-old Oshkosh man was put on trial for illegally seducing a woman called "S" who claimed at least 18 personalities. The state intended to prove that the man broke a state law forbidding sexual relations with someone too mentally ill to monitor his or her own conduct.

The prosecution maintained that the man knew perfectly well that S spontaneously shifted from one alternate personality to another. Indeed, according to the district attorney, on the day of the alleged crime, S had assumed three different personalities while she was catching a single fish! The district attorney also contended that the defendant knew that if he asked a younger, free-spirited, and even reckless personality named "Jennifer" to take control over S, Jennifer would promptly appear. In this way, the prosecution alleged, the man misused S's MPD to gain access to Jennifer, who then acquiesced to sex.

But another alter named "Emily," a six-year-old, happened to witness the act. She told a neighbor, who then told S. S was irate that her "body" had participated in sex with the defendant, and charges were then brought. On the witness stand, several of S's personalities were separately sworn in.

After four days of testimony, the defendant was convicted of rape. A month later, however, the judge threw out the verdict on a technicality and awarded a new trial. For reasons of their own, perhaps due in part to the media circus surrounding the original trial, S and the district attorney decided not to proceed any further.

The strangeness of these cases has made them fodder for the tabloid market. As such, the very real dilemmas faced by the courts in justly serving defendants and victims with MPD are often trivialized. Additionally, it should always be remembered that behind these burlesque displays are real people with real disorders who are living tormented lives.

False Claims of MPD

The term *malingering* refers to medical deception in the service of accruing an external gain. Examples include exaggerating back pain to acquire prescriptions for narcotics and simulating intractable seizures to gain disability payments. In a psychiatric variation, alleged mobster Vincent "Chin" Gigante was ruled sane after feigning disorientation and psychosis in an effort to evade prosecution—a psychiatric spin-off. And malingered MPD emerged in the late 1970s during the criminal trial of Kenneth Bianchi, who was charged with the notorious Hillside Strangler murders in Los Angeles. Initially, his defense team claimed that he was a victim of MPD and that an alter—"Steve"—had committed the crimes. Though experts were divided, the jury ultimately accepted the testimony of psychiatrists such as Dr. Martin Orne, who stated that Bianchi was faking the disorder. Ultimately, Bianchi pled guilty to seven murders.

In another legal case, the defense argument was patently absurd, and the jury knew it. Herbert Napier, on trial for murder, claimed that he could not be held accountable because of his "split" personality. His alters, he said, included not only a woman, three men, and a boy (reasonable enough so far), but also a god named Zygor and a dog named Demolition. In a primitive attempt to mimic a disorder he knew little about, Napier created a courtroom display that was less compelling than silly.

The Bianchi and Napier cases highlight the myths and misconceptions surrounding mental illness and the unjust stigma it bears. The mistaken belief still prevails among many that homicide and other violent crimes are likely to stem from mental illness. Attempting to capitalize on this flawed view, Bianchi and Napier used the courtroom as center stage. Thankfully, the jury found their performances unconvincing.

Court cases such as those just described provide an urgent motivation for malingering. But false claims of MPD can also arise from unmet emotional needs. In 1991, a teenager from Massachusetts falsified MPD simply to win attention and sympathy that she felt unable to get in any other way. This 15-year-old girl initially described four other personalities in addition to her own, including three girls and a boy. Later, she presented two others: a 78-year-old woman and another boy. Her portrayal of MPD was so persuasive that she was referred for specialized inpatient treatment. However, during follow-up outpatient care, her hoax began to unravel. It was learned that the patient had been preoccupied with the book *Sybil* and the movie based upon it and even mimicked the sketches that Sybil drew.

After weeks of therapy, she revealed to her therapist that she had been keeping a journal, and she was asked to bring it to her next session. By that time, another personality had emerged, this one a paraplegic individual who turned up on the floor outside the therapist's office, crawled inside, and presented the journal. Entries intimated that the patient was feigning the MPD, and when confronted by her therapist, the girl seemed relieved that the truth was finally known. After a further year of therapy that taught her to use words, not bizarre actions, to get her needs met, she no longer showed any signs of MPD.

Few situations are as unsettling to a health professional as the discovery, as in this case, that a patient has been feigning his or her ailment. Sorting out what's true and what isn't is especially difficult when such a patient presents with a number of different maladies. The task then is not simply to uncover the deception but to understand why the patient felt the need for it in the first place.

Barbara (as told by Marc)

Barbara, a petite 35-year-old woman, had shown up late one night at the emergency room. She had been distraught, holding her head in her hands, and sobbing as she told the ER doctor she was hearing voices and was battling strong impulses to commit suicide or even to kill someone else. The decision to admit her to the psychiatric ward was instantaneous. When the doctor let Barbara know a room was available, she appeared relieved and grateful.

The next morning, I met Barbara for the first time. She seemed relaxed, and I was surprised by how forthcoming she appeared. As I explored her background, she told me without hesitation that she had had 10 psychiatric hospitalizations in the past. Sometimes she had been treated for major depression or bipolar disorder ("manic depression"), but the most consistent diagnosis had been multiple personality disorder. Our staff had rarely encountered MPD. Barbara seemed pleased when I asked whether I could bring the rest of the treatment team into her room during the interview. I felt that a team approach would not only provide a teaching opportunity for the staff but also result in the best possible treatment plan for Barbara. When the staff assembled, I asked Barbara to describe her symptoms for us.

" 'Alexis' is my other personality, but the person you're talking to now, Barbara, is the 'core' personality, the 'host.' Alexis takes over when Barbara can't handle the stress. Barbara is a reasonable personality but not an assertive one, so it's pretty easy for Alexis to take over. Barbara isn't that emotional either; Alexis is the one who explodes into rage, and she can definitely be dangerous. And Alexis is the one that wants to hurt somebody, especially if they mess with her."

I admired Barbara's insight and her knowledge of MPD terminology but was confused by the detached, even clinical way she talked about her own potential for violence. Carrie, a medical student, whispered in my ear, *"What about the hallucinations?"* She had noticed that the ER doctor had written down that Barbara specifically reported hallucinations, a psychotic symptom. When I asked Barbara about it, she denied them, saying only that Barbara was able to hear whatever Alexis said. I figured the ER doctor hadn't asked enough questions to detect the difference.

I queried Barbara about why she thought the previous night had been so difficult for her. Had she been under more stress than usual? Had something awful happened? She told the group with a surprising, almost conspiratorial smile, "The answer's in my head." Barbara seemed to be presenting us with a riddle. Intuitively, I felt that she was inviting us into a game in which she would purposely hold back something essential and watch to see how we would go after it. This nagging doubt persisted throughout the session.

Barbara finally explained that she often had headaches so severe that she felt like killing herself . . . or even someone else. She had been in terrible pain when she was seen in the ER. She then mentioned and spelled out the name of the only medication—a narcotic—that had ever fully alleviated the headaches and thus the dangerous feelings that went along with them. She mentioned several other medications, including milder narcotics, that we "shouldn't even bother with. I can tell you already, they don't work." As the group's empathy toward her rose, Barbara claimed that at times she would go eight agonizing days without sleeping for a moment. Although eight days without sleep was unlikely, I knew that serious insomnia altered one's perception of time. Severe, unrelieved head pain coupled with insomnia might cause a person to consider suicide, but, I thought to myself, "Do your headaches make you homicidal, too?"

It seemed doubtful in my experience, and later I continued to wonder about a few more of Barbara's statements. Most of all, I was disturbed by her stated need for a specific and remarkably potent narcotic and the vague threat that she would become intensely destructive without it. I thought of patients who exaggerate their stories or symptoms, believing that hyperbole is needed in order for them to be taken seriously. I wondered whether this were true in Barbara's case, but I said nothing, preferring to watch and wait.

During our subsequent meetings, Barbara fleshed out her background. She had been married and divorced four times; each husband had been alcoholic, and two were now in jail. After receiving her bachelor's degree in psychology, she had worked as a substance abuse counselor but hadn't been able to work at all for some time, subsisting first on unemployment compensation and then on handouts. I admitted to her that I was still struggling to understand more about her MPD. She then shared her secret: she had first become aware of Alexis in her early teens, and MPD was her only way to cope with a devastating childhood. As she held her hands over her eyes, she whispered that she had constantly been sexually assaulted as she grew up.

Clearly, Barbara's past held some awful secrets that brought her to this place in life, but by now my doubts about the true nature of Barbara's behaviors were extending to her stories. I was finding it difficult to remain nonjudgmental, and it disturbed me deeply that my unconfirmed doubts were intruding upon our sessions at every turn. I believed that getting at the truth was essential if I were really to help Barbara. I decided to follow her lead with some questions that might bring us to the truth.

"Do you remember who assaulted you?" I asked. She revealed that there had been 10 different perpetrators, including most of her male relatives and immediate neighbors. During Barbara's initial physical examination, an internist had discovered a scar on her abdomen.

"Why is it there?" I asked her. "Is it related to the assaults?"

Barbara then revealed a problem she hadn't mentioned before. "I'm recovering from cancer. Cervical cancer. They diagnosed it two years ago and immediately did a complete hysterectomy. But it had already spread. The surgeon couldn't believe it at first; he was sure he had caught it early enough. He ended up having to go back in three different times. He removed my appendix and part of my colon because of the 'mets' in them, and then I had chemotherapy. Now they think I'm in remission but I still feel like there's a clock ticking over my head. You can never be sure."

Barbara had evidently been betrayed by several husbands, a host of sexual molesters, and now even her own body. This escalation of tragic events continued to feed my misgivings. I remembered how effectively Barbara had garnered sympathy from the treatment team in her initial interview. I sensed that Barbara's enormous need for love and nurturance was producing these suspicious stories.

I had not yet shared my misgivings with the staff. Over the next few days of observation and assessment, however, Carrie and some other members of the treatment team expressed their own doubts. It struck all of us as odd that, almost immediately following admission, Barbara had abruptly dropped her complaints of powerful suicidal and homicidal impulses. Yet the terrible headaches had persisted; indeed, Barbara talked about little else but her headaches and her need for the particular narcotic medication. Initially giving her the benefit of the doubt, I did in fact prescribe several doses. But when she denied any benefit whatsoever and demanded higher and higher doses despite her already-slurred speech, I was forced to question the extent of her pain. In the past I had worked with cancer patients, some of whom were in the final stages of the disease, and I had been able to remedy their pain—but not Barbara's. I could no longer brush aside the possibility that an addiction was driving Barbara's desperate behaviors, at least in part. If it were indeed an addiction, I worried that I was only fueling it by prescribing potent narcotics. After discussing options with the staff, we agreed to stop the narcotic on a trial basis.

Barbara's reports of pain escalated phenomenally. Sometimes she "swooned" with pain in the dayroom, upsetting other patients who then rallied around her, presenting the staff with a tremendous dilemma. *Why were we being so withholding,* they said, *when Barbara was obviously in excruciating pain? Weren't we human?*

We held our ground, believing that this maneuver was truly the most therapeutic thing we could do for Barbara. The next morning, Barbara awoke, got up, and suddenly began to speak unintelligibly. Wearing only her nightgown, she wandered into other patients' rooms, seemingly unaware. Had the stress on the unit gotten to her? Had Alexis emerged? I was on a seesaw of doubt and belief. Just when I had convinced myself that Barbara was malingering for drugs, I was now doubting my own doubt. I felt the inner struggle of every therapist who works with "feigners."

Regardless of what the truth might really be, I felt that I had to transfer Barbara to a higher-security unit because I was concerned about her safety in this state of apparent dissociation. If she wandered into other rooms, might she wander out of the hospital and into the street? Holding her arm, I guided her toward the elevator and accompanied her to the sixth-floor unit. When the doors opened, Barbara's grip tightened and I felt her stiffen. Like most units of its kind, the new ward was notably less plush than the original "open" unit.

The instant she saw the new accommodations, Barbara "came to."

"I'm fine now," she said. "I'm back. It's me, Barbara. That other person was Alexis. I need to go back to my own room now. My room is on the other unit."

Barbara's immediate transformation told me that she had total command over the comings and goings of her two personality states, a level of control that would be absent in authentic MPD.

Back on the open unit again, our doubts only increased as we continued to observe Barbara. She consistently ate and slept well, laughing and socializing freely with other patients. But whenever she saw a staff member approach, she suddenly became deeply subdued or grimaced and braced her head because of the "pain." We were now reasonably certain that Barbara was feigning her symptoms as well as her stories. Thinking that we might gain some insight from Barbara's previous clinicians, we placed a call to the surgeon who had treated her "cancer." Barbara had not been forthcoming with us about her medical history either. Although she had indeed had a hysterectomy, it was prompted by uterine prolapse (a laxity in the muscles that hold the uterus). She had never had any form of cancer and had not undergone any other operations. She had never had chemotherapy. Furthermore, the surgeon—who had known her family for years—said Barbara had never received a psychology degree or worked as a substance abuse counselor.

I knew from my work with other patients who have falsified psychological and/or physical problems that direct confrontation of the patient rarely works. Even when they're confronted with incontrovertible evidence that they've misrepresented the truth, they will convolute their stories to absorb the new evidence. In such cases, to remove their mask is simultaneously to force them to "lose face," to lose the personae that have been so carefully crafted. It leaves them adrift, sometimes even shattered. Gentler methods are required to keep the patient in therapy long enough to get to the root of the real problem.

Disappointingly, we did not get the chance to work further with Barbara. Perhaps she recognized a subtle shift in our attitudes or maybe she had simply tired of the game. She insisted on discharge, now saying that she felt entirely well.

In retrospect, I can see that Barbara had found remarkably creative ways to get her wants and needs met. Her story of "Alexis" afforded her a ready explanation for the episodes of rage and impulsivity that were, in reality, attributable to a personality disorder that she didn't understand herself. By presenting the reason for her surgery as cancer and exaggerating the extent of the subsequent treatments, she was seeking the nurturance that a report of cancer is likely to elicit. And she used specious pain complaints, displayed selectively and abandoned promptly when she wished to be discharged, to obtain narcotics and possibly to reduce her own disappointment in how her life had turned out.

Ultimately I felt very sad for Barbara. By misleading those who were in a good position to help, she diverted attention from her actual life problems and missed an opportunity to get the help she truly needed. I also felt sad for myself and my colleagues, left feeling helpless and unsure of our own judgments.

Consolidating the Identities

Psychotherapy has long been a mainstay of the treatment of MPD, but valid success rates are impossible to come by: there have been no controlled, randomized trials of treatment for MPD despite its formal recognition by the American Psychiatric Association almost two decades ago. Nonetheless, in case reports and small case series, therapists have advocated strategies such as teaching the patient how to self-soothe; mapping out in writing the system of alternate personality states; facilitating communication among the alters and with the therapist; and gently encouraging emotional expression while also helping the patient manage the strong feelings that threaten to trigger renewed dissociation. The overall goal is the fusing or consolidating of the personalities. Judicious, noncoercive use of hypnosis is often incorporated into the psychotherapy, sometimes to activate a hidden personality and make it accessible for contact and communication.

Less conventional approaches are supported by some people and lambasted by others. One approach views the various identities as a *family of the self* for which family therapy should be prescribed. The strategy here is for the therapist to employ a kind of "internal diplomacy." Another tactic is to draw on *natural trance therapies* in other cultures, redefining the alters as potential resources rather than problems (an approach Roseanne has embraced, as we have seen). Recently, *therapeutic writing* exercises have found a few advocates in the professional community. In therapeutic writing, the patient writes letters to him- or herself as a way to enhance communication among the various identity states. Ideally, writing out the thoughts, feelings, and urges of the identity states will empower the patient, encourage more mature approaches to everyday life, and help expand the patient's self-healing skills. Because these novel techniques do seem to help some patients, we advocate selective use of them for patients in therapy who fail to show the expected improvement over time.

But just as the jury is still out on how common MPD really is, we also do not have a solid grasp of what treatment works best and most consistently. As with all uncertainties in medicine, we need quality research that goes far beyond the current idiosyncratic, shoot-from-the-hip approaches. Effective treatment will come only through the formation of collaborative research networks among psychiatric centers, not through militancy for and against the diagnosis.

▌ Dissociative Fugue

Each year thousands of Americans simply disappear, joining the rolls of the vanished. Their families distribute flyers and plaster billboards with their pictures. Within a day or two, the local media may report expectantly that the person's abandoned car has been located or that sightings have been phoned in to the authorities. But all too often, these clues seem to lead to dead ends. Fears of foul play usually arise, but there may be little actual evidence to suggest an abduction. Ultimately, as time passes, media and finally even police interest fades. Another missing person case is added to the tally even as families struggle to keep up their hopes.

Some will never return: they may indeed have been crime victims, or they may have ended their own lives. But most of those who vanish do eventually come back. At one end of the spectrum are elderly people with Alzheimer's disease who have simply wandered off and were later located. At the other end of the spectrum are those who have chosen deliberately to flee and establish new lives elsewhere.

Individuals who have chosen to disappear are usually desperate to escape crushing marital, financial, or occupational problems. The abandoned husbands and wives may have been genuinely unaware that the level of stress had become unbearable for their spouses. In a Milwaukee case, for example, the sudden, agonizing disappearance of Brett Pabst's newlywed husband Michael was followed by a number of disturbing revelations. Among the most startling: he had left behind massive numbers of surreptitious financial deals gone sour. With his disappearance, his new wife—a member of the Pabst brewing family—was forced into the quagmire of debts and lawsuits. Only later did she learn that the man she thought she knew had vanished under nearly identical circumstances once before: during his first marriage. None of his relatives had told her about this episode, perhaps fearing she would call off the wedding, and so the same events unfolded, with another bride victimized.

In this case, the "spontaneous disappearance" was actually premeditated, a calculated way for this man to escape responsibility for the financial and legal mess he had created. Individuals who choose this route to evade the consequences of their own behavior may go so far as to select a new name (perhaps from a tombstone or obituary), create a false Social Security number, obtain a new driver's license, and even design a phony handwriting style.

But in rare cases, none of these explanations for the disappearance applies—not crime, suicide, loss of intellectual faculties, or willful planning. Instead, the answer is found in a psychiatric condition called *dissociative fugue*.

The Phenomenon of Fugue

In dissociative fugue, a person suddenly travels away from home or workplace and, during this time, is unable to recall some, or even all, of his or her own past. The travel can range from a brief trip lasting hours to extensive wandering lasting weeks or months. Indeed, in the most extreme cases, individuals experiencing dissociative fugue have literally crossed national borders and covered thousands of miles.

A case lasting only a couple of hours was reported by our colleague from the University of Alabama at Birmingham, Dr. Charles Ford. A confused and dehydrated middle-aged man was found sitting silently in his car at a truck stop. When concerned travelers questioned him, he denied knowing who he was, but his car registration provided the answer. He was 35 miles from his home and had no idea how he had gotten there.

The man was admitted to a medical ward, where a drug screen disclosed that he had taken sleeping pills. During a series of psychiatric interviews, the man was able to piece together the reasons for his sudden travel and amnesia. He was a fundamentalist Christian who had been depressed for some time. He became overburdened when job stressors multiplied and he simultaneously became aware that his daughter had been highly promiscuous. He had simply had enough, and his unconscious protected him from his intolerable frustration and sorrow through dissociation—this time, dissociative fugue. His strict religious beliefs would have forbidden such behavior, but in the fugue state he was able to flee his work and home situations and even attempt suicide through use of the sleeping pills.

Though the fugue had already ended, the man was offered ongoing psychiatric care. It was explained to him that treatment of his depression would increase his resilience when stressors intruded and that treatment was an investment that could help prevent the fugue from developing again. He gratefully accepted, and his unplanned journeys have come to an end.

Fugue, then, results in a kind of "wandering John (or Jane) Doe," a person who, even as he or she travels, is thoroughly unaware of his or her personal identity, including name, family, and occupation. In especially remarkable cases, these patients assume brand-new identities, as in the Woody Allen film *Zelig*, without having consciously decided to do so. Taking up a new residence and career, they give no outward appearance of having a mental disorder.

Although the vast majority of cases of fugue have occurred among adults, children and adolescents are not immune. In 1985, for example, a 16-year-old boy was found lying tangled but unharmed in shrubbery along a state highway. He had road maps and food with him but carried no personal identification. When police brought him to the hospital, he could not recall any details of his past—his family, residence, schooling, medical history, not even his personal interests. He also had no idea why he had embarked upon his journey in the first place.

Physically, the patient checked out fine. After his photograph was shown on television, his parents quickly came to the hospital. They said that their son had suddenly disappeared from home almost two days earlier. They admitted that he had been a quiet, reclusive youngster and a marginal student. Although nothing like this fugue episode had ever occurred before, there had been a number of recent problems within the family that had been stressful to them all—a close relative had recently died, and the mother herself had just been diagnosed with cancer. The hypothesis was that this youngster, who had always had trouble verbalizing his feelings, literally and figuratively ran away from home and forgot a situation with which he couldn't cope.

Fortunately, with reassurance from his family and the staff and gentle reminders of the facts of his life, the boy was soon able to recognize his family. Although his memory for the events leading to his being discovered along the highway always remained limited, he—like the fundamentalist man—consented to ongoing therapy to help prevent fugue from ever recurring in his life.

Fugue and Its Causes

True dissociative fugue does not stem from physical causes. Head injuries, seizures, chemical abnormalities in the body, and street drugs can all result in confusion, wandering, and amnesia. However, such physical explanations are lacking in dissociative fugue. Instead, everything checks out, and the cause is thus considered to be "psychological."

As we've explained, fugue generally stems from overwhelming events and intolerable stress. This degree of stress leads to feelings of personal powerlessness and loss of control, a breeding ground for a number of psychiatric problems, including fugue.

One of the most interesting opportunities to study fugue emerged during World War II, when the number of cases swelled among soldiers as a result of the stress of military service. But researchers also recognize that even stressors much milder and more circumscribed than war can provoke the extreme emotions that can spiral into dissociative fugue. The discovery that one's spouse is having an affair or a violent argument with one's child can serve as the impetus. At such times, what fugue patients are fleeing isn't the horrible situation itself so much as their own impulses. They may have such powerful feelings, perhaps even suicidal or murderous ones, that they become frightened of themselves. As if to ensure a break with the past, patients may adopt personalities that are diametrically opposed to their former selves—for example, an incorrigible partygoer becomes a shy and reserved wallflower. By moving on to new places and even forgetting who they are, they unconsciously seek to escape these forbidden emotions. When they assume brand-new identities, they move even further away from the Mr. (or Ms.) Hydes they fear they could become.

Finding the Way Back

Dissociative fugue rarely ends as a result of intervention by a psychiatrist or other health professional. Rather, a chance encounter or idle comment provides the magic key that, sometimes instantaneously, unlocks the past. In other cases, the events and feelings that precipitated the fugue ultimately resolve through tincture of time; with the monster no longer looming, the person can safely reassume his or her former identity.

As we will demonstrate in the chapter on false memory syndrome (FMS), the techniques sometimes advocated to help patients "recover" memories and identities are controversial. A variety of these techniques, including hypnosis, intravenous barbiturates, "automatic writing," "urgent questioning," and "persuasion," had been advocated by earlier scientists to treat fugue patients. However, the recognition of FMS has proved that in trying to restore "lost memories," therapists may inadvertently create false ones. And because no single medication has emerged as a reliable aid in the treatment of fugue, clinicians usually end up treating fugue *ex post facto*, offering psychotherapy to help the patient withstand the kinds of conflicts that originally provoked the fugue state. With enhanced coping skills, the risk of a recurrence is theoretically reduced. But patients, families, and therapists should also feel reassured that, regardless of the type of treatment offered, fugue tends to be a one-time (though sometimes lengthy) occurrence in a person's life.

▌ Dissociative Amnesia

Forty-five-year-old criminal defense attorney Lucy was sure something awful had happened following a visit to a client at the Central Jail in San Diego County. She certainly knew she had left with a sprained wrist and aching shoulder. Another attorney had filled in a few details: he had found her on the floor, a deputy standing over her. After retaining a private investigator who helped her piece together the facts, Lucy surmised that the deputy had wrestled her to the floor when she had tried to leave but could not produce any identification.

Although subsequently she moved to a new city to find some sort of escape, Lucy was persistently troubled by the experience. She went on to develop depression and anxiety and even had trouble continuing to practice law. Finally, although she still could not actually remember the events, she decided to sue the county. As her own attorney put it, "How do you win when your own client doesn't remember what happened?"

But win she did, to the tune of $114,880. Almost exactly three years after the incident, a jury found that the deputy had engaged in "intentional, unlawful, and harmful" contact with her. The client whom Lucy was visiting that day said he had seen it all, and the jury believed him. They also found Lucy's expert witness convincing. He had testified that the trauma caused Lucy to block out much of that ignoble day, and he had added that the formal term for her condition was *dissociative amnesia*. Because of this condition, he reasoned, it would have been a catch-22 to expect her to be able to describe for the jury an experience so upsetting that her mind refused to allow her to bear it.

Dissociative amnesia is a stripped-down version of the two other dissociative disorders we've presented in this chapter—MPD and dissociative fugue. An inability to remember events and behaviors is common to all three. But whereas patients with MPD have two or more personality states, and dissociative fugue patients unexpectedly travel, dissociative amnesia patients simply find themselves unable to retrieve important autobiographical information such as their names and dates of birth.

Amnesia, because of its inherent drama, has long been a staple of entertainment. Movies old *(Mirage* and *Spellbound)* and new *(Overboard* and *The Long Kiss Goodnight)* incorporate amnesia as a plot device. TV soap operas use it constantly to keep viewers hooked, and recent novels such as Kazuo Ishiguro's *The Unconsoled* and Jodi Picoult's *Past Perfect* buffet their principal characters with the winds of profound amnesia. Amnesia has even been a plot device in the popular Internet soap opera *The East Village*.

Dissociative amnesia, as in Lucy's case, is not caused by a medical problem or by alcohol or drug use. Instead, the loss of memory—the very linchpin of identity—is psychologically induced in these cases. It is far too extensive to be explained by the ordinary forgetfulness that plagues us all and instead seems to arise from trauma or stress.

Dissociative amnesia patients do not behave in a confused or disorganized way. Rather, they retain their IQs, their vocabularies, their skills, and their ability to learn new things. They appear perfectly fine to others even though they themselves are usually aware that they've lost pieces of their memories. Surprisingly, only some get upset by this recognition; the rest are relatively unconcerned about the missing information.

Because dissociative amnesia usually arises out of a highly unpleasant situation or psychological conflict, it, like fugue, seems to increase during times of war and natural disasters. But severe interpersonal conflicts, such as the one leading to Lucy's winding up on the floor of the jail, can provoke the amnestic episodes too.

Degrees of Forgetfulness

The two most common subtypes of dissociative amnesia are *localized* amnesia and *selective* amnesia. In localized amnesia, the individual can't recall the first few hours following a profoundly disturbing event. This is precisely what happened to Lucy. In selective amnesia, the person can recall some, but not all, of the events during a personally trying period. For example, a soldier with selective amnesia may recall only snippets of the combat missions in which he fought.

Fortunately, a third subtype, *generalized* amnesia, is much less common than these two. Here, the person has forgotten everything about his or her whole life. Finally, in *systematized* amnesia, also rare, the patient forgets entire categories of information—such as all information relating to his or her family.

The duration of the events for which there is amnesia is typically hours to days, but in unusual cases it may be years, resulting in a *Back to the Future* scenario that is all too real. In one such case, a 55-year-old man insisted in 1984 that it was actually 1945 and that he was 14 years old. He had no idea that he was now a middle-aged man and that his parents and various other family members had died years earlier. His treatment involved essentially reacquainting him with the intervening four decades. And such treatment requires painstaking work, patience, and extraordinary sensitivity on the part of the therapist. In helping this patient to reclaim life in the present, for example, he was essentially robbed of his past: if therapy is successful, he "awakens" like Rip Van Winkle to a life without the people he loves. He has lost his youth and half his vital years. Treatment for bereavement and depression are essential therapeutic extensions.

Unlocking the Mind

Because dissociative amnesia is more likely than fugue to occur multiple times, therapists work hard to intervene before a pattern gets established. We worry that if the original traumatic events, feelings, and impulses are not brought to light, the episodes will snowball and amnesia will become an increasingly persistent protective device in the individual's psyche.

Although the caveats about the risk of inducing false memories clearly apply to dissociative amnesia as well, patients who seek to recapture the forgotten material do sometimes respond to hypnosis or to drug-assisted interviews performed with exceeding care. When hypnosis is used, it is suggested to the patient while in a trance that he or she go back in time to the period immediately preceding the memory loss. In this way, the goal is not only to restore the lost memory but to identify the life stress that precipitated it. During drug-assisted interviews, a sedating medication (such as amobarbital [Amytal]) is administered intravenously to a patient who is then able to relax enough to talk openly. (This technique is illustrated in the chapter on phobias and described more fully in the chapter on FMS.)

Even without such techniques, acute amnesia may resolve over time once the traumatic circumstances have passed. To assist in this process, either the individual must be removed from the upsetting life situation if it is ongoing or steps must be taken to reduce the stress so that further episodes of amnesia are not triggered.

Who? Where? What?

Can amnesia itself, like MPD, be faked? Could a defendant attempt to evade responsibility for a criminal act by feigning amnesia for the period during which the crime was committed? Could a recruit aiming to avoid military service suddenly drift wide-eyed through the barracks, claiming not to know who or where he is?

Fortunately, most people are not exceptional actors, but the direct answer to these questions is "certainly." There are no foolproof ways to distinguish between real and malingered amnesia. Clinicians need to balance any skepticism with the recognition that authentic amnesia does occur, albeit rarely. In the absence of scientific ways to ascertain the truth, we have to look broadly and dispassionately at the context in which a claim of dramatic memory loss arises. Our suspicions will mount, however, when we can discern a possible motive, and avoidance of prison or combat have indeed been the goals in some cases.

The following example, albeit disturbing, will clarify some of the difficulties that clinicians face.

Miss Arlie (as told by Jackie)

In North Carolina, I was asked to testify in the case of Miss Arlie, a middle-aged white woman who had been charged with the murder of a fellow tenant. Miss Arlie had previously had some run-ins with the law for disorderly conduct, but she had never committed an overtly violent act. A long-term psychiatric patient, she had been hospitalized many times over the last 15 years.

I had treated her on an inpatient unit after the murder she was alleged to have committed. Throughout the hospitalization, she consistently denied any involvement. Instead, she said that the only thing she remembered about the evening of the murder was hearing some noises. Otherwise, her mind was a complete blank.

In the hospital, Miss Arlie typically sat calmly in the dayroom. It was only when the treatment team made its visits that she appeared agitated. She would suddenly take to her room, wring her hands, roll her eyes, and pace as if it were impossible for her to be still. During those times, she would claim to be hearing voices making statements such as "You are a fish" and "You can walk all the way to Antarctica" and "You are a fine black woman." Although her face showed little emotion, she often pled for us to give her some medicine.

When several team members wondered out loud about the sudden change in her behavior when they approached, Miss Arlie would magnify her symptoms. We all pitied her even though we doubted her. However, on the day of discharge, when she learned that she was definitely going back to jail, Miss Arlie dropped her facade, and we, her caregivers, saw her true colors:

"Yes, I killed her," she snarled. "Get someone here to take a confession. She was a dirty dog and I hated her. She deserved to die. I planned it and I did it. I stabbed out her eye and cut off her breast and stabbed her a hundred times."

All of these grisly details of the murder were true but not yet publicly known. She was taken back to jail.

Almost a year later, her case came to trial. Miss Arlie appeared docile and pathetic, almost an exact replica of the first few days of her hospitalization with us. Her attorney proclaimed that Miss Arlie may indeed have killed the victim but that she was compelled to do so by her mental illness. He added that her amnesia was authentic, persistent, and only confirmed the extent of her psychological compromise. He asked the jury to decide that Miss Arlie was not responsible for her actions.

After considerable testimony from the clinical staff about her perplexing hospital behavior and her confession, Miss Arlie was found guilty of murder and sentenced to 30 years in prison. She had tried to run and hide by denying her own recollections, but Miss Arlie's memory of her own terrible acts persisted. Untrained in psychology, the members of the jury could still behold the gruesome story behind Miss Arlie's blank eyes.

▌ Summing Up

Perhaps no mental phenomena better illustrate the sheer resourcefulness of the human mind than the dissociative disorders. In its effort to defend itself from realities too ruthless to endure, the mind barricades itself behind walls of amnesia or clones fresh identities with virtual lives of their own. But the price for this self-protection is heavy and something most of us take for granted: a sense of continuity to our lives. In dissociation, the mind shields itself from the anguish of the moment, only to shoulder a different kind of burden—one of perpetually feeling incomplete. As French philosopher and Nobel Laureate Henri Bergson wrote, we are free only when "our actions emanate from our total personality, when they express it, when they resemble it in the indefinable way a work of art sometimes does the artist."

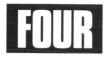

FALSE MEMORY SYNDROME

Accurate Recollections or Implanted Histories?

The difference between false memories and true
ones is the same as for jewels: it is always the false
ones that look the most real, the most brilliant.

—Salvador Dalí (1904–1989),
The Secret Life of Salvador Dalí

IN 1990, EILEEN FRANKLIN-LIPSKER took the witness
stand, and solely on the basis of her testi-
mony, her father, George Franklin, Sr., was sentenced to prison for the rest of his life.
The brutal rape and murder of eight-year-old Susan Nason had perplexed authorities for years with its elusive leads, and thus the crime had remained unsolved. Now,
20 years later, Franklin-Lipsker had come forward with the startling claim that she
alone had been an eyewitness—a terrified child who had remained huddled in the
back of Franklin's van where the crime allegedly occurred. So traumatized was
young Eileen that she supposedly repressed all memory of the event, until, with the
help of her therapist, she was able to reconstruct the grisly scene in lucid detail. It

was, in fact, the extraordinary precision of Franklin-Lipsker's descriptions that moved the jurors to convict Franklin of first-degree murder. They concluded that an individual would not be capable of concocting such complete and vivid scenarios through imagination alone.

▌Behind the Scenes

At the time that her memories began to surface, Franklin-Lipsker's therapist had been plumbing her subconscious for a repressed memory of childhood trauma. Incorporating techniques such as induced relaxation, the therapist seemed able to lift Franklin-Lipsker's deeply sequestered memory into the bright light of conscious thought. The initial images—vague, shadowy renderings—were gradually transformed into the clear pictures and descriptions that supposedly only an eyewitness could have produced.

In dusting the remote corners of her mind, Franklin-Lipsker and her therapist discovered George Franklin's prints everywhere. Her "recovered" memory thereby verified what Franklin-Lipsker had always suspected: that it was her own father and not some drifter who had murdered young Susan. Over time, Franklin-Lipsker was able to produce ever more detailed images of the crime scene, which she confidently narrated to the jury: Susan Nason's startled eyes as George Franklin raised the rock that would fracture her skull; Susan's small hand lifted in self-protection; and then the hand, still and lifeless, with a crushed silver ring bearing witness to the attack. She even claimed to recall the brand of cigarettes and beer that George Franklin had carted to the murder scene in his Volkswagen bus.

The jury was riveted by Franklin-Lipsker's dramatic story and seemingly uninterested that the details she recited were either already known or were unverifiable. There was evidence enough that George Franklin had indeed been an abusive father, prone to violence and fits of rage. But Franklin was not being tried for these past actions. He was on trial for murder, and in the final analysis there simply were no hard facts upon which to base a conviction. Even Franklin's junked van, which was exhumed and examined for evidence, did not produce a single incriminating clue. Franklin-Lipsker's late-recovered memory was thus solely responsible for George Franklin's life sentence. In April 1995, five years into his sentence, Franklin's conviction was overturned, with the judge concluding that "the risk of an unreliable outcome in this trial is unacceptable." Yet George Franklin remained in jail, unable to post $1 million bond, and San Mateo County prosecutors announced in January 1996 that they would retry him. Finally, in July 1996, Franklin's six years of incarceration came to an abrupt end: the prosecution's house of cards collapsed as vital information that Franklin-Lipsker had provided was proved false, and all charges were dropped. At the end, the complaint voiced by Franklin's attorney—that Franklin had been a victim of "voodoo psychology" all along—enjoyed a level of credibility that far surpassed the testimony of Eileen Franklin-Lipsker.

▌ The Appeal of the Psyche

With its blend of theory and theatrics, the Franklin case has captured our imagination as effectively as a murder mystery and renewed our interest in an old fascination. Our intrigue with repressed memory dates back to Sigmund Freud, whose ideas about the unconscious eventually transformed psychiatry. But to popular audiences, Freud's theories had been all but incomprehensible until Hollywood helped translate them to the silver screen. Merging Freudian theory with intriguing plots, Alfred Hitchcock's *Spellbound* and *Marnie* began shaping a public awareness of repressed memory and childhood trauma. Years later, when *Sybil* exploded onto the scene (see also Chapter 3 of this book), the theory of repressed memory moved from fiction to reality in the public mind.

But if the American public was all too thoroughly persuaded by Sally Field's stunning performance as Sybil, scientists were trying to take a more investigative approach. Their sober research into the nature of memory, and whether repressed memory is a verifiable phenomenon, may never have rekindled public interest if not for a surprising trend: a burgeoning of allegations beginning in the late 1980s that were based on recovered memories, specifically memories of childhood sexual abuse that the accused vehemently denied.

This alarming increase in accusations coincided with the rising popularity of a book that gave the recovery movement the spotlight among mental health therapies. This publication, *The Courage to Heal* by Ellen Bass and Laura Davis, was instantly anointed by self-proclaimed recovery therapists as the incest survivor's bible. Not even its authors—who have no training in psychology—could have predicted such phenomenal success, which to date has included sales of over 800,000 copies.

Although grounded in the good intention to help those who have experienced actual childhood sexual abuse, the recovery movement appears to have created a monster. Since the original publication of *The Courage to Heal* in 1988, reports of recovered memories have snowballed, resulting in a veritable industry of self-help literature, seminars, workshops, support groups, and sex abuse therapies. An avalanche of charges has been leveled against fathers and mothers, grandparents, neighbors, ministers, teachers, and even former therapists. The recovery movement is now seen by many as a threat to the falsely accused; to the truly abused, whose needs are overshadowed by the circus atmosphere the movement has spawned; to the accusers themselves, many of whom have been terribly misdiagnosed and misled; and to mental health professionals as a whole, whose credibility is tainted by bad therapeutic practices that are recovering counterfeit memories in record numbers.

■ Creating False Memories

Correct or Corrupted?

The nature of memory fascinates us, but research tells us little about this mysterious mental property. What we do know is that memory is not an objective recording of events; rather, it is easily contaminated by many factors.

Consider, for example, the family stories you have heard or repeated over the years with various spins and embellishments. Consider too that when part of a story is vague or incomplete, we commonly—either consciously or unconsciously—create scenarios to fill in the missing pieces and give the story coherence. Over time, it is easy to lose track of what was remembered and what was created, and thus our memories become distorted or corrupted.

Sometimes the memories of what we believe to be our own experience are nothing more than memories of mental images we create upon hearing an often-repeated story. A classic example of this complicated phenomenon comes from the renowned Swiss psychologist Jean Piaget, who falsely recalled a traumatic incident from his childhood. Throughout his life, Piaget had often heard the story of his attempted kidnapping at the age of two. He told the story himself many times, detailing his recollection of how his nanny bravely fended off the attackers. But years later, Piaget learned that the story was a complete fabrication. His nanny admitted that she had concocted the story to garner attention and admiration for herself. Piaget's vivid "memory" of the incident was in reality only a memory of the stories he had so frequently heard. Through the power of suggestion and repetition, Piaget's mind became fertile ground for an implanted memory.

Studies show that false memories can be implanted through other forms of repetitive suggestion as well. For example, people who initially deny a specific memory that has been suggested to them by an interviewer have been known to change their minds when questioned repeatedly about the same matter. Berkeley's Frederick C.

Crews, Ph.D., who has analyzed the litigation involving recovered memories, describes a scenario in which repeated questioning elicits the desired response:

> In such prosecutions [such as those involving day care workers accused of perpetrating satanic abuse against children] . . . a vengeful or mentally unhinged adult typically launches the accusations, which are immediately believed by police and social workers. These authorities then disconcert the toddlers with rectal and vaginal prodding, with invitations to act out naughtiness on "anatomically correct" dolls with bloated genitals, and, of course, with leading questions that persist until the child reverses an initial denial that anything happened and begins weaving the kind of tale that appears to be demanded.

Having reviewed the world's scientific literature on children's suggestibility and memory for their book, *Jeopardy in the Courtroom*, psychologists Stephen Ceci and Maggie Bruck find support for each of Crews's concerns: the natural suggestibility of children   particularly when combined with suggestive interviews, insistent questioning, and overzealous use of anatomically detailed dolls—can entirely destroy the validity of their reports and court testimony.

Adults enrolled in "trauma survivors" groups can be subtly manipulated in the same way: the repeated theme of sexual abuse and the explicit objective of acknowledging an abuse history can exert extraordinary pressure on members to dredge up an incident. Group members are usually encouraged to explore their inner experiences through intensive autobiographical writing, art renderings, and/or visualizations that are then shared with the group. The respect of the group is earned insofar as members are willing to show progress in their recovery work. As one group participant has described it, "I found myself making more and more dramatic and condemning interpretations of my recollections of the past, for which I was rewarded by the group for showing 'the courage to heal.' " In some groups, only those individuals who can "remember" and recite instances of sexual trauma in their lives are permitted to retain their membership. Clearly, then, there can be considerable group pressure to secure the trophy of a formerly lost memory of childhood abuse.

In the above examples, the implantation of false memories derives from repetitive questioning or immersion in discussions about abuse. But less flagrant forms of suggestion can be just as powerful. Even the undeniably passive act of watching television can evoke false memories in suggestible individuals. In 1988, after Geraldo Rivera hosted two specials on the subject of satanism, an Indianapolis outpatient clinic for dissociative disorders reported that 29 patients showed up claiming to be victims of satanic ritual abuse. There was no evidence to suggest any truth to these reports, and clinic staff were mystified by the sudden rush of claims. When some of the patients revealed that they had seen the *Geraldo* series, the show was credited with implanting the suggestion of ritual abuse.

Experimenting With Memory

In demonstrating that suggestion plays a prominent role in false memories, we can point not only to anecdotes but to experiments documented in the professional literature.

A now classic example of experimentally induced suggestion comes from the well-publicized court case of Paul Ingram. A devout Christian who was accused of satanic activities that included incest and sodomy, Ingram readily confessed to a sexual crime against his children that he did not commit. The confession arose after the suggestion was purposely implanted by a talented and respected psychologist, Richard Ofshe. Ofshe had been troubled by the tentative nature of Ingram's previous confessions and believed the man to be highly suggestible. He therefore decided to test Ingram's suggestibility by instilling an idea. Ofshe falsely reported to Ingram that, in talking with the Ingram children, he had learned about an incident in which Ingram had forced his son and daughter to have sex with each other. The alleged episode was a pure fabrication but, amazingly enough, the accused man probed his "memory" until he was able to supply a detailed account of the crime. Even more astounding is that when Ofshe informed Ingram that he had made up the story as a test, Ingram tenaciously stood his ground, initially refusing to believe that his memory could be so clear about something that had never happened. Only much later, having finally accepted that the crimes never happened, did Ingram seek a pardon. Granting a pardon is a risky and unpopular move for any governor, and Ingram's request was denied.

Based upon her own research, psychologist and memory expert Elizabeth Loftus has discerned that potent suggestion can elicit detailed "pseudomemories" in about 10% of the adult population. Another 15% can be convinced that the proffered event did occur, even though they cannot recall the details.

The False Versus the Repressed

However compelling the evidence proving the existence of false memories, it does not automatically negate the phenomenon of repressed memories. We take strong issue with the extent to which repressed memories are reported to exist: if we are to believe some recovery movement proponents, at least 50% of all women are victims of childhood sexual abuse, even though they may have no memory of it at all. Additionally, although no serious investigator denies that people sometimes forget parts of an experience, are we really to believe that entire traumatic experiences so commonly and completely vanish from conscious memory? If so, why isn't there pervasive memory repression among children who survived the Holocaust? In a study of children who witnessed a parent's murder, why is it that—though the children's memories were sometimes distorted—not in even one case were they lost entirely? Considering all the forms of childhood trauma, why should repressed memories be unique to sexual abuse?

However a counterfeit memory emerges, the outcome is a literal lie of the mind: a real belief in a false event. Thus, the sincerity of the person who suddenly "recovers" a false memory is not in question. Similarly, therapists who have unwittingly produced false memories in their clients are, for the most part, genuinely interested in their clients' well-being and are motivated by a sincere desire to help. But the fact remains that false memories do real harm and that the effects can be far-reaching and long-lasting.

■ The Role of Therapy in False Memory Syndrome

Therapists Who Believe Too Much

Although false memories can be the product of media suggestion, misinterpretation, or group pressure, most cases of false memory syndrome (FMS) can be traced directly to the therapist whose prejudgments drive the therapy sessions and treatment plans. We have already observed one of these guiding beliefs: that childhood sexual abuse is an almost routine experience. When a therapist embraces this notion, the goal of therapy centers on rooting out the memory of abuse so that real healing can begin. In this way, the therapist's entrenched ideas become the mechanism by which memories are "recovered."

Suggestion can also occur when a therapist has resolute preconceptions about the meaning of a particular symptom or diagnosis. Many recovery therapists, for example, believe that psychiatric maladies such as bulimia or depression are strong indicators (or even proof positive) of childhood sexual abuse. The recovery literature is replete with checklists by which therapists can measure the current symptoms of their clients against the likelihood of childhood sexual abuse. For example, in E. Sue Blume's *Secret Survivors*, the following medical problems are listed as potential indicators of past incest: "gastrointestinal problems, gynecological disorders including spontaneous vaginal infections, headaches, arthritis or joint pain." Although there has never been a study linking any one medical or emotional condition to childhood sexual abuse, the myth persists among many recovery therapists that a particular symptom can be scientifically classified under precisely this rubric.

Karen (as told by Marc)

After many months of individual psychotherapy with a social worker in town, Karen was referred to me for a medication evaluation. Before I saw Karen for the first time, her therapist told me that she probably needed an antianxiety medication because the recall of sexual and physical abuse by her uncle, the central issue they had been working on, was becoming more and more disturbing to her. Karen had been a brilliant student in high school, demonstrating academic excellence and a highly developed creative ability. Indeed, by the time she was 15, Karen had received professional recognition for her writing talents, particularly her poetry. According to her therapist, her present state of decline was the result of "unprocessed abuse during childhood" This, he claimed, was the reason she could no longer write poetry and was solely responsible for her deteriorating college performance. By the time I met Karen, her work had become so poor that she had dropped out of school and had been unable to handle even a part-time job since then.

During my first meeting with Karen, I observed that she was immaculately groomed, but somehow something was "off"; for example, she interrupted the interview at various times by peering off at a corner of the room, as if searching for someone she knew. These behaviors interested me and I wondered whether Karen might be dissociating even as we were talking.

"Are you looking for someone?" I asked her.

Karen's eyes remain fixed on the empty corner and she did not respond.

"Karen, what are you experiencing right now?"

At the sound of her name, Karen seemed to snap to, and she explained away her pause with the answer "Nothing, really"—but she still appeared troubled and distracted. As we chatted further, most of Karen's responses struck me as idiosyncratic, not quite in tune with the situation. For instance, when I mentioned that I understood that her hobby was growing orchids, she replied, "Oh yes, I love to, even when the sun is disconnected." Her conversation was like a train that kept leaving the tracks.

As Karen and I met over several sessions, she began to talk openly about the symptoms she had diligently tried to conceal—first at college, then on the job, and now as a young woman who was demoralized by having had to return to her parents' nest.

"Please don't think I'm crazy," she said, leaning forward and lowering her voice. "But sometimes early in the morning, when my parents are still asleep, I hear voices."

With this new revelation, I was beginning to discern a clinical picture that was very different from the one reported by Karen's therapist.

"And what do these voices tell you?" I asked her.

"They call out my name, as if they want me to pay attention, but then I can't hear what they're saying. They mutter in low voices and speak words I don't understand, like nonsense words. And something else," she said, nervously rubbing her hands. Her voice was now a whisper. "When it is quiet at night, I have visitors in my room. I think they're. . . ."

Karen hesitated, as if considering whether she could trust me with this strange revelation. ". . . I think they're ghosts," she said. "They stand at the foot of my bed and then rise up and glide over the wall. I don't know what they want. They scare me."

Like her mind, Karen's body seemed to betray her at times. Her arms would suddenly rise as we spoke, hovering over her lap as if they were as light as helium balloons. They would just as suddenly fall again, now heavy as bricks. This bizarre posturing, and the auditory and visual hallucinations that Karen described, were characteristic features of psychosis. Combining these findings with the normal physical exam and lab results her internist had reported, I was now sure that Karen was exhibiting symptoms of schizophrenia.

Though she seemed genuinely to enjoy our meetings, I still felt that we were not in synch. She was never unpleasant, hostile, or suspicious toward me—just different, subtly but undeniably different. I would become aware of how penetrating her gaze became at times; though our conversation would proceed as it had, Karen would suddenly start to stare at me so unblinkingly that I would find myself squirming in my chair. Or the faint sound of a distant siren would make her literally leap from her seat. Or she would lean into me far too close as she spoke and run over my own remarks, seeming unable to adhere to the tacit rules that govern usual social interactions. I could readily understand that these features alone would have had vast consequences for her ability to function in school and at work.

My initial impressions were only confirmed over time. I could not escape the conclusion that Karen's abnormalities in thinking, actually stemming from schizophrenia, had been misattributed to abuse. Indeed, struggle as she might, Karen could not recall any details about possible abuse by her uncle or anyone else. She mentioned, for example, that her fear of fireplaces over the past year or two must have been due to someone's having seriously burned her in childhood, and she thought that "maybe" she could remember "that something like that happened"; but she herself pointed out that she had no scars or medical records to suggest that she had actually experienced such a trauma. After months of therapy by an avowed recovery-movement therapist, Karen did believe that at times she could recall snippets of sexual abuse, but I felt sure that, unconsciously, this gentle, cooperative patient was simply trying to please her therapist and be a "good" patient.

With Karen's permission, I met with her parents, neither of whom had ever met her therapist. The meeting went well over the hour scheduled as they tearfully shared their sorrow at her failed effort at college and their worry about what the future might bring. They had been befuddled by her allegations of abuse and could see Karen's own indecision and confusion whenever they had tried to discuss it. I talked with her parents about the diagnosis of schizophrenia and the fact that Karen's high intelligence and rich creativity would still allow her to reach her goal of working in health care, although most likely in a less ambitious capacity than she and they had originally hoped. I gave them reading materials about schizophrenia and arranged for a member of the local chapter of the Alliance for the Mentally Ill to give them a call.

Just as Karen's parents left the session better informed but still faced with major challenges ahead, I wrestled with a difficult dilemma. Although Karen and I enjoyed a warm working relationship, she truly adored her outgoing, charismatic therapist. I suspected that if I were as direct with her as I had been with her parents, I might alienate her. Instead, I shared my impressions with the therapist. During a tense telephone call, I tried to mobilize his support in offering Karen an antipsychotic medication; eventually, he did reluctantly agree that it made sense. Although I didn't convince him that Karen suffered from schizophrenia, he concurred that an antipsychotic drug might help Karen with her feelings of distress—which he still blamed on percolating memories of abuse.

Since then, there has been remarkable improvement, and Karen has eagerly absorbed an impressive amount of lay and professional literature about schizophrenia. Karen has also reported that the feelings that her uncle must have abused her have entirely vanished. She assertively told her therapist that she no longer believed that recovered memory therapy was appropriate for her, and, to his credit, her therapist has also revised his opinion. He has curtailed the frequency of his meetings with her and has altered his focus to issues in the "here and now," such as Karen's finding her own apartment and obtaining work as an occupational therapy aide.

The waning of the FMS and the provision of proper therapy and medication have allowed Karen's abilities as a poet to resurface. This selection, presented with her permission, is a joyful picture of a flower opening in spring—an apt metaphor for Karen:

The Amaryllis

She begins a brown bulb
in the paper white of winter.
Outdoors,
she has slept through
light dances of spring rain,
long drums of summer sun
and cooling strokes of autumn wind.
Indoors,
she bursts into the world
an apple green shoot bearing an apricot babe.
She opens like a stretching hand,
one finger at a time,
melon or orange or sweet tangerine.
Blooms swell two at a time,
four in a day,
until twenty five sisters
sing like a hillside of lilies.
They smile
radiant as dew,
clear as a moment
and joyous as the birth of a moonbeam.

Winter returns
from slinking under the hedges—
frosts the windows,
sticks the door.
The amaryllis goes to sleep again,
still as the first rose,
quiet as a fir tree
and dreamy as an early rising snowflake.

Guidance or Guise?

Suggestion can be overt or subtle. Overt suggestion occurs when the therapist openly expresses to the patient his or her belief that childhood sexual abuse is responsible for the patient's problems. But a therapist's bias may be just as effectively conveyed in a more subtle fashion. For example, a therapist who has arrived at certain premature judgments about the patient's symptoms might say, "It has been my experience that patients with your problems often have been sexually abused as children. Can you remember a time in your childhood when you were particularly unhappy?" In this gentle, often inadvertent way, the suggestion is planted, and probing continues until at last the patient uncovers a "memory" that verifies the therapist's early impressions.

A core tenet of recovery therapy is that one may count on current feelings as strong indicators of abuse. However, one may not count on the fact of having no memory of abuse because this feature could very well stem from denial. This tenet is exemplified in the original edition of *The Courage to Heal* when the authors state,

> Assume your feelings are valid. . . . If you think you were abused and your life shows the symptoms, you were. If you don't remember your abuse you are not alone. Many women don't have memories. . . . This doesn't mean they weren't abused.

Adopting such approaches, recovery therapists write themselves an intellectual blank check.

Although feelings are indeed always valid, the patient's memory for what has produced a particular feeling may be well off the mark. Therefore, patients may seek to corroborate their memories. This is what Karen was attempting to do when she observed that she had no scars or medical records to suggest she had been burned as a child. But recovery therapists, by and large, reject the value of corroboration, believing that the "narrative truth" (the patient's understanding of his or her past) is more important than "historical truth" (events as they actually transpired). Eileen Franklin-Lipsker's therapist spoke for many recovery movement advocates when he testified in court that "it wasn't important whether her visualizations were real or not" and that they "could sort that out later." The problem is that "later" seldom comes. Accused families understandably reel at such comments, registering their outrage at what seems to be total disregard for them.

False Memories in Command

Once false memories are implanted and take root, they can hold great power over an individual. Patients themselves may resist reclaiming the truth, their convictions reinforced by the emotional ties that bind patients to their therapists. As a result, false memories may endure even when the patient is offered another interpretation of his or her symptoms.

Christopher (as told by Jackie)

What I had viewed as a simple effort to supply a little medical objectivity in a case of FMS actually led to a permanent rupture in the relationship. I had seen Christopher for almost a year. He had come to me with a severe anxiety disorder that was rapidly ripening into agoraphobia. He had been seeing a therapist on a regular basis who asked me to evaluate whether short-term medication use might impede the looming agoraphobia.

Shortly after we met, Christopher let me know that he was struggling in therapy to recover memories of childhood trauma.

"My therapist thinks that I was sexually abused as a child," he told me. "I feel so nervous all the time. My therapist says that sexual abuse as a child causes a lot of anxiety in adulthood and that I have to deal with it if I want to get better."

"What do *you* think?" I asked him.

"Dr. Feldman, I feel scared all of the time. I can't sleep at night. I can't make decisions about my life. Lately I can't even go outside my house without feeling panic. I have no other explanation for my anxiety. I think my therapist is on to something."

Christopher's poignant expression sent up a red flag for me. A patient so desperate for answers might easily be persuaded to find a false solution. I decided to explore Christopher's beliefs further.

"Have you identified any facts about your abuse?"

"Well, I know that I must have been very young, and that my father was the one who did it."

Christopher stumbled over these words but continued narrating what was obviously a difficult concept.

"I have symptoms," he continued. "Like lately I've been finding some blood on the toilet paper now and then. My therapist says that this is my body reliving the trauma of what my father did to me. He says I'm having 'body memories.' "

Looking into his eyes, I saw the extent of his emotional pain. I wanted to assure Christopher that there was help for his anxiety, that he was not required to accept this disturbing belief in order to get better, that there are many explanations for pervasive anxiety in adults.

As for the bleeding he described, the trauma of anal penetration to a young child certainly *could* result in bleeding. But to assume that Christopher's adult symptoms naturally stemmed from such an experience was a leap of logic I could not accept. Observing that Christopher was firmly convinced of his therapist's interpretation, I gently offered him another perception. Could it be that he was experiencing a mundane case of hemorrhoids? Had he tried using a hemorrhoidal cream as a straightforward way to test this theory?

Christopher appeared thoughtful, as if considering that I might have a point. But he didn't show up for his next appointment and never called to reschedule. Later, I learned from a colleague who knew Christopher personally that he had been offended by my inability to accept what was "really" causing the bleeding and that he was continuing to explore his beliefs about abuse in his therapy. I suspected then that my medical explanation was offered too early in our work together and that it had been viewed as a betrayal.

Almost a year later, at a social function, Christopher's therapist approached me. Amidst the small talk, he admitted sheepishly that he had actually been the one to encourage Christopher to find another, more "understanding" psychiatrist following the "hemorrhoid incident." But he was no longer treating him either; their efforts to reconstruct the abuse had led nowhere, and their work together ended by mutual agreement. Christopher declined a referral to another therapist.

Christopher's psychological problems had been disabling and required serious treatment, but he had been encouraged to chase after false leads. In such cases, patients can wind up disillusioned with therapy and quit out of frustration before receiving the help that brought them to the office in the first place. Christopher deserved better, and I remain hopeful that he will secure it.

Even when a patient's recovered memory has been countered by irrefutable evidence, the patient will sometimes attempt to make sense of this new evidence by holding fast to the belief and simply altering a few details to support it. In an essay titled "Psychiatric Misadventures," psychiatrist Paul McHugh tells of a young woman who, with the help of her therapist, recovered a memory of sexual abuse by her uncle. So powerfully forged in her memory was this childhood trauma that she could even disclose the precise date on which the abuse occurred. When her mother confronted her with the fact that she could not possibly have been raped by her uncle at that time because he had been serving overseas, the daughter thought for a moment and then replied, "Well, then, if your dates are right, I suppose it must have been Dad."

In a case cited by researcher Richard Ofshe and journalist Ethan Watters, a 38-year-old woman recovered memories of being raped repeatedly as a child. Under hypnosis, she also recalled her sisters' having been raped. When she met with her sisters to offer her assertions about the assaults, they dismissed the allegations as mere fantasy. Embracing the circular logic of many recovery advocates, the patient then accused her sisters of being in denial. She stuck confidently by her own personal "truth."

The Motives for Believing

For the casual observer, it is difficult to understand why patients cling so fiercely to a "truth" that is immensely painful. When the evidence points them toward a clean exit, why would they willingly choose their torment?

This is exactly the question that haunted the jury in the Franklin case. The possibility that Eileen Franklin-Lipsker had chosen suffering countered everything the jurors thought they knew about the self-protective instincts of human beings. Franklin-Lipsker's willingness to take the hard road was accepted as a powerful indication of her credibility.

But the jury didn't recognize that by the time a patient has acquired "recovered" memories, he or she has walked through fire to reach them. The memories are the long-sought prize that has kept the patient coming back to therapy in the desperate hope of getting better. Many personal accounts testify to the anguish patients have experienced in the recovery process—paradoxically enough, all in the hope of achieving release from their suffering. Having bought their recovered memories at such a high price, patients are not easily persuaded to relinquish what they believe to be their only hope for wellness.

Another motive for believing derives from the relationship forged between a patient and therapist. Unable to surmount life's problems on their own, patients in treatment look to the therapist to lead them out of deep psychic pain. Patients who have bonded with their therapists typically work hard to demonstrate progress: "If I work hard," the insecure patient may think, "my therapist will like me." Within this web of vulnerability and unconscious motivation, the patient becomes ripe for suggestion.

The problems facing any patient are inevitably complex, yet human nature leads us to seek simple solutions. In arriving at a scenario of abuse, patients may initially feel overwhelming relief in understanding, at last, that they are not to blame for their problems. If they are already harboring anger toward a parent, it seems to them that their anger is now vindicated. Therefore, in accepting the false memory as a true event, the person actually solves two problems: the venting of long-held anger toward a parent becomes justifiable, and the patient now has a ready explanation for the problems in his or her life. In an article published in *Modern Woman*, 38-year-old Elizabeth Godley, who was led to believe that her mother had sexually abused her, provides this insightful account:

> Certainly I was desperate for answers—a drowning woman grasping at anything to keep afloat. On the surface I appeared to have everything—a promis-

ing career, intelligence, attractive looks—but I was miserable. My temper was explosive, my relationships with men stormy; I was extremely vulnerable to criticism; my self-esteem was non-existent. At work, I couldn't get along with my supervisors or my colleagues. So when I was offered an explanation for my depression and problems, I lunged at it. It was easier to blame my mother than to accept responsibility for my unhappiness.

Some experts have put forth the theory that false memories of sexual abuse are really a metaphor for the feeling of being ill-treated as a child. They add that the unconscious translation of these nebulous feelings into the dramatic scenario of incest elicits great sympathy from others. In this way, the patient starts to feel that the suffering (which is genuine) has finally and effectively been acknowledged. Furthermore, such claims are reinforced by a society that links the role of victim to the virtues of strength and stoicism—implied, for example, by the word "survivor." For persons with self-esteem deficits, the acceptance of victimhood can be a badge of honor, a sign of their innate strength that they had never before recognized.[1]

▌ The Methods Controversy

Review any court case involving recovered memories of incest. Read any article involving claims of satanic torture and cannibalism or of sexual molestation by space creatures. Do so and you will detect an almost universal pattern in these seemingly disparate situations. The recaptured memories did not rise up from the natural process of talk therapy. On the contrary, the memories were facilitated by any of the methods favored in recovery therapy: visualization, age regression, abreaction, eye movement desensitization and reprocessing, journaling, dream analysis, hypnosis, drug-assisted interviews, and still others. Some of these methods are denigrated as quackery, psychofads, or pseudoscience. Other techniques are criticized not for any inherent weakness, but because they are misapplied or misinterpreted in the service of "refreshing" memory. We'll consider three of them: *hypnosis; drug-assisted interviews;* and *symptom checklists.* We'll also end with one, *facilitated communication,* that was initially heralded as invaluable for autistic individuals but has recently emerged as the methodological equivalent of snake oil.

---

[1] In 1996, the on-line service CompuServe established a "Survivors Forum" (GO SAFEPLACE) for "survivors, their caring friends, and non-offending family members" within its "Home & Leisure" section.

Hypnosis

Under the guidance of skilled and experienced practitioners, hypnosis has long been used to delve into the subconscious. The information uncovered in this way often reflects themes significant to the patient. It may express the patient's fantasies or fears, or it may be a modified or distorted reenactment of some event in the patient's life. This material can then be explored further in the therapy if its factual limitations are respected.

At the same time, hypnosis is known to heighten a patient's suggestibility, making the method vulnerable to any agenda the therapist might have. Under hypnosis, for instance, the therapist may call for the patient to produce certain images that will bring a spurious trauma to light. That mere suggestion can result in distinct images of sexual trauma that are then wrongly interpreted as liberated memories. In a case that galvanized Catholics around the world, Steven Cook accused Chicago's Joseph Cardinal Bernardin of sexually abusing him after hypnosis "liberated" Cook's memories of the assault. Eventually recognizing the unreliability of his memories, however, Cook retracted the accusation and apologized to Bernardin.

Although in other cases people have actually been convicted on the basis of hypnotically induced "memories," there is simply no question about the unreliability of hypnosis in producing factual material. One psychiatric clinician and researcher, Dr. Philip Coons, was struck by an experience involving a female defendant who, while under hypnosis, appeared to develop an alternate personality and then confessed to a crime she did not commit. Since that time, Coons says, he rarely relies on hypnosis as a method for reconstructing memories; when he uses it at all, he maintains that independent confirmation is mandatory.

Two researchers, Hollida Wakefield and Ralph Underwager of Minnesota, have sought to correct some of the myths surrounding hypnosis. In reviewing the literature, they arrived at the following conclusions, many of which are bound to be disconcerting to recovery movement therapists. First, hypnosis increases the vividness of imagined experiences. Second, people who are highly hypnotizable are also easy to persuade. Third, hypnotized subjects are likely to "remember" traumatic incidents that are suggested during hypnosis. And fourth, hypnotized subjects experience these "memories" as real, which may increase their confidence in them as well as their persuasiveness when they report them to others.

Wakefield and Underwager conclude that since hypnosis tends to produce a mélange of fact and fantasy, outside corroboration is the only recourse for the responsible use of hypnosis that leads to recovered memories.

Drug-Assisted Interviews

For the past 50 years, sedatives such as amobarbital (Amytal) have been used credibly and responsibly to assist psychiatric patients in producing narratives that can help target key psychotherapeutic issues. Amytal and its pharmacologic cousins—like hypnosis—continue to be of some value as adjuncts to therapy, and we illustrated an appropriate use of Amytal in a case of conversion disorder in the chapter on somatoform disorders. But, again like hypnosis, the misapplication of the drug-assisted interview (also called *narcoanalysis)* has undeniably resulted in the production of false memories.

Amytal, which has been erroneously labeled a "truth serum," is actually nothing more than a barbiturate belonging to the same family of drugs as pentobarbital (Nembutal) and secobarbital (Seconal). Administered intravenously, it produces effects similar to those of alcohol intoxication: drowsiness, warmth, relaxation, and often a feeling of personal closeness. Unfortunately, Amytal also produces other effects: memory disturbances, for instance, and a distorted sense of time. Patients under the influence of Amytal (or the related medications some physicians prefer to use) are highly suggestible and cannot reliably discriminate between fact and fiction.

Nevertheless, the drug-assisted interview has become the method of choice for many recovery therapists who commonly err in two important ways: by administering the drug inappropriately and by interpreting the results incorrectly. In a highly publicized case, the therapist and psychiatrist for Holly Ramona were successfully sued for implanting or reinforcing false memories that her father had molested her in childhood. The plaintiff's attorney in the case charged Ramona's therapist and psychiatrist with misrepresenting the validity of the Amytal that had been administered as part of her treatment: they were accused of calling it a "truth serum," of informing Ms. Ramona that no one could lie while under its influence, and of insisting that a recollection of abuse while a person was under Amytal's effects was proof that the abuse had occurred. Denouncing these falsehoods, the attorney claimed that the Amytal interview was used not to produce a useful narrative but simply to verify the clinicians' own belief that Holly Ramona had been the victim of childhood sexual abuse.

The Ramona case serves as an excellent example of the misuse of the drug-assisted interview. Of considerable concern is the added fact that, too often, patients—and therapists—are awed by the technique. Whenever they resort to such dramatic interventions, therapists convey the tacit but mighty expectation that their patients will produce something valuable. In many cases, say the experts, the patient is just dutifully rising to the occasion.

Nancy (as told by Marc)

Nancy's story is a murky mix of truth and lies, accurate perceptions and false memories. That Nancy had lost control of herself while under hypnosis and Amytal plagued her long after the fact. Ever since, she waffled between furious expressions of anger at the therapists who had "tricked" her and staunch denials that they had ever been able to do so. After treating Nancy for more than two and a half years, I was finally able to understand her experience in therapy.

Nancy was a highly intelligent young woman burdened with a severe personality disorder. She felt chronically demoralized, yet she always managed to remain aware of her own bright mind. She prided herself on using it to stay one step ahead of her doctors and create minor chaos among the members of her inpatient treatment teams.

Since early adolescence, her life had entailed frequent bouts of rage, episodes of self-harm in which she lightly cut or burned herself, and continual blame of others for her failures in school and work. Seeking external causes for her unhappy life, Nancy bounced from one psychiatrist to another, firing them when the work of therapy became too challenging. I was the latest in a long succession of doctors charged with the formidable task of solving Nancy's problems.

Nancy's inveterate doctor shopping had led predictably to fragmented care and little therapeutic success. If progress were ever to be made, I knew that it would first be necessary to help Nancy break the cycle of starts and stops that had characterized her therapy. It seemed important, therefore, to see through Nancy's eyes what experiences had led her to the office of yet another psychiatrist. This became our starting point, and it was during this process of exploration that Nancy's story was revealed.

Medications had done little to quell the turmoil so characteristic of her personality disorder, and at times Nancy had been hospitalized to contain her angry and self-destructive behaviors. During her most recent hospitalization—an especially prolonged one—Nancy's psychiatrist enrolled her in a newly created group for sexual trauma survivors. Although Nancy had always denied any history of sexual or physical abuse, in this new setting she began dutifully narrating stories of sexual abuse.

It is possible that Nancy found the drama of an alleged history of abuse too much to resist, too useful an explanation for her lack of fulfillment and accomplishment. Or perhaps she longed for a group identity, a sense of belonging where before there had been none. Revelations of abuse were the only currency with which one could retain membership in her therapy group, a forum that Nancy seemed to have found highly alluring.

In all probability, a mixture of conscious and unconscious motivations led her to buy into the program. But to hear Nancy tell it, she had only one. Her stories, she said, were purposely cast out as bait, and she watched with pleasure as her therapists eagerly went after them in what she termed their "feeding frenzy": "I knew they wanted a good story and it was so easy to humor them. My stories were totally invented. I told them that when I was six, a neighborhood boy forced me to have oral sex with him. I could see this interested them, so I spiced it up with plenty of details. They kept wanting more, so I told them that the neighborhood boy was really my brother, and that my brother and a gang of his sex-crazed friends took turns abusing me for more than two years. They always wanted more details. They believed everything I told them without question. I made complete fools of them."

In the hospital, these ostensive episodes of depraved abuse had become the entire focus of her treatment. Nancy was transferred to an abuse specialist who listed her symptoms (mood swings, self-harm, impulsivity) and stated incorrectly that only a long history of extreme abuse could have produced this clinical picture. By this circular reasoning, her revelations were "confirmed," and—in the interest of building upon her "awakened memories"—her therapy was stepped up with more frequent sessions and greater pressure to produce fresh memories.

Nancy soon began to feel that the game she had started was out of her control: "It was like *I* had become the one being played for a fool," she told me. Trying to backtrack, she first told her therapist that she had just meant to describe "possible" memories of abuse. Finally, she admitted to her doctor that she had made up the stories to garner attention.

Like the boy who cried "Wolf!" Nancy left her truth at the feet of her disbelievers. The psychiatrist and therapist reassured her that unconsciously she was trying to protect herself from recollections too painful to bear. And although research tells us that it is virtually impossible to discern from a patient's appearance whether he or she is lying, Nancy's psychiatrist told her he "could tell" that she spoke the truth when she first leveled the allegations. Thus firmly "corrected" and a bit intrigued by the certainty and passion of the two clinicians, Nancy acquiesced to the first of many hypnosis sessions, during which she added the names of three other relatives who had abused her.

The "success" of Nancy's hypnosis was the impetus for an ever-increasing reliance on memory-enhancing methods. During lengthy interviews using Amytal or hypnosis, the number of alleged abusers quickly and dramatically escalated. A female teacher, the family gardener, and her grandparents were now perpetrators; her breasts had been burned with a cigarette lighter; she had been raped with a vibrator and assaulted with a knife. By this time,

Nancy had lost her mental mooring and could no longer discern which of her stories were purposely contrived and which were artificially induced. Under the wavy warmth of Amytal, for example, Nancy felt her mind drift into a deep pool that offered up dim, distorted images. These vague images in turn formed the armatures upon which finer features were shaped and molded with each succeeding session. Drifting in and out of the dreamy states produced by Amytal and hypnosis, Nancy experienced false memories mingled with the conscious embellishments she produced until what was a false belief and what was a knowing lie became indistinguishable.

Each time a new trauma was recounted, her doctor documented the session as a success. Conversely, whenever Nancy expressed doubts about her recovered memories or admitted to embellishing her accounts, she was told she was "losing ground." Nancy recalled that her psychiatrist explained that her doubts were probably induced by her past use of antidepressants, a remark that she found bizarre based on her own readings about the medications.

Eventually, Nancy was discharged from the hospital. No longer receiving the daily therapy, Nancy saw her entire experience as a hoax—albeit one to which she had contributed. She went on to write a letter to all of the members of her hospital treatment team. In it, she stated that she found it "warped" that they were so enthralled by her claims of abuse (especially the most graphic ones) and that she was disgusted by their recalcitrance when she attempted to set the record straight. She added that it had become clear that the only way to get an Amytal interview or hypnotherapy session to end in a reasonable length of time was to fabricate a new tale. She ended by writing that the greatest trauma she had experienced came not from abuse or even from her own self-harm but from her own misstatements about the past and the single-mindedness of those whom she termed "abuse groupies."

If Nancy's story contains deeply disturbing questions of what constitutes therapy, it also presented me with a troubling paradox. Nancy had a long history of criticizing and blaming her therapists, an attitude that had short-circuited her progress and that formed the basis for my first therapeutic objective with Nancy. How could I hope to help her develop and sustain trust in me—indeed, in the value of therapy at all—while accepting her position that she had been ill-served by all of her previous therapists?

Ultimately, my approach was to help Nancy understand that doctor shopping was only worthwhile if she knew what she was shopping for. Drawing on Nancy's analytical strengths, I worked to help her identify and write down her own therapeutic goals—goals that were realistic, concrete, specific, and measurable. She then drew up a list of attributes, general therapeutic skills, and specialized training that she believed would satisfy her in a therapist. We reviewed what she had written—compromising, clarifying, and at times debating. This process of negotiation and alliance building was as important as the content of the list. In performing these tasks, Nancy discovered that she had the power to make choices for as well as against and to be in control without being controlling. With this first small step, Nancy began the long journey toward reclaiming responsibility for her own life.

Survivors' Symptom Checklists

Of all the methods used in recovery therapy, there may be none more unsound than the survivors' checklists. The checklist approach has done more to create specious abuse victims than has any other strategy. Developed as a quick means of assessing whether one might have experienced incest, the checklists have been promoted in *The Courage to Heal* as well as many other publications on incest recovery. These lists of reputed "abuse symptoms" are actually compilations of generalities that could describe almost anyone who has successfully made it to adulthood. Note that some symptoms are opposites, proving that whether you *do* or you *don't*, you probably *are!* Here is a sampling from Renee Frederickson's book, *Repressed Memories:*

- I am preoccupied with thoughts about sex.
- I have had a period of sexual promiscuity in my life.
- I have had periods in my life when I couldn't eat or had to force myself to eat.
- Sometimes I binge on huge amounts of food.
- I often have nightmares.
- I have difficulty falling or staying asleep.
- I have taken foolish risks with my safety.
- I can't seem to control myself when it comes to spending money or gambling.
- Nothing seems very real sometimes.
- There are certain things I seem to have a strange attraction or affection for.
- I hate going to the dentist more than most people.
- I do not take good care of my body.

In an article in *Esquire* titled "The Lost Daughter," John Taylor compares modern checklists to those from the distant past. His research led him to a list from mid-17th-century France that was used to identify witches. The haziness of Renee Frederickson's list is apparently nothing new, for if you lived in 1644, any of the following could have implicated you as demonically possessed:

- To think oneself possessed.
- To lead a wicked life.
- To live outside the rules of society.

- To be persistently ill.
- To blaspheme.
- To be tired of living.

The popularity of checklists among recovery therapists is symbolic of the unscientific approaches used. As a crude home test kit of sorts, it is also representative of the deceptively simple (and simpleminded) solutions promoted by some abuse-recall advocates.

Facilitated Communication: Messages From the Autistic Person?

Upon learning of a new, startlingly simple technique for communicating with their 17-year-old autistic son Matt, the Gerardis felt immense hope. But shortly after Matt was introduced to *facilitated communication*, they began to have serious doubts about its reliability. For one thing, their son's schoolwork improved so suddenly and dramatically that such a change seemed flatly impossible. And Mrs. Gerardi could not understand why the technique worked so well at school but so poorly at home—what could explain such a difference?

Facilitated communication (FC) emerged in 1989 as an exciting breakthrough in work with autistic and other disabled children. Initially, it seemed miraculous that such an uncomplicated device could have such transforming powers. With the help of a facilitator, children whose thoughts had been locked away in stony silence now seemed to be freely expressing themselves. Best of all, anyone could learn to use FC with just a day or two of training. Facilitators were taught gently to guide the child's hand over a keyboard and wait for the child to begin pointing toward letters. The results of this method were often astonishing. In some cases, the cogency of the elicited messages seemed far beyond the child's age and ability. Questions such as the one raised by Mrs. Gerardi started to arise: Whose hands were doing the pointing? Who was really authoring the messages?

These questions may have remained within therapeutic circles if not for what happened next. With the assistance of facilitators, some autistic children began producing messages about sexual abuse. Matt Gerardi "shared" such a message with his teacher, who immediately went to the authorities. The events that followed swept the Gerardi family into an emotional and legal maelstrom. Although investigations could uncover no evidence of abuse, Mr. Gerardi was forced to leave his home, and for the next six months he was denied all contact with his son.

During this time, however, Mr. Gerardi made an amazing discovery. Conducting an investigation of his own, he found that many other families were sharing his predicament. All over the country, FC had produced similar claims of sexual abuse, usually implicating a family member.

As with the false-memory accusations described earlier, litigation brought this issue into the realm of public debate. Accused families demanded legal redress. James Randi, an investigator of unusual claims, charged that FC simply turned autistic children into "human Ouija boards." Others called FC a cruel and reckless hoax that played on parents' dreams for their children.

Medical professionals also entered the arena by studying the FC phenomenon experimentally. In a controlled study at Children's Hospital in Boston, a facilitator and an autistic student were individually shown pictures; they were then asked to use FC to type out what the student had seen. The researchers found that whenever the pictures were different, the printed message conveyed what the facilitator—not the child—saw. The Boston study proved that the messages were authored, albeit unconsciously, not by the child but by the facilitator. This test has been repeated more than a dozen times in three countries with over 100 subjects, and in every case the results have been the same. The American Psychological Association has formally stated that FC has no known value.

In view of such evidence, the Gerardi family was finally reunited; but, with unconscionable commitment to the technique, Matt's school continued to use FC. In this case as in others, FC proponents have been loath to accept the scientific findings that have discredited it. By the time the controversy erupted, many therapists had built their entire careers upon facilitated communication. More than a few stated openly that FC had become their whole lives. Parents too were understandably shaken. For many, dreams for their children were forever lost, whereas others clung fiercely to their hope.

A 1995 book, *I Don't Want to Be Inside Me Anymore*, purports to be a landmark work by a nonverbal autistic patient. Only in the introduction, written by a journalist, does it become clear that the material was created through FC. Readers are also left to guess how the "first-person account" of the patient, Birger Sellin, might have been affected by its having been "selected," "arranged," and partially "corrected" by the same journalist.

The courts remain just as perplexed, as revealed by some perplexing decisions. In March 1995, for example, the Kansas Supreme Court upheld the use of FC "testimony" to support the conviction of a school staffer for the sexual abuse of a 12-year-old autistic boy.

Supplementing the intellectual and emotional investment of some is a more tangible one. FC is now practiced in at least 38 states, and millions of tax dollars fund the centers. With the added force of this political backing, it is unlikely that the case for or against FC will be decided on purely objective grounds. Although advocates and adversaries continue to take shots at each other, the method endures, leaving parents, taxpayers, and disabled children caught in the cross fire.

■ False Memory Syndrome Variants: From Satan to Space Aliens

Although FMS is associated mostly with the incest survivors' movement, other phenomena have emerged as FMS variants. Two of these—satanic ritual abuse and space alien abductions—are so bizarre that they occupied a central place in the talk show and tabloid markets even before they emerged as subjects for clinical debate. Because neither phenomenon has been irrefutably proved or disproved, the controversy surrounding the credibility of such claims continues to sizzle. On one side are those who dismiss such stories as pure fabrications. On the other are those who are convinced that they reflect real experience, and clinical treatments for satanic ritual abuse and alien abductions have even become self-proclaimed therapeutic specialties.

Satanic ritual abuse (SRA) and alien abduction claims are linked to false memories of incest and other childhood abuse in several ways. Among the features they share are the individual's report of abuse of a sexual nature, the snowballing of the story as more shocking memories are supplied over time, the fact that the information commonly arises out of suggestion, and the induction of an altered state of consciousness—often through hypnosis or Amytal—as part of diagnosis and treatment. In the case of alleged SRA, as with incest, long and costly investigations, legal proceedings, and even criminal convictions have resulted from claims based solely on recovered memories (but no one has yet tried to sue a space alien).

Satanic Ritual Abuse

In Hanover Park, Illinois, a quiet Chicago suburb, a case of satanic sex abuse was dismissed last week for lack of evidence. The charges against 28-year-old John [F.] were made by the five-year-old girl next door and entailed, apart from oral sex, forcing her to witness the murder of five identical young girls in his upstairs bedroom and a basement ceremony of devil worship where a man was murdered and then partially eaten by Mr. [F.], his wife and several others. No physical evidence was ever found for such crimes and last week the court judged the girl—the prosecution's only witness—"incredible." The girl had been "counseled" by Pamela Klein, a self-appointed expert in satanic and ritual abuse. The Chicago court had already ruled that Ms. Klein was "not a legitimate therapist." . . . The judge in the Hanover Park case said the five-year-old girl was "unable to distinguish between reality and fantasy," in part because she was "coached over and over and over again." . . . Ms. Klein, who runs a consulting business on ritual abuse, says that the criminal justice system is not accommodating enough to child witnesses.

In 1991, this story appeared in a British publication, *The Economist*. It was of special interest to its overseas readers because of what had happened just two years before when Ms. Klein had been lecturing in Britain. The chaos that ensued in two English towns following Klein's lectures was still fresh in their minds. After the citizens of Rochdale and Orkney had heard her tales of satanic abuse, they became convinced, to their horror, that their towns were populated by satanists. As in the cases of mass hysteria described in Chapter 7 of this book, reports of abuse flourished, and when the final tally was in, 32 children had been removed from their homes. Their sordid stories became the subject of judicial inquiries and many of the children were made wards of the court.

If this were an isolated occurrence, it would scarcely be worth noting. But for the past 10 years, reports of SRA—including murder, cannibalism, sexual perversion, and forced human breeding—have been filling more and more police files. In California's McMartin Preschool scandal, which launched the most expensive trial in U.S. history, seven employees were arrested and imprisoned for the alleged sexual abuse of children. In 1984, after the allegations were already under investigation, some of the McMartin children began mentioning "secret rooms" beneath the school that were joined by dark passageways. These strange tales led some parents to believe that satanists were using the children in bizarre rituals. A dig was organized to locate the tunnels, which would supposedly verify that the McMartin teachers were incarnations of Satan.

In 1985, the first search for the mysterious tunnels yielded two tortoise shells that the parents believed were evidence of animal mutilations. After investigators determined that the shells had been purposely planted, the tunnel issue died down, only to resurface five years later. Another dig was organized. This time, tunnels were indeed discovered, generating much excitement, but they appeared nothing like those described by the children. Contractors and construction workers studied the site, finally concluding that the tunnels were probably simple plumbing channels from earlier construction projects. Eventually, no one tried in the McMartin cases was found guilty.

Less fortunate were the accused staff members of the Fells Acres day care in

Malden, Massachusetts. In 1986 and 1987, three of them were convicted of the rape and indecent assault and battery of small children. Various reports by the children included a secret room, a "green and yellow and silver robot from 'Star Wars,' " "bad clowns," and a "magic wand." At trial, the prosecution argued that 19 children had been assaulted and raped with knives as long as 14 inches—somehow without injury and without anyone noticing. Although freed on a technicality in 1995, the elderly proprietor of the day care, Violet Amirault, had been denied parole months earlier for the sole reason that she continued to proclaim her innocence. In March 1997, the State's Supreme Judicial Court reinstated the convictions, refused staff members' request for a new trial, and ordered Mrs. Amirault and her daughter to return to jail. A *Wall Street Journal* columnist called the court's written opinion "so larded with reasoning in support of the unreasonable as to be worthy of study by generations of law students to come."

Were the McMartin and Fells Acres children exhibiting false memories or were they demonstrating vivid imaginations? The term *false memory syndrome* is generally reserved for adults whose memories have supposedly been in suspended animation—sometimes for up to 40 years. But children are even more imaginative and suggestible than adults and, as the McMartin, Hanover Park, and other stories illustrate, kids can produce counterfeit memories too.

Kenneth V. Lanning, an FBI investigator who wrote the book *Investigator's Guide to Allegations of "Ritual" Child Abuse*,[2] attempts to bring logic and common sense to the subject of satanic cults. He reports that not one of the 300 reports of SRA that he has personally reviewed has ever been corroborated. As he noted in the professional journal *Child Abuse and Neglect*,

> We now have hundreds of victims alleging that thousands of offenders are murdering tens of thousands of people. . . . Any professional evaluating victims' allegations of ritualistic abuse cannot ignore the lack of physical evidence (no bodies or physical evidence left by violent murderers), the difficulty in successfully committing a large-scale conspiracy crime (the more people involved in any crime conspiracy, the harder it is to get away with it), and human nature (intragroup conflicts resulting in individual self-serving disclosures are likely to occur in any group involved in organized kidnapping, baby breeding, and human sacrifice). . . . Mental health professionals must begin to accept the possibility that some of what these victims are alleging just didn't happen

---

[2] Available on the Internet at http://www.ieway.com/~csukbr/juslib/abuse.html.

and that this area desperately needs study and research by rational, objective social scientists.

Despite these persuasive remarks by an acknowledged expert, the pervasive belief in satanic cults remains a strong influence in eliciting fantastical accounts from suggestible individuals. Indeed, in a television documentary titled "The Search for Satan," a woman named Patty B. came forward to state that—assaulted by heavy medications and constant, aggressive therapy crossing over into interrogation—she came to believe she was part of satanic royalty, a "high priestess" controlling a nine-state network of individuals programmed to kill. An insurance company reviewer discerned an interesting pattern that suggested an odious ulterior motive in such florid "discoveries" of SRA: patients targeted as SRA victims also had unusually rich insurance coverage. Patty's insurance company paid out almost $3 million for the damaging treatment of her and her two sons.

Alien Abductions

On the surface it would certainly appear that alien abduction stories have little to do with spurious reports of childhood sexual abuse. To suggest that these two experiences are even remotely linked risks trivializing real and reprehensible acts perpetrated against children. Let us go on record as stating the obvious: the sexual abuse of children is a real and provable phenomenon. It leaves deep emotional scars on its victims and sometimes has long-term physical consequences as well. But although no reasonable person doubts the existence of sexual crimes against children, many reasonable people doubt tales of space-creature abduction. And the specious memories that lead people to believe they've been abducted, examined, and inseminated by aliens have unmistakable parallels with the faulty memories driving other forms of FMS.

In the past few years, alien abduction accounts have proliferated. An "Abductees Anonymous" page has even been established on the Internet. Harvard psychiatrist John Mack's popular 1994 book, *Abductions: Human Encounters with Aliens*, contains 13 such personal accounts. The narratives, which are often quite similar, tend to have dreamlike overtones: the person has vague impressions of unease that give rise to anxiety or fear, and he or she feels stalked or hunted and often experiences a lapse in time. Common sensations include physical paralysis and floating through space. A nearly universal theme of abduction stories is medical experimentation, usually of a sexual nature. The Hollywood B movie stereotypes of big-eyed, translucent humanoids arriving on circular spaceships often figure prominently as well.

The following account from *People Weekly*, describing the experience of a 32-year-old Massachusetts woman, illustrates many of the common elements of abduction stories. Jerry's first memory of abduction took her back to the age of two, but it was not until adolescence that she remembered experiencing real terror. It was during this time that the aliens began subjecting her to painful gynecologic procedures. She recalls, for example, that when she was 13, her captors began inserting embryos into her womb only to extract them when they got to the fetal stage.

Jerry estimates that she has been abducted more than 50 times. The abductions usually occur at night, when she is taken from her bed and made to float up into the aliens' spaceship. The visits are preceded by a ringing in her ears and an electrical energy that causes her hair to stand on end. She feels awake when the aliens come for her, yet she is unable to move and completely under their control. In this state of paralysis, she is then transported to the spaceship, where a team of space creatures performs excruciating medical procedures. Her abductions end almost as quickly and mysteriously as they begin. She seldom remembers being returned to her bed but usually discovers her husband beside her in an unnaturally deep sleep, which she believes is induced by the aliens.

Such colorful anecdotes have intrigued popular audiences, such as the readers of *People Weekly*, but they have done little to capture the interest of mainstream researchers. Dr. John Mack, for example, has eschewed psychological testing of his abductees as too expensive—although the Human Potential Foundation, a UFO watchdog group, has funded his work with almost $200,000. Therefore, the information we have is limited and largely speculative. Still, we do know from the personal accounts of alien "experiencers" (as abductees prefer to call themselves) that, as with FMS, suggestion—particularly while under hypnosis—sometimes plays a key role in their retrieving detailed memories.

New York artist Budd Hopkins, a hypnotist and the author of the books *Missing Time* and *Intruders*, has said that most of the abductees he knows remembered their encounters only after being hypnotized. Hopkins does not question the validity of hypnosis in eliciting memories nor does he speak to the suggestibility of his clientele. Instead, he simply summarizes their experiences, pointing out, for instance, that some abductees have felt as though they had been "marked" or "tagged" and were now being tracked by aliens as though they were an endangered animal species. This observation is of particular interest in that it suggests that some of these abductees are dealing with issues of paranoia, which requires serious treatment, not pseudoscience. The overzealous approach of abduction therapists, like that of some in the recovery movement, tends to perpetuate problems by requiring the troubled person continually to pry out greater detail about his or her terrifying experiences. Such an approach can contribute to the person's anxiety, reinforce his or her belief in a false memory, and delay or prevent accurate diagnosis and treatment.

▌ False Memory Syndrome and the Multiple Personality Disorder Debate

The diagnostic label of multiple personality disorder (MPD) has become a central issue in the false memory debate. As we discussed more fully in Chapter 3 of this book, skeptics have questioned how it is that such a previously uncommon phenomenon is now so frequently observed. Prior to 1980, the entire world literature contained about 200 MPD cases, but by 1986 there were 6,000 diagnosed cases in North America alone. Not lost on the skeptics of recovered memories is the fact that this unlikely epidemic of MPD parallels precisely the rapid rise in abuse allegations.

A number of concerned professionals track the exponential increase in the MPD diagnosis to the untrained therapist's leap of logic: if a patient demonstrates symptoms that could be related to sexual abuse, then MPD is a likely diagnosis. And if MPD is a likely diagnosis, the patient's barricaded memories—and the alters responsible for repressing them—must be rooted out. Believing that through this process—and this process alone—the patient can be healed, the therapist feels a moral obligation to assist the patient in every way possible to recover the memories of his or her abuse.

A reverse problem exists when the therapist incorrectly assumes that MPD is proof positive of sexual abuse. Within this scenario, a patient already diagnosed with MPD is led by the therapist to uncover memories of abuse and to discredit memories that don't fit.

The risk stemming from such faulty beliefs is that people in need will grow increasingly disillusioned and cynical about therapy and the knee-jerk diagnoses of abuse and MPD. In this atmosphere, the public might retreat to an earlier state in which abuse claims were trivialized and widespread denial took precedence over the needs of victims.

▌ False Memory Syndrome Backlash

From Office to Courtroom

There was a time when what happened in the intimate atmosphere of therapy remained strictly between patient and therapist. The therapist's office represented a safe harbor where secret thoughts and feelings could flow freely, protected from the harsh judgment of the world outside. The therapist was generally the only one privy to the patient's most menacing fears, lurid fantasies, and wretched emotions. The trust forged by this deeply private connection has historically ensured that problems worked out within the four walls of a therapist's office would remain there forever.

Enter the recovery movement. As litigation involving charges of sexual abuse has grown, expectations have changed. In court proceedings and even congressional hearings, the most intimate moments of therapy have been dragged into public view. Is confidentiality being violated? Technically not, because such disclosures occur only with the consent of the patient; indeed, it is the patient who, upon advice from a trusted therapist, is the one responsible for going public. But at the same time, the patient's judgment has been tainted by a perverted logic that holds that total healing requires the patient to open his or her wounds before the world—to publicly disown any happy memory of his or her childhood, to charge his or her abuser, to face the abuser in court, and to disavow his or her family forever.

While recovery movement therapists have been marching their wounded soldiers into battle in increasing numbers, another force has been quietly gathering. Wrongly accused parents are no longer willing to stand by and watch their children being snatched away. Alarmed professionals are also beginning to take aim at what they call the "junk science" of recovery therapists. In March 1992, a concerned group of parents and professionals gathered in Philadelphia to discuss the problem, and thus the False Memory Syndrome Foundation came into being.

The FMS Foundation is a nonprofit organization that seeks reasons for the spread of FMS and works for its prevention. It also aids victims of FMS, attempts to reconcile families when appropriate, and promotes and sponsors competent research, the results of which are shared with mental health professionals. Acknowledging that the sexual abuse of children has historically been underreported, the foundation evaluates each case on its own merits through monitoring boards. The foundation, which has among its members many concerned educators, psychiatrists, and medical researchers, is one of the few bodies collecting ongoing data that may ultimately help us to better understand and respond to the FMS phenomenon.[3] Correlates to the foundation have been established in Canada, England, Australia, The Netherlands, and elsewhere.

---

[3] The address for the FMS Foundation is 3401 Market Street, Suite 130, Philadelphia, PA 19104-3315. The URL is http://iquest.com/~fitz/fmsf.

Largely because of the foundation's work, sued parents have become emboldened to use the legal system to fight back. In a case alluded to earlier, patient Holly Ramona charged her father with sexual abuse after, with the aid of Amytal, she reconstructed memories of abuse. Outraged by the charges, Gary Ramona sued his daughter's therapists and the medical center where she received the Amytal treatments. Ultimately, Mr. Ramona was awarded a half million dollars in damages. But this verdict could not resuscitate the failed marriage, alienation from his other daughters, and loss of a $400,000-a-year job that had befallen him in the wake of the original allegations.

More recently, a Texas psychiatrist was convicted of slander for telling his patient's daughters that, based in part on information elicited during an Amytal interview, he believed their grandfather had sexually molested their mother as a child while their grandmother looked on. The grandparents, horrified by this unfounded accusation, took their case before a jury, which agreed that their "great mental anguish" and "loss of reputations" were deserving of hefty compensation. The grandparents were awarded $350,000 despite the jury's determination that the psychiatrist had not acted with malicious intent.

As of this writing, the FMS Foundation is tracking more than 800 civil and criminal lawsuits against alleged perpetrators resulting from recovered memories, but more suits against clinicians are being filed as well. Of 300 families in which patients had later retracted their accusations, 60% to 70% informed the foundation that they were or would be taking legal action against the therapists. Two such cases against the same Minnesota psychiatrist have already resulted in verdicts totaling almost $5.2 million, and out-of-court settlements were reached with four other former patients.

Thus, the Ramona case has been a harbinger. The accused are recognizing that they can mobilize the impressive force of the law behind them. Stirred by the false memory controversy, at least two states—Illinois and New Hampshire—have reexamined their laws in regard to therapeutic practices and informed consent. In Illinois, an FMS information booth was set up at a public exhibition, and families in both states have been writing to legislators and the state consumer fraud division.

Nonlegislative forums have been equally active in helping to create public awareness about false memories. In Seattle, a group of mothers and sisters formed the Women's Brigade to raise the consciousness of the public about FMS. They have asked a powerful question: "Why is it that this generation of . . . [therapists] assume[s] that there are hundreds of women—grandmothers, mothers, and sisters—who are too weak, lazy, or stupid to have noticed that their daughters or sisters were subjected to horrific sexual abuse for years in their own homes?"

If the recovery movement is experiencing a backlash from families, it is also feeling the sting of the damage it has done to the very population it was designed to serve. Patients who have leveled and then retracted accusations are struggling to rebuild their lives out of the rubble of therapy. The intensity of the emotional fallout is illustrated in the following letter from a daughter:

> My mother died in January 1992, and I never had a chance to tell her how sorry I was for the accusations. I now have to make my apologies at her grave. . . . This past year has been very painful to me as I've really begun to acknowledge what I lost as a result of therapy. I went from being a very productive woman who was raising three children and was serving on a school committee to a dependent, depressed, regressed, and suicidal woman.

■ Informing the Debate

The issues surrounding false memories are inherently sensitive. Whereas medical science tackles questions about the evidence for repression, the need for corroboration of memories, and the reliability of "memory-enhancing" methods, the patients are left to negotiate an emotional minefield. Similarly, falsely accused parents, child care workers, teachers, and ministers must deal with the reality of the loss of children, jobs, reputation, financial security, and emotional well-being—in essence, their former lives as they knew them.

For authentic victims of child abuse, any discussion of FMS ignites feelings of outrage and concern for the next generation of abused children. With so many patients and therapists jumping on the incest bandwagon—and with all the attendant media hype, ludicrous claims, infamous court cases, and circuslike atmosphere—will we become saturated with the subject and shut our eyes to even valid allegations of abuse? Will we bury the important issue of how to protect and support the truly abused?

In FMS, as in all areas, education is the key to understanding and proper perspective. In the past five years, there have been a number of responsible books published for popular audiences on the subject of recovered memories. The American Psychiatric Association (APA) has also published an official position paper. It states in part,

> It is not known how to distinguish, with complete accuracy, memories based on true events from those derived from other sources. . . . Psychiatrists should maintain an empathic, nonjudgmental, neutral stance toward reported

memories of sexual abuse. As in the treatment of all patients, care must be taken to avoid prejudging the cause of the patient's difficulties or the veracity of the patient's reports.

Despite such cautionary statements, however, professional organizations such as the APA, the American Psychological Association, and the American Medical Association have not offered clear, specific guidelines on how clinicians should proceed when questions about recovered memories arise. As rigorous experiments enter the arena, however, such guidelines may be forthcoming. Early work has shown, for example, that physical arousal signs such as increases in skin conductance, heart rate, and blood pressure may be useful in differentiating true from false memories. Positron emission tomography scanning, which measures changes in cerebral activity, is also showing promise; Harvard psychologist Daniel Schacter and colleagues have demonstrated that true and false memories seem to activate slightly different areas of the brain.

At the same time, individual experts have come forward to offer advice to patients that will help them determine the validity of a memory. In the hard work of therapy, there are no easy answers; both patient and therapist must apply intelligence as well as intuition, reason as well as emotion. For patients involved in memory work, we endorse the following caveats and considerations:

1. True memories should arise spontaneously and not be coaxed out. Patients should be wary of therapists who take an authoritarian approach and who persist in attempting to retrieve memories that the patient claims not to have.
2. Professionals disagree about the importance of corroborating memories. But when a patient desires corroboration to still his or her doubts, the request should evoke a serious discussion. A good therapist will not brush off a patient's concerns about the validity of a memory by claiming that doubts prove that the patient is in denial.
3. Hypnosis, drug-assisted interviews, dream interpretation, and many other techniques can be wellsprings of unreliable memories.
4. Patients should be aware that some states do not require licensure for counselors, hypnotherapists, and other classes of clinicians. When licensing laws are absent, patients should attempt to gain a referral from a trusted professional. Additionally, patients should not hesitate to ask a clinician what credentials he or she has.
5. Therapists who instruct their patients to take harmful actions against others should be considered suspect. Examples of such actions are bringing suit

against a family member or publicly accusing an individual of abuse. A good therapist will assist patients in weighing the pros and cons of any potentially damaging action and encourage patients to decide for themselves.

6. Patients should be leery of therapists who urge them to make dramatic changes in their interpersonal relationships, such as leaving a spouse or cutting off contact with a family member, based upon recovered memories.

Beyond this listing, and perhaps most importantly, all of us need to resist the urge to find simple solutions to the captivating mysteries of human behavior. We need to recognize, as media commentator Tom Shales has put it, that "those who cannot remember the past are inclined to invent it. . . . Truly, the human mind is a wondrously mysterious thing. So is the human imagination."

DELUSIONS

Miss Annie's Bucket and Other Unrealities

> "But he hasn't got anything on," a little
> child said.
>
> —Hans Christian Andersen (1805–1875),
> "The Emperor's New Clothes"

DESPITE THE DRAFTY FEEL of his "new clothes," Andersen's naked emperor maintained that the fabric was divine and that anyone worthy could see that His Majesty looked grand indeed. The story leaves us smiling and secretly satisfied. Who among us doesn't know at least one arrogant person who needs a reality check now and then? In fact, we often complain that such people (usually our bosses) possess "delusions of grandeur."

Most of us have experienced false, yet firmly maintained beliefs at one time or another. It sometimes happens when we want something so deeply, so desperately, that our minds leap from a belief in its *possibility* to a belief in its *reality*. An illustration of such thinking is the following story of adolescent devotion. It came to a bitter end when the ardent heart discovered that the actions of the beloved had been grossly misinterpreted—a faulty belief fostered by nothing more than personal desire. One of Jackie's friends wrote about it this way:

He was a senior, after all, and I was just 14. I had adored him from a distance
since I was 12. He approached me at a party, put his strong arm around me,
and asked me if I'd like to dance. Might as well have asked me if I wanted to get
married. It was much the same, in my mind. As we moved slowly and dreamily
across the dance floor, I was aware of his profound presence—the cool scent of
his cologne, his starched collar against my cheek—and every whispered word
spoke directly to my heart. "Will you be going to the football game on Friday?"
he asked. This was the invitation I had always dreamed of. "Oh yes!" I said, in
eager acceptance. The next day I proceeded to tell all my friends that I had
been personally invited by *the* Evan Daniels to be his date for the homecoming
game. What a grievous blow when I discovered that what I had come to believe
had been nothing more than my own airy wishes. Though I had been Evan's
dance partner for a few minutes, it was a senior girl who received the much
longed for invitation; his question to me had amounted to nothing more than
small talk. I was left to nurse my wounded ego.

Such unfounded convictions are not uncommon, and they might more correctly be
called "mistaken beliefs." Usually the misguided thinker will succumb to reason
when the evidence is convincing enough.

In contrast, delusions that are truly "psychotic" are immutable beliefs that
nonetheless are completely contradicted by every shred of physical evidence. With
psychotic delusions, the false belief overwhelms all other considerations. What seems
to be obvious contradictory evidence to anyone else can be easily molded to or explained away by the patient's personal view of what is "real." Delusions are the most
common psychotic symptoms psychiatrists encounter.

Although delusions can present in many forms, the war between a person's conviction and all the evidence at hand is perhaps best captured by the so-called
somatic delusions. Somatic delusions also epitomize the dramatic interplay between
the mind and the body, a phenomenon that we see repeated in all the chapters of this
book.

Miss Annie (as told by Jackie)

The very first patient I ever encountered who had a somatic delusion was Miss
Annie. I met her early in my medical school training, when I was only beginning to juggle the options about which type of residency to enter after gradua-
tion. Miss Annie's dilemma, and her dramatically successful treatment,
helped crystallize my initial thoughts that no medical field would hold more
fascination and gratification than psychiatry.

The emergency room had called the psychiatric consultation service in the middle of the night. The ER doctor was extremely irritated because the patient was carrying a hefty wooden bucket she would not surrender. He refused to try to perform a physical exam when he might suddenly be bonked with a bucket, and, indeed, she had become ferociously agitated whenever anyone asked her to put it down. Eager to impress on one of my first clinical tours of duty and intrigued by this unusual story, I quickly dressed and ran down the back stairs. I expected to hear a loud commotion and anticipated a cadre of security officers ready to wrestle the bucket free of the patient's grip.

Instead, I saw Miss Annie, a scrawny but feisty 78-year-old woman, clinging to her bucket. As I introduced myself, I could see that Miss Annie still was tentative, but she relaxed as she came to realize that I wasn't going to snatch away her treasure. I was less preoccupied with her bucket than her appearance: her hair was dirty and matted, her clothes were in disarray. Her two sisters buzzed about, apologizing for the way she looked, claiming she had "been on the go-down for several weeks." I settled back and asked Miss Annie to tell me why she might need this bucket, especially considering it was raising such a ruckus.

"Well, about four months ago I slipped and fell and hit the back of my head," she replied. "Broke all sorts of bones, got all sorts of chips and pieces there."

By this time, her nephew had sauntered in. It was apparent that he'd heard this before. Behind her back he circled his index finger near his temple and rolled his eyes to indicate that she was "crazy."

"These bones," she continued, "they been workin' their way down. First they settled here in my throat. I couldn't swallow or nothin', but the doctor said there wasn't nothin' wrong with my throat. Then the bones, they slipped again into my chest. Oh, darlin', I thought the Lord was coming to get me for sure. The bones was interfering with my heart. I pert' near died with them then."

Her sister interrupted. "I'm sorry, doctor, we know there's nothing wrong with her heart."

"Lorraine, hush! Of course, there's nothing wrong with my heart," Miss Annie said. "The bones passed on to my stomach. They's eatin' it alive, and it hurts so bad I cain't stand it."

"But Miss Annie, why do you have the bucket?" I asked, still baffled.

"So when I pass these bones, I can catch 'em and show 'em to everyone. Won't nobody say I'm crazy then 'cuz I ain't."

With that, Miss Annie huffed and turned away, rocking a bit with the bucket and talking to herself now and then. It seemed she could derive comfort only from the container that would "catch" the bones that had been causing all her problems. Her loved ones had been at best quizzical, at worst taunting and unkind.

Her sisters filled in a bit of the picture.

"You see," Agnes said, "Annie has always lived such a full life. Not much schooling, but married, and raised some beautiful children. Worked cleaning houses. Harry ['That's her husband,' said the other sister] died last year and her children have moved away. Really only us oldsters here, except for that sorry nephew of hers."

Agnes continued. "Annie has always kept herself neat and clean, upright, righteous, churchgoing. But about two, no maybe three months ago she changed. Got sadlike, and kept to herself. Every ache and pain meant she had something. Then this fall . . . It wasn't serious, but she's gotten so focused on it, all she talks about are her moving bones. She got so many aches and pains, she cain't eat or sleep, her energy has got up and went." Agnes shook her head in disbelief. Her sister started to cry.

As I confirmed after discussing this dilemma with the psychiatric resident, Miss Annie was indeed experiencing a classic somatic delusion. Furthermore, it was a delusion probably fueled by depression, a depression that had hit her subtly and insidiously, finally swallowing her up. She didn't notice her changed mood nearly as much as her increased bodily discomforts; she searched for a reason for these new pains and became convinced that her moving bones were causing all her troubles. Even reassurance from many doctors and exhaustive testing could not convince her otherwise. She was a woman with no tolerance for self-pity, and we guessed that unconsciously Miss Annie couldn't tolerate being "depressed"; in her mind, it was probably equated with being "weak." Being "sick"—having a "real" illness—was a more acceptable way to retreat from life. And something really was "rattling around" inside her: her jumbled and forbidden thoughts and feelings.

The tenacity of her delusion was amazing. We admitted her to the hospital only by suggesting we might be able to piece her bones back together—which, figuratively, we did plan to do. We began to treat her depression. I tried, as an earnest but naive medical student, to show her the error of her ways by holding up the X rays of her head and chest and viscera, pointing out that they were all normal.

It was to no avail. She patted my hand. "Never mind, chile, Miss Annie knows. Those bones float. It's hard for the rays to pick 'em up, but they's there."

After three weeks of therapeutic doses of medication, her depression was no better; in fact, it, and her somatic delusion, had worsened. Her "pain" became so awful that she refused to eat.

"Ooooh, I cain't," she cried when I tried to cajole her with some broth. "It just pushes the bones down."

I attempted to argue with her, using the delusion. "But maybe it will push them on out," I said.

"No, they's stuck. I wish the Lord would take me away."

She huddled in her bed. No amount of arguing or convincing was going to change her mind, and she was wasting away.

The depression, and the delusion it had spawned, were now life-threatening. The treatment team finally recommended electroconvulsive therapy, or ECT, the "shock therapy" that usually succeeds—often remarkably—where other treatments for depression have failed. But Miss Annie's family felt that this idea was far too extreme. They realized she was, as one niece put it, "looking like death eating grits," but to "shock" her? Never!

I couldn't decide who was more frustrating, Miss Annie or her family. We couldn't just let her starve to death based on the misconceptions people have about ECT. To break the impasse, the social worker and I held a family conference (they didn't want to talk with "them highfalutin doctors"). They began with a prayer; then we spoke for an hour about the reality of ECT as it is currently practiced. The two sisters, whose signatures we sought on the consent form, remained unconvinced until their "sorry nephew" told a story.

"Aunties, we need to let the doctors help Aunt Annie with the electricity. The other day I was feeling down, you know how I get, and I put my fingers into a wall socket and got a big shock! I felt so much better after that! Think what a jolt could do for Miss Annie."

The two women put their graying heads together. They *had* noticed an improvement in the boy. Maybe it would be okay?

"Well, all right, you can do it." The weird wall outlet story had succeeded where a scholarly medical review did nothing. Now to convince Miss Annie.

It was easier to persuade her than I had imagined. Although we were administering intravenous fluids and using a thin tube to deliver food directly into her stomach, she was still so weak that all the fight had gone out of her.

"Oh, hon, I don't care, whatever you can do to help with the bones, just do it."

With fingers crossed, we proceeded with a course of ECT. By now, we were all very attached to Miss Annie. To get her to eat, the dietary staff was buying her special foods her family suggested and trying out different recipes. Anything to entice her to take in a few calories.

To our colossal relief, the ECT succeeded. Miss Annie began to perk up, and her color returned, as did her appetite. She began to push at her stomach; she told me she was trying to find the bones. With a mixture of perplexity and satisfaction, she said, "I musta passed 'em and not knowed it. They's gone." Her sadness gradually lifted and her thinking cleared. She regained

John Dewey Library
Johnson State College
Johnson, Vermont 05656

some weight. After her course of ECT was completed, Miss Annie was started on maintenance medication to help prevent a recurrence of her psychotic depression. She declined our offer of follow-up psychotherapy—too explicitly "psychiatric," I guessed—but did state her own hypothesis about her depression, one that rang true: "That fall some months back . . . I been healthy as a horse all my life, and then one day I become an ole woman who cain't take a flight of steps and no husband to help. Never thought of myself as an ol' lady before but that's who I am." She paused, then gave me a wink and chuckled. "Unless I decide different!"

Miss Annie hugged me before she left—a big, wonderful bear hug—and told me she had something for me, that it was in her room and not to get it until she had gone. After many good-byes, she left with her elated family.

I noticed immediately how quiet the ward was without her. Once she had improved, she was vivacious and into everyone's business. I walked into her room to get my gift, and there was a box with a bow on it. I opened it up. It was her bucket. For better or worse, now it was mine.

I still keep it to remind me of Miss Annie . . . and her illness. That bucket had been a metaphor for Miss Annie's feeling that the very essence of her life was flowing out of her. Now it's my reminder of how feelings and thoughts can be so powerful that they propel patients to behave in such idiosyncratic, yet strangely understandable ways.

In cases such as Miss Annie's, in which the somatic delusions arise from deep depression, treatment is often extremely effective because depression itself is such a treatable illness. But the sad fact is that in many other cases of somatic delusions, the treatment options are more limited and less successful. When the brain has been harmed in some way, for example, the delusions may be as lasting as the effects of the damage itself. Marc remembers just such a situation; it involves a woman whom he met only once:

Kathryn (as told by Marc)

I was asked to evaluate Kathryn to see if she still qualified for state funding based upon a mental disability. Such requests were hardly unusual. New to private practice, I found that these Social Security disability reviews were a way to meet people and learn more about the community into which I had just moved.

Kathryn walked into my examination room with obvious strain. She was remarkably obese, so much so that it was difficult for her to walk. As I helped her to the couch, I thought it likely that she would have physical problems—such as diabetes or hypertension—caused by such ponderous weight, and I hoped Social Security had arranged a medical evaluation as well. The records showed that she was 45 but she looked 20 years older—a hard life, no doubt.

Only weeks earlier, I had spent five hours at furniture stores on a mission to find the perfect office sofa: the one among hundreds that would instantly help my patients feel at ease. The one I had selected, of deep burgundy leather, was overstuffed, even squishy, a feature my patients seemed to love. But this very quality made it unsuitable for Kathryn. As she sat, she gradually tipped back into the softness more and more; her chest and abdomen began to settle onto her rib cage and, before I knew it, Kathryn was struggling to breathe. My own breathing grew more rapid as she flailed her arms. Using an end table for leverage, I pulled her out of this unexpected quicksand. She and I then spent several minutes trying different chairs and arranging pillows until the examination could proceed.

This momentary problem seemed in a strange way to have broken the ice, and Kathryn was ready to talk right away. She told me that she knew she was on disability but had no idea why: "There's no reason. I'm not disabled. My daughter set it up and made me come today. She put me in the state hospital too, but I'm fine. Is that how a daughter should treat her mother? Is that what you get?"

I was intrigued whenever I met patients who didn't want the monthly checks from the state. It had been my experience that such people usually were very deserving but that they resisted any kind of dependence on others; their strong work ethic was in total opposition to an official determination of disability. I pressed Kathryn a bit to try to understand more.

"So you feel you're ready to go back to work? There's nothing really stopping you?"

"Nothing but this weight problem. And there isn't a thing I can do about that."

I was surprised that even though Kathryn acknowledged her profound obesity, she simultaneously spoke of it as if it had been forced upon her. I asked her about diabetes, which she denied, and about her typical meals: did she favor the deep-fat frying for which the South is both famous and infamous?

"Has nothing to do with it. It's that other woman."

I was baffled. "What other woman?" I asked.

Pandora's box had been opened. Kathryn seemed relieved that I had finally tapped into the area that troubled her most, and she shared her story eagerly. She explained that another woman, a nameless person, was living inside her. This living, breathing woman had moved in years ago and wouldn't leave. She was jealous of Kathryn—Kathryn didn't know why—and took up residence to embarrass her. How else could she have wound up so fat? How do you think you'd look carrying around another person?

"Every time I try to lose weight, she pooches out her stomach and it makes my own stomach stick out," Kathryn said. "I'll look just the same no matter how much weight I lose. No point in trying. And she tricks me into eating the wrong foods anyway, so the nutritionist couldn't help."

I had treated patients with other types of somatic delusions. Some patients with severe depression expressed extreme negativism toward themselves, an abandonment of even a fragment of self-esteem. When they would talk at all, they described themselves as despicable and hopeless, not worthy of the treatment team's attention and sometimes not even of food and water. Such patients commonly reported delusions that they were physically "rotten" as well. They saw themselves as grotesque or withering, and they would hide in their rooms to avoid offending others. They would claim that suicide was the only possible option. But Kathryn seemed satisfied with herself and her life except in this discrete area. She had a twinkle in her eye, a ready smile, and an undeniable charm. An isolated somatic delusion? Why?

Kathryn's daughter, Anna, had driven her to the appointment and helped her to my door, and Kathryn allowed me to meet alone with her. Anna reported that her mother had had six psychiatric hospitalizations over the past 15 years, often through commitment by the courts. She had been a responsible single parent and diligent factory worker until her drinking got the best of her, and then she became suspicious and withdrawn. She had burned down half the house and saw nothing wrong with it. That's when the hospitalizations began, but Kathryn continued to drink immediately after each discharge. Following a circuitous course through five different hospitals, Kathryn was finally sober but unable to live on her own or care adequately for herself. Now living at Anna's home, she was little trouble, but she ruminated as she had for years about the unnamed presence inside her.

An antipsychotic medication called haloperidol had helped a bit. When she remained on it for at least a few days, Kathryn would remark that the other woman inside her had "died," but then she would add that she now had to go through life with a "corpse" inside her "still making me fat." Anna no longer had the heart to fight this battle over medication, and it had been months since Kathryn took her last pill.

Kathryn now spent most days watching TV and helping out a bit with the housework. The doctors had told Anna that her mother's drinking had caused an "organic delusional syndrome"—that the alcohol had damaged her brain in ways that made her believe this story of "the other woman"—and that there was little else to be done.

I felt frustrated, but I knew that the doctors had been right. Such conditions are notoriously refractory to treatment, and, when I brought Kathryn back into my office, I realized that the disability payments were all too necessary. On the other hand, there were a few bright beacons in her case: she was now sober, she had broken the disruptive cycle of hospitalization and rehospitalization, and she had a home and the love and support of her daughter.

And clearly flashes of her old self had survived. As I escorted her to the door, Kathryn suddenly turned to me with enormous urgency.

"Did you do it? Don't tell me you did it."

"I'm sorry? Do what?" I was aghast. It seemed that another delusion—this time incorporating me—was about to emerge.

"You know, " she said. "Make Anna sit on that awful couch." She smirked. "Looks like I pulled your leg pretty good, huh, doc?" She started to laugh. "If I can hook you that easy, I'm smart enough that I don't need to be on disability, now, do I?"

▌ The Pregnancy That Never Was

One of the most dramatic of the somatic delusions is *pseudocyesis*, a person's faulty conviction that he or she is pregnant. Variations on this theme that fall short of actual delusions are fairly common; they can even be considered a sign of empathy. Consider this letter sent in to a popular medical columnist:

> My husband acted like he was pregnant. Are men physically affected by their wives' pregnancies? This sounds crazy, but when I was pregnant, it seemed every time I felt nauseous or dizzy, my husband did too. Then when my morning sickness cleared up, so did his. Finally in the last months of my pregnancy, my husband actually started gaining weight and getting a paunchy stomach. What in the world was going on?

First for Women, August 22, 1994

It is likely that this "Mr. Mom" did not suffer from a delusion that he was pregnant. If asked, he would instead be likely to answer that, even at the time his belly was ballooning, he knew perfectly well that he wasn't pregnant. He might say that his body had assumed a "mind of its own" and that his concern for his pregnant wife had affected him in a profoundly emotional and ultimately even physical way. No harm done. Indeed, some wives might be gratified by this somatic display of spousal empathy, also called *couvade syndrome*, which has been reported among expectant fathers all over the world.

In certain cultures, couvade syndrome may find the father fully "experiencing" the pregnancy and even going through all the motions of childbirth and postpartum exhaustion. In its most dramatic form, the mother, following her delivery, returns to work while the father remains at home to bond with the child and rest from his birthing experience. However delusional this practice may seem, it is culture based and therefore not a true delusion. In other words, the participants have no confusion about which gender is physically birthing the child. People within these cultures would tell us that this ancient tribal tradition ensures a tight family unit with the father's full involvement in raising and nurturing his child to maturity.

Throughout the world, healthy young women may also develop symptoms of pregnancy without being delusional. In some instances, arising from a mixture of fears and wishes, a woman's menstrual period stops, she experiences "morning sickness," and her abdomen and breasts enlarge. And then these changes and sensations pass. This phenomenon is observed in the popular Mexican film *Like Water for Chocolate* when the young heroine Tita, whose true love Pedro has married her sister, initially believes that she is pregnant. In reality, it is her sister who is carrying the longed for child. As her sister's pregnancy progresses, Tita finally fully understands the reality, but her body refuses to accept this fact. Mingling elements of mysticism with her profound love and longing, she begins to develop an extraordinary ability to produce milk for her sister's newborn child.

Contrast our "Mr. Mom" and these healthy young women with those who have actual pseudocyesis. Despite all the evidence to the contrary, such people have an entrenched belief that they are pregnant when they clearly are not. For example, one woman's false pregnancy lasted *almost 10 years*. This patient's pseudocyesis was part of a larger psychotic disorder, and, fortunately, she improved after she began to take an antipsychotic medication called pimozide.

In other cases, patients keep the central delusion of pregnancy aloft by affixing the frail support wires of other mistaken beliefs. A 39-year-old woman, for instance, contended that she had become pregnant when her dancing partner kissed her at age 19 and that the same kiss had been repeatedly impregnating her ever since. How did she explain her never having delivered any children? The pregnancies were "supernatural," she believed, and her father had somehow "withdrawn them."

A type of "contagion" was responsible in part for one *man's* pseudocyesis. Already prone to psychotic thinking and to the power of suggestion, he was admitted to a ward on which several patients happened to be pregnant. He dutifully began to order double meals, drink all the milk he could find, gain weight, and wear oversized clothing. Patting his abdomen, he would say, "I shouldn't be smoking these cigarettes. They're bad for the baby." He quizzed the baffled but affable staff about how labor might be for him and spoke of looking forward to having a baby of his own. His delusion did clear with medication, and his bout with pseudocyesis became an opportunity for insight. In therapy, he recognized that his delusion fulfilled a wish for him, that of being a nurturing and understanding parent. He was able to realize that he could make this wish come true by being a much better father to his two real daughters from whom he had been estranged.

This case is not so unusual as it might seem. Remarkably, pseudocyesis has been reported more commonly among men than women. And yet, these gender differences may be less pronounced than they appear at first glance. For obvious reasons, a man claiming to be pregnant is far more likely to be noticed than his female counterpart. Pseudocyesis in women, therefore, may be just as common, but underrecognized. When a woman's claim of pregnancy fails to materialize, we are likely to conclude that her pregnancy test gave a false result or that she miscarried.

Just as a Y chromosome confers no protection against pseudocyesis, the delusion certainly knows no age limit. At one extreme, a 60-year-old man insisted that he was pregnant; at the other, a 6-year-old girl did the same. Not only can there be the conviction of multiple pregnancies, but some patients report deliveries that never really occurred. Sometimes clinicians will know that afflicted patients are finally recovering when they announce, occasionally with a surprising nonchalance, that for some reason the pregnancy has come to end.

Conceiving of the Causes

Many researchers believe that life stressors and underlying personality characteristics serve as the templates shaping pseudocyesis. Certain psychological and sociological factors—such as sexual abuse in childhood, social isolation, medical naiveté, the loss of a child, and membership in a religious or cultural group that emphasizes childbearing (such as Catholicism)—have played central roles in individual cases. In patients who have had truly deprived childhoods, the delusion of pregnancy may represent the unfulfilled longing to carry, to bear, even to be someone's much-loved baby, a role sadly denied them in the past.

Clinicians must be ever mindful of all the forces bearing upon a particular patient before drawing a firm conclusion. Consider, for example, the case of a teenage girl who, by all appearances, seemed to be demonstrating a classic case of pseudocyesis. Her periods had stopped not because she was pregnant, but because she had developed an ovarian cyst, an outpouching of fluid that occurs commonly and is usually readily corrected surgically. Why did she refuse to accept this straightforward physiologic explanation and insist, definitive negative tests notwithstanding, that she was pregnant?

A deeper analysis of the girl's condition revealed the immense anxiety she felt over her diagnosis and her impending surgery. To this young person, an ovarian cyst represented a highly traumatic, even devastating condition. It was more reassuring to imagine that she was pregnant: in claiming pregnancy, she was simultaneously restoring herself to reproductive wholeness and overcoming her fears. A compassionate approach ultimately helped her to accept her condition and understand that, with surgery, her health would be completely restored.

Although culture, religion, and emotional defenses do play a role in pseudocyesis, we must always be aware that, as in delusions as a whole, underlying brain abnormalities, hormonal and chemical imbalances, and overarching mental disorders such as schizophrenia or severe depression may be at the root as well. This same constellation of factors has in rare cases led to the reverse problem: psychotic denial—sometimes even through delivery—of a pregnancy that really does exist.

▌ Delusions and Mistaken Identity

As almost any parent of a teenager will tell you, somewhere around the age of 14 his or her child became a stranger. "From angel to anarchist," bemoaned one mother. "He had always been a sweet child—affable and kind," said another, "but on his 13th birthday, someone else moved in and took up residence in his body. Surely this could not be our Gerald!"

These statements reflect parental consternation over the child's sudden transition into (as one father aptly put it) a "*mean*ager." When Gerald's mother stated that her son's body was inhabited by someone else, she obviously meant it metaphorically. But people suffering from the delusions called *misidentification syndromes* believe that such transformations are literal—that undesirable tenants move into bodies as easily as though they were vacant apartments.

Delusions surrounding identity generally take one of two forms. In delusions of *self*-identity, extremely disturbed patients believe they are someone else, no longer recognize themselves, or become inordinately fearful of the "strangers" who are taking over their bodies. When the delusion involving identity applies to *another*, the patient comes to believe that a familiar or beloved person has been dispossessed and that an impostor, usually malevolent, now inhabits the body of the once-familiar person. A number of writers, including Edgar Alan Poe (in *William Wilson*) and Dostoyevsky (in *The Possessed*), have featured this phenomenon in their works, making riveting fiction out of a desperately real psychiatric disorder.

Delusions of identity richly reflect the patient's fears, conflicts, and deepest longings. Like a road map, the character of the delusion will often guide psychiatrists past all the bright lights onto the byways and back roads of the patient's mental processes. Although treating the delusion is always the first and highest priority, understanding the symbols and signs allows the physician to speak in the patient's own language, to convey a depth of compassion and understanding, and thus to help greatly in the healing process.

Ultimate Makeovers

The most common of these syndromes, and one of the most distinctive in all of psychiatry, is *Capgras's syndrome*, named for the doctor who first reported this phenomenon. The patient with Capgras's syndrome insists that a spouse or other relative has been replaced by a double who may look just about the same—save perhaps for a minute difference in the nose, the skin, the way the hair is combed—but who nonetheless is a charlatan with a wholly different personality.

In 1923, Dr. Capgras described a 53-year-old woman who believed that her husband and children had been replaced by identical doubles as part of a plot to steal her property. As we shall see, misidentification syndromes and paranoid thinking often occur together. Although the nature of this connection is not entirely understood, it is likely that when the paranoid beliefs are primary, the patient may feel compelled to create a scenario that does not implicate the people he or she loves. Thus, in the case of Dr. Capgras's patient, contemptible doubles became responsible for the plot against her, and her family was thereby vindicated.

The permutations of the misidentification syndromes are as varied as the human imagination. Patients show astonishing creativity in painting colorful scenes to support their delusions. For example, a 52-year-old woman claimed that her husband's "twin brother" (who had never existed) would take his place from time to time. The substitution first occurred on their wedding day, she said, when her husband went to the men's room and the twin returned in his place. She was appalled by his intermittent reappearances and especially by his sexual advances, which she firmly rejected. Understandably, her husband was bewildered and frustrated when his wife told her doctors that all she really needed was a hospitalization so that she could get some rest. At the core of this delusion may have been the woman's fear of sex. What better protection than to transform her husband into a perfect stranger, someone with whom sex would be improper and immoral—she was, after all, a married woman!

As with this patient, delusions involving identity can reveal a great deal about the person's inner conflicts. If the psychosis can be medically treated, these revelations can form the basis for continuing psychotherapy. For example, issues of power and control were central to the delusion of 48-year-old Donald. Donald emphatically insisted that the woman who claimed to be his mother was a despicable substitute bent on his ruin. He argued that this woman looked and acted nothing at all like his real mother who, he erroneously claimed, had died decades earlier. Growing increasingly agitated, Donald maintained that this "faker" was out to control his life, that he could no longer abide her interference, and that he planned to kill her. With this threat, Donald was immediately hospitalized.

Donald's long history of utter deference to his mother had led to a growing self-abasement that helped to precipitate his delusion. Understanding this history helped the staff in devising his treatment plan. Donald was first treated with mood-stabilizing and antipsychotic medications. Psychotherapy then provided him with the support, advice, and even tangible assistance that he needed to help resolve his feelings of powerlessness. As Donald's case demonstrates, psychotherapy can indeed be beneficial to many people—but when psychosis is this severe, powerful medications are among the most important selections we can make from our treatment armamentarium and will almost always compose the first line of attack.

Clinicians will occasionally discover patients whose delusions make up a veritable combination platter. Given the variety of their symptoms, it may seem that these patients will require spectacularly complex treatment approaches. However, the successful treatment of one delusion will often take care of virtually all of them. In a case combining somatic delusions such as Miss Annie's with the Capgras's syndrome, a lovely adolescent girl claimed that her entire body was covered with coarse, ugly hair—"a terrible deformity," she said. Simultaneously, she was sure that her mother and siblings were impostors. She referred to them openly as her "fake mother," "fake brothers," and "fake sisters." Fortunately, as in some of the cases mentioned earlier, antipsychotic medication treatment led to a resolution of both the somatic and misidentification delusions.

In the examples we've cited, the delusions revolved around the mistaken identities of other people. In some severely psychotic individuals, delusions manifest as the disintegration of one's own personality. Patients suffering from the delusion of *reverse intermetamorphosis*, for example, believe that they have assumed entirely new identities. Although in some cases these identities extend to nonhuman forms, such as a robot, grasshopper, or snake, most often these deluded patients adopt alternate human forms. Sometimes they believe themselves to be famous historical figures.

Harold (as told by Jackie)

Recently, I was asked to see a middle-aged man named Harold. I had never met him before, but the nurses, some of whom have worked in our clinic for many years, knew him well and fondly described him to me. They knew that Harold was chronically psychotic and that he had a persistent delusion in which he claimed to be Moses.

One of the seasoned nurses pulled me aside. "But he's a little different from before," she said. "I've never seen his conversation so loose; I can barely follow what he's saying. I asked him about being Moses and this time the story just poured out of him. He's usually more focused and coherent."

I pulled up a chair and asked Harold to talk with me. He was dressed in old, dirty clothes, and I could see that he obviously hadn't bathed in a long time. Hygiene often abruptly deteriorates as a patient's psychosis worsens, and this finding alone supported Sarah's apprehensions. Nonetheless, I found Harold to be thoroughly pleasant and engaging once he realized that I wasn't going to harm him or, in his words, throw him in the hospital.

"I hope you can tell I am Moses," he volunteered. He pointed to the urban skyline out my window. "In 1991, I destructed this city, and my body died, and I left it in the gutter." He picked up a pencil and placed it on my desk. "I left my body there, in the gutter, laying straight like this pencil, and plucked out my old eyes. These are new eyes, and a new body, a resurrected body I have now."

Harold's reference to plucking out his eyes alarmed me. He had picked up the sharp pencil, a potential weapon, once again. As we'll describe later, some patients with acute schizophrenia or other psychoses impulsively mutilate themselves, and I didn't like the fact that Harold was "armed," even if it was just a pencil.

He went on. "The woman I live with, she says she's my mother, but she's not. I made her over when I destructed the city. So she stays with me."

The specificity of his delusion seemed matched only by its intractability. He wasn't God or Jesus Christ. He was Moses, and this city had arisen at his behest, from the ruins of the city he had "destructed."

When he put the pencil down again and looked away, I swiftly snatched it. No need to tempt fate.

Although I knew that it would be futile to argue with the delusion, I thought I could get a read on its tenacity if I challenged it a bit. "But Harold, I've lived in this city for years. I don't recall it ever getting destructed," I said, taking care to use his own choice of words.

He looked at me askance. "Well, then maybe you ain't been destructed and resurrected. Or maybe you've come to challenge the way of Moses, which is the way of the Lord. And the way of the Lord is the way of the world. Peace and destruction. Love and hate. Good and bad. And Mrs. Doctor Feldman, I can't understand why you can't see my point!"

Harold was getting more agitated, his thoughts careening and derailing as he went on. He knew who *he* was. As he saw it, *I* was the one with the problem. His stance was immutable. The nurse had mentioned that Harold wouldn't budge even when faced with a punishment that many chronic psychiatric patients would view as extraordinarily harsh: his mother had threatened to stop his cigarette money unless he stopped talking about "this Moses nonsense." For reasons psychiatrists don't fully understand, a tremendous number of seriously mentally ill patients are nicotine addicted. When behavioral changes are needed, the threat of ending a patient's cigarette supply typically gets results, at least temporarily. But not even this threat had been potent enough to bring Harold's constant chattering about Moses under control.

At this point, Harold was being treated with a "depot neuroleptic," an injection that releases antipsychotic medication gradually into the body. Administered in this form, patients require the shots only one or two times per month, and they are better able to lead lives unconstrained by continual pill taking and office visits. I checked his chart; Harold was about due for his shot. Maybe that's why we were seeing such a decompensation: the effects of his last dose were wearing off. It made sense either to increase the dose or the frequency of his shots, and I recommended the former. Although the Moses delusion was absolutely impenetrable, perhaps a higher dose would restore a more logical flow to his thinking.

Harold wasn't happy about my recommendation: "Mrs. Doctor Feldman, why you doing this? You think I'm worse off? You trying to deconstruct my body again?" His voice was getting louder and he had risen halfway out of his chair. Before he could explode, I lowered my voice and leaned in close to him.

"Harold, I think being Moses is a hard life, and it's working on your last nerve. Admit it, it's hard, hard work."

He sat back down and smiled. An ally! "It is! I work and work, no one works harder, and don't nobody appreciate it."

"Well, I appreciate hard work. And I'm a nerve doctor. Let me increase your medicine a notch to help your nerves, that's all."

This logic appealed to him. He rolled up his sleeve and said, "Okay, doc, give it your best shot!" He paused and then burst out laughing at his own pun.

There is always the risk that using a patient's delusion to win his or her cooperation will endorse the distorted thinking; after all, a doctor has now apparently adopted the same beliefs. In Harold's case, however, the pressing need to reach him meant conversing in the only language he was prepared to understand. Rather than bolstering his delusion, the medication change, combined with more frequent clinic visits, averted an otherwise inevitable hospitalization.

In some cases, such as Harold's, the treating physician may never learn just what spawned the unique delusion, and, indeed, understanding the cause is sometimes the physician's last concern. When a patient is in an acutely psychotic state, controlling the symptoms is the preeminent goal of treatment. Only then can more comprehensive therapies be applied to enhance the effects of the medical intervention.

Kelly's story that follows illustrates the phenomenon of *reverse subjective doubles*, in which patients believe they are becoming someone else or are in the process of being replaced. In Kelly's case, the triggering event was clearly known, and it became an important part of her treatment program.

Kelly (as told by Marc)

Kelly, a neighbor and personal friend of mine, was a devoted mother who loved both her children dearly. Still, she couldn't conceal her preference for 17-year-old Steven, on whom the sun rose and set. He was, at the same time, her greatest heartache. He continually flirted with danger, experimented with drugs, and got into minor scrapes with the police. Kelly lived in a state of constant anxiety over Steven's self-destructive behaviors. In her misguided effort to set him on the right track, she wound up being wildly oversolicitous: whatever Steven wanted, Kelly gave. But nothing Kelly did for him could alter the course of Steven's reckless life. When I learned one night through a frantic phone call that Steven had taken his life in a drunken game of Russian roulette, I knew this terrible tragedy would be Kelly's undoing.

But oddly, following Steven's death Kelly appeared transcendent—not as though she had lost a child, but ironically as though she had just given birth. At the funeral, her face was radiant, her manner calm and poised. All of the mourners, including Steven's many friends, passed through Kelly's arms, where she bestowed reassuring hugs and maternal words of comfort. "Don't blame yourself," she told them. "You couldn't have known. Please be happy, for Steven's sake." The teenagers found her attitude amazing: "Incredible. Absolutely awesome," they marveled. At the same time, I was feeling immense concern that her sunny facade was blocking any fragment of the normal—and necessary—grieving process.

My concern turned to alarm when Kelly appeared at my front door two weeks after the funeral. She did not look herself. Indeed, she was not herself at all, although I did not yet know how accurate this thought really was. Dressed in one of Steven's T-shirts and carrying his baseball cap in her hand, she asked if she could come in and chat for a while.

Kelly's grief was still barely evident—she was betrayed only by some tender reminiscing, a brief trickle of tears, and haunted eyes behind a too-bright smile. When I spoke Steven's name, a grateful look came over her face, followed by a changed affect.

At the sound of her son's name, Kelly paused thoughtfully, tucked up her long dark hair, and placed Steven's cap on her head backwards: the way he used to wear it. A smile spread unevenly across her face—as if looking for the right place to settle—until it formed one of Steven's characteristic crooked grins. In this eerie transformation, there was no doubt about what was happening, and yet I was totally unprepared for the voice that issued forth—unmistakably Steven's. She had captured his intonation and pitch, even his characteristic choice of words.

Too close a friend to serve as her psychiatrist as well, I referred Kelly to a colleague who saw her that very day. He hospitalized her the next morning, having determined that Kelly had suffered a psychotic break characterized by delusions involving her identity. A hypothesis we shared was that Kelly had dealt with her son's death in the only way she could possibly bear. Maintaining her commitment to giving Steven all that he desired, she gave him her body to inhabit after his death. At the same time, this strategy enabled Kelly to protect herself from the unendurable pain of Steven's death by keeping him alive within her.

In the hospital, Kelly was medically treated for her delusions and received therapeutic help in processing her enormous grief, which she could finally start to release. After her discharge, I talked delicately with her about her experience.

"I really believed," she told me, "that I could call him back. I would look in the mirror at myself and I'd literally see Steven." Her face softened and her eyes filled with tears. "At those moments, I could actually feel his spirit passing through mine, *becoming* mine."

She paused, looking deeply into my face for some sign of understanding. "I wish it could have been that easy," she said, tears now flowing freely. "Oh, how I wish it were that easy."

I put my arms around her while her grief poured out openly and without restraint in an unmistakable sign of healing.

Understanding the cause of Kelly's delusion was invaluable in assisting her to find an appropriate and healthy expression of grief. Medication and continuing therapy also helped her to resume her life, however changed. But such an understanding does not necessarily ensure a successful and satisfying outcome. In another case of reverse subjective doubles, 27-year-old Donna believed that part of her body had been overtaken by a new, hostile persona. She was hospitalized after threatening her neighbors. When she appeared on the ward, Donna was carrying a telephone through which, she said, she made telephone calls from one side of her body to the other. She believed that the left side of her body had become an angel who had arrived to "heal" her. The right side of her body was the "immoral" side that acted aggressively toward others. She hoped that the supernatural being controlling the left side of her body would eventually also control her right side, so that her aggressive behavior would end.

Donna's records showed that her delusion started two years earlier, shortly after she suffered a head injury in a car accident. The accident, however, had left her with no overt physical damage. Because she had been emotionally well prior to the accident, it was assumed that a brain injury caused the delusion. Unfortunately, despite the best efforts of the treatment team, the delusion failed to abate: Donna continued to struggle between her "good" and "evil" sides.

In many ways, Donna wrestled in a concrete way with a central dilemma of human existence—the struggle between good and evil, which has eternally challenged philosophical minds and contributed to the world's great religions. It strikes us as both poignant and profound that, even as psychosis undermines our patients' best efforts to get along in the world, their struggles, at the core, are little different from our own. It is only their expression of those struggles that sets them apart and weighs so heavily upon them.

▋ Delusions and Distrust

A colleague of ours told Marc the story of a young female patient who had been referred to him for psychiatric evaluation. In recent weeks, her bizarre evening ritual had escalated from annoying to nasty, and it was beginning to make her neighbors edgy. Before setting foot inside her apartment, the young woman would turn toward those passing in the hallway and, in a strange variant on the hex sign, thrust her middle finger toward them while delivering obscene epithets. Perplexed by these unprovoked assaults, the psychiatrist directly questioned her about this unneighborly practice: "But why would you *do* such a thing?" he asked her. "Because," she hissed, "they are always talking about me behind my back."

No doubt!

Paranoid thinking, as we have seen, is a common feature of delusions. In many cases, the patient's delusion incorporates the belief that he or she is being directly harmed—or, at the very least, observed with malice by others. These thoughts, ironically enough, can lead to the very circumstances the patient imagines, thereby reinforcing the delusion. The woman above, who assaults her neighbors with obscenities, has undoubtedly perceived correctly that they often talk about her.

Physicians who treat elderly patients note that paranoia is also commonly observed in persons with hearing loss. As some individuals can no longer easily discern what is being said, they begin to feel isolated from group discussions. At some point, this sense of isolation translates to alienation as they perceive themselves to be the subject of conversations that sound to them like whispers. They start to believe that they are the butt of jokes they can no longer hear. This suspicion then creates a self-fulfilling prophecy as confused friends and family members discuss among themselves how to cope with the person's new and upsetting attitudes toward them.

When Belief Becomes Behavior

James (as told by Marc)

It's disturbing enough when paranoid patients believe things that are patently untrue and can't be dissuaded. But it's even more worrisome when they act on their delusional ideas.

One of my patients, a dockworker who was a productive employee and excellent husband and father, had for over a year harbored the belief that his neighbor was repeatedly putting sugar into his gas tank. This was, he maintained, the only explanation for the repeated failures of his car. He refused to "give in" by buying a new car: "He'll just do the same thing to the new one anyway," he said.

His wife was understandably frustrated by his insistence that an innocent neighbor was to blame ("His '78 Chevy is going bad. 'Deal with it,' I say."). Still, he had never accused the neighbor to his face. Realizing that no amount of discussion would convince him otherwise and suspecting that medications could be avoided in this case, I had proposed to James that he simply keep his concerns to himself and not trouble the family or the neighbor with it. If he felt the need, he could call me and we could meet and review the matter again.

This passive approach worked well for a year. Then I received a call from his wife.

"James isn't just 'talking' anymore. Now he's 'doing,' " she said.

"What do you mean?" I asked.

"The Chevy went bad again and he won't just give it up. He's gone and put sugar in the neighbor's car. And he poured Clorox on the man's flowers. He keeps talking about not taking it anymore, 'doing something worse,' he says, 'an eye for an eye.' "

James's delusion, which for so long had been confined, had burst the dam and was now spilling over into his behavior. This new and ominous development meant that the family and I needed to intervene much more actively.

Fortunately, James still trusted his wife and his doctor. He accepted the advice to enter the hospital. During his time there, his wife junked the old car and got a newer one. After his discharge, James would wonder aloud about every momentary squeak and rattle, but his claims of malice by another never resurfaced to the point of his destructively acting out his concerns.

I could not identify any single biological, psychological, or social factor that pushed James over the edge into mental illness. As in so many other cases, it seemed that multiple factors conspired. For example, although he generally felt satisfied with his job, it was nevertheless very stressful, and a change in bosses—to one much younger and harsher than the last—played a role. In addition, we discovered that James's father, whom he had thought had abandoned the family, had actually died after years of institutionalization for schizophrenia; thus, genetic factors could be implicated as well.

▎ Erotomania: The Sinister Side of Celebrity

In 1976, rocker Bruce Springsteen jumped the fence at Graceland in an effort to meet his idol, Elvis Presley. Instead, he met Elvis's security patrol and was summarily escorted out.

That was that. But at times a fan's admiration can deteriorate into obsession and even delusion. Through newspaper and television accounts, we've all become aware that, sadly, in some cases such delusions can lead to overt violence, including murder. John Hinkley, Jr., shot President Reagan because he believed it would impress Jodie Foster. The promising young actress Rebecca Schaeffer was shot and killed by an obsessive fan, Robert John Bardo, in 1989.

Movie stars, sports heroes, and other celebrities know that sometimes a fan's admiration becomes twisted into a complete preoccupation. Stephen King depicts such warped devotion in the story and movie *Misery*, in which a disturbed fan rescues her idol, a famous author, then takes him to her remote cottage and resorts to terrifying methods to prevent his escape. Obsessed fans are typically people who have always had trouble establishing normal friendships and who may divert the need for relationships into a single-minded devotion to a celebrity. Such people may compile an exhaustive accounting of the star's comings and goings and even proceed to stalking. British gymnast Lisa Grayson moved to the United States largely to escape such a stalker; over the span of six years, the misguided suitor sent her nearly 6,000 letters and over 500 songs he had written himself. And it took the threat of an arrest warrant for otherwise-imperious Madonna to face in court the stalker who twice invaded her Hollywood Hills home.

When this type of preoccupation advances to overt delusion, clinicians diagnose *erotomania,* or *de Clerambault syndrome* for the doctor who first reported it. Although we generally think of paranoia as encompassing delusions of *persecution,* erotomania is a type of paranoia that encompasses delusions of *grandeur.* Fans with erotomania are not just fascinated with a particular public person: they become convinced that they share a special love relationship, a love that—although unspoken and possibly even forbidden—is nonetheless passionate. One such person, who calls herself "Billie Jean Jackson" (taken from the hit song "Billie Jean") has appeared on national television to implore the performer Michael Jackson to admit publicly that they are secretly married. David Letterman has spoken of his fright of a mentally ill fan who has repeatedly broken into his home, claiming that she is his wife and that she belongs there.

In erotomania, the desired person represents all the fantasies for power and success that the delusional person has never been able to realize in his or her own life. Over time, erotomania can deteriorate into a consuming rage as the passion is unrequited, a setting in which violent impulses emerge. As Bardo wrote in a letter to his sister before murdering Schaeffer, "I have an obsession with the unobtainable. I have to eliminate [what] I cannot attain." Recognizing the possibilities of stalking and erotomania, a number of celebrities now check into hotels under assumed names, surround themselves with bodyguards, charter air flights rather than travel publicly, and share absolutely nothing of their private lives.

Although we have focused on famous people, delusions of obsessive love have resulted in the harassment and stalking of men and women from all walks of life. It is the famous personalities, however, who have called public attention to stalking and erotomania and who have created the impetus for legislation to protect against potential acts of violence. Following the murder of Rebecca Schaeffer, California became the first state to pass an antistalking bill, and almost all the other states have followed with similar legislation.

We know from the work of noted researchers such as Dr. E. Fuller Torrey that, although uncommon, violence by psychiatric patients is more likely to arise when they are not receiving the treatment they need. Patients who comply with treatment and whose families and friends encourage attendance at therapy sessions, proper use of medications, and abstinence from drugs and alcohol are generally much less likely to engage in any kind of violence. We also know that a history of violence is the single best predictor of violence.

▌ Religion's Beleaguered Believers

If you have a religious affiliation and were asked to identify its place in your life, you might say, "My religion helps me to be a better person" or "My faith brings me great comfort." Some people might answer that religion alone is the factor that carried them through a particular life crisis or that for them an act of faith produces an immense feeling of joy. Many delusional patients, however, experience their religion as an oppressive burden, a legacy of emotional torment, the earthly bequest of a punitive and unforgiving God. For them, the "hound of heaven" of Francis Thompson's 19th-century poem pursues not with love but with lips curled and teeth bared. Some of the most tragic cases that we have encountered have been those involving religious delusions: patients who have misinterpreted biblical injunctions and carried them to extremes or who have tried through ultimate acts of self-abasement to render themselves acceptable to God.

Berryl (as told by Marc)

When I was a junior resident in psychiatry, I admitted a middle-aged woman with a history of bipolar disorder, or "manic-depression." Berryl and her family had noticed that her medications were not stabilizing her well enough. She was having trouble sleeping, always seemed in a rush, had started applying excessively thick and colorful makeup, and had often appeared deeply preoccupied. We all viewed the hospitalization as a way to intervene before her symptoms progressed any further.

But we couldn't move fast enough. Within hours of admission, after Berryl had been given a tour of the unit and was supposed to be unpacking, I noticed a small puddle outside her door. I figured that a patient had spilled a glass of water and I alerted the housekeeping staff.

A minute or two later, several patients began to call out.

"Something's wrong! Look at this!"

The puddle had turned into a stream and was rapidly enlarging into a river. Beyond the closed door we could hear the sounds of splashing water and a woman cursing. As Amy, a seasoned nurse, and I threw open the door, we had no idea what we would find.

"Get out! In the name of Jesus, Mary, and Joseph, in the name of Christ himself, get out!" Berryl yelled.

Berryl was standing in the middle of the shower as the water, and all her heavy rouge and mascara, came pouring down. Although I could tell that she was clothed, I could actually see only a part of her body because she had stacked most of the contents of her room in the shower as well. The linens, the end table, the Janet Fish print from the wall: everything was soaked. And like an ant trying to carry a gigantic crumb, Berryl had her arms around the mattress, seemingly trying to hold it steady and scrub it down at the same time.

"I beseech thee!" she screamed, mumbling religious invectives and four-letter words. It was as though the Bible and *Tropic of Capricorn* had been superimposed.

In a remarkably short period, Berryl had gone from mildly delusional to overtly psychotic, and there was no time to try to "talk her down." Joining with the staff that had amassed, Amy and I pulled Berryl from the shower. Transformed by her psychosis, she growled like a cornered animal and began to claw at the nurses and aides, making frenzied efforts to bite anyone, everyone. Someone grabbed her head to keep it steady and to protect it as she flailed. Everything else on the unit had stopped: *how could any treatment proceed during the equivalent of an air raid?*

Now held aloft by five of us, Berryl was carefully carried to the seclusion room, a bright but bare room with reinforced walls and a Plexiglas window. Once there, I ordered an emergency injection of a potent antipsychotic medication to help calm her and to allow her to regain some semblance of control over her own behavior.

The medication appeared to work almost immediately. Within moments Berryl was quieter, and one of the staff members relaxed his hold on her arm. Seizing the moment, Berryl suddenly came alive, reaching up and ripping the gold crucifix from her neck. As she began again to yell out epithets and scripture, she managed to shove the necklace into her mouth and gulp it down. Twenty or 30 seconds later, she was finally asleep.

Several weeks later, when she had responded well to further treatment, Berryl told me that she fully remembered and was mortified by her outburst. She also apologized to the staff and the other patients, although we all understood that she had been the victim of her own delusions.

"I just got scared that I wasn't saved," she explained. "That I needed to be baptized, that *everything* needed to be baptized. It was like I feared for my life. I just knew I had to wash, wash, wash. And then I got to thinking that if I swallowed that crucifix, I'd have Jesus inside me and I'd be saved and no one could take that away from me."

In reality, we did have to take the crucifix away from her. Our initial fears that the crucifix might become lodged in her breathing passages subsided when we could verify with a stethoscope that her respirations were normal. But we also worried about the size of the crucifix—no one was quite sure about that—and whether it might lodge somewhere in her gastrointestinal system.

An X ray had proved that our fears were founded. There, amidst the landmarks of her heart, lungs, and ribs, was the startling white outline of a crucifix, firmly lodged in the middle of her esophagus. It was going nowhere, and we knew it could cause bleeding, infection, or ulceration if it stayed. While Berryl had still been groggy from the injection, we asked the GI service to insert an endoscope, or lighted tube, into her esophagus, and they pulled it out.

I have always been impressed at my patients' innate strength. They often display a surprising ability to laugh at themselves even after recovery from a situation that has been demoralizing and painful. As a discharge gift, Berryl's sister had had the extricated crucifix encased in Lucite: "It's partly a 'Get Well' present," she had said, "but mostly it's to be sure it won't fit in your mouth anymore." I have to admit that I didn't find her sister's notion of a keepsake very amusing, but Berryl seemed to enjoy the ribbing, and that was all that really mattered.

Keith, Amos, Merritt, and Jonathan (as told by Marc)

Over a period of years at hospitals in the South, two colleagues and I came across four patients, each of whom made the same statement: that their current anguish was the result of their having committed the "unforgivable sin." Three of the patients were Southern fundamentalist Christians for whom the Bible represented the literal word of God. The last was a Northerner whose Christian experience did not include fundamentalism. Was their shared statement a delusion in each case or not?

Trying to understand these patients, we had asked each to explain just how he had committed the worst sin imaginable. The responses were enlightening: each man reported a different behavior as having been the unforgivable sin.

The first, Keith, revealed that his sin had consisted of a secret four-year intimate relationship with a younger stepsister. The second, Amos, responded that his unforgivable sin was the "adultery in my mind" that he had committed 32 years earlier when he watched a pornographic film. The third, Merritt, feared that he had unintentionally blasphemed God and spent hours each day occupied with bathing and cleaning rituals "so it doesn't happen again." The fourth, Jonathan, had heard a sermon in which the term *unforgivable sin* had been mentioned, and he worried that by his merely contemplating what this awful sin could be, he might inadvertently have committed it.

What we learned from these patients was that our initial question— "Which of these patients is delusional when he says, 'Doctor, I've committed the unforgivable sin'?"—was the wrong question to ask. The possible delusionality of each of these common statements became academic when we saw the agony each patient was experiencing. Each man was distraught and anxious, each utterly disabled, each isolated from family and friends. Three could scarcely eat and two had suicidal feelings. They were all undeniably mentally ill, and we soon recognized that a much more important question was "How can we help relieve their dreadful pain?" Treatment did in fact reduce or abolish the ruminations of guilt in each case without undermining the patients' general religious beliefs. In fact, all four men felt freer to participate in religious practices than they had in years.

Later, Jonathan was able to share an amusing anecdote. Once, when he had called his pastor yet again after midnight to ask, "Do you think I've committed the unforgivable sin?" the exhausted clergyman replied that yes, by calling him at such an hour the man had just done it. The humor had absolutely escaped Jonathan at the time, but now he thought it was pretty funny.

The guilty feelings of these four men resulted in delusions that were dramatic by any standard. But some patients, in an effort to follow the letter of God's law as they interpret it, carry their behaviors to even greater extremes. Engaging in the ancient religious practice of self-flagellation, for example, these patients inflict harm on their bodies in an attempt to set things right with God.

They may even cite the Bible as the very reason for their self-aggression. In the King James Version, Matthew 5:29 does state in the words of Jesus himself, "And if thy right eye offend thee, pluck it out, and cast it from thee, for it is profitable for thee that one of thy members should perish, and not that thy whole body should be cast into hell." And Matthew 5:28 asserts that "everyone who has looked at a woman lustfully has already committed adultery with her in his heart." Some psychotic patients, concretely interpreting these biblical injunctions, decide to remove or destroy one or both of their eyes (an act called *self-enucleation*, or *oedipism*, after the story of Oedipus Rex). But they almost always grieve the irretrievable loss once their delusions have abated.

Religious overtones have also been noted among psychotic patients who mutilate or amputate their genitals. For example, one patient who was admitted to the hospital following self-amputation of the penis explained that he was trying to atone for a sexual transgression by getting rid of the "guilty" part of his body. Other cases of genital mutilation have resulted from the patient's inability to draw conceptual and abstract meaning from biblical exhortations. Thus, to the literal-minded psychotic patient, a verse in Matthew 19:12 suggests self-castration as a means of gaining God's favor: "For there are some eunuchs which were made eunuchs of men, and there be eunuchs which have made themselves eunuchs for the kingdom of heaven's sake." In sacrificing their own body parts, these patients seek spiritual emancipation; instead, they suffer debilitating and devastating loss through egregious punishment at their own hands.

The following case study illustrates the complexity of disturbed thought processes in which elements of religion merge into an emotional whirlwind of anger, control, and revenge. The result was one of irreparable self-harm.

Johnny (as told by Marc)

An 18-year-old high school senior named Johnny was brought to our emergency room after a particularly gruesome attack on his own body: he had deliberately shot himself in the right eye with a BB gun. Despite the best efforts of the ophthalmologists, the eye couldn't be salvaged. Once the acute medical crisis had passed, he was referred to psychiatry by a treatment team still struggling to understand how anyone could harm himself in this way.

Johnny was surprisingly eager for psychiatric treatment when he arrived on our ward. A handsome young man who was now permanently disfigured, he felt terrified that he had actually shot himself. He recounted his reasoning at the time. He had had a bitter argument with his mother and had sought a way to get even with her. He had become convinced that shooting himself in the eye would not only upset his mother, a given, but "through strange spiritual forces" would also guarantee his ultimate entry into heaven. It was to be his way of "capturing the divine," he remembered.

As we continued to assess him, Johnny was seldom as cooperative and clear as he was on that day of transfer. By seizing the moments when he could be engaged, talking with his family, and reviewing the outside records, we learned that Johnny had started receiving psychotherapy for depression when he was 13. However, he had often skipped his appointments, and the sessions were finally stopped. His family said that he had never harmed himself in the past and that there was no warning before his self-directed attack; Johnny and his mother had indeed had an argument, but after it he had seemed sullen rather than agitated or violent.

Such arguments were commonplace now that Johnny's grades had dropped precipitously. Teachers reported him to be increasingly distracted, his attendance at class had become sporadic, and he had twice been suspended for truancy during the six weeks before his hospitalization.

There was never any evidence to suggest that Johnny had been abusing drugs, a natural concern in the setting of such dysfunctional and unpredictable behavior. My working diagnosis became schizoaffective disorder—a diagnosis used when a patient's depression and psychosis are so intertwined that neither seems primary. Although I continued to try to engage him in psychotherapy, he often was suspicious and reluctant to talk about himself at all. The staff also observed him to be talking to himself, whether walking around the gym or lying down in his room, although he would always deny it when asked. He did consent to antidepressant and antipsychotic medications as part of his treatment regimen in order to target the two elements of his psychiatric ailment.

Over the next few days, although Johnny no longer had overt delusions, the suddenness of his assault on himself still worried everyone involved. He and his family agreed with the need for continued treatment, although we all sought a less restrictive environment than continued inpatient care. As a result, we discharged him to a residential program in which monitoring, medication adjustments, and therapy could continue in a setting more like home.

▌ Delusions and Culture

As we have seen vividly, then, delusions can spring from commonly held religious beliefs gone awry. But how do we distinguish where a normal belief ends and a delusion begins? When is a belief odd or extreme enough to constitute a delusion?

To answer this question, we must evaluate the patient in the context of his or her culture or subculture. Ethnic, religious, and other sociocultural factors influence our belief systems. Taken out of this context, unusual beliefs that are nevertheless standard within a particular culture may appear delusional to the naive observer.

For example, among some African Americans in the South, *rootwork* is a culturally appropriate belief. Those who believe in rootwork ascribe illness and even "voodoo death" to witchcraft, sorcery, or the evil influence of another person. They may consult "root doctors," or traditional healers, to remedy the "hexes" that have been put on them. This same belief is common in Caribbean societies, and it is known as *mal puesto* or *brujeria* in Latin American countries.

Similarly, in the trance state known as *spells*, individuals "communicate" with deceased relatives or spirits. Also found mostly among Southern African Americans, spells may be associated with interludes during which the individual's personality appears to change. In folk tradition, spells are by no means medical or psychiatric abnormalities, however. A related phenomenon, *zar*, occurs in many parts of the Middle East and North Africa. The term refers to possession by a "spirit." Persons dominated by such a spirit may suddenly shout, laugh, sing, or weep; yet, zar too is not considered delusional in the societies in which it occurs.

On the other hand, some syndromes largely confined to particular cultures are acknowledged as delusional even within the cultures themselves. The best known example is *koro*. Koro, also called *suk-yeong* or *suo-yang*, refers to sudden, intense anxiety that the penis (or, in females, the vulva and nipples) will recede and vanish into the body. The panic often results from the belief that a ghost (who has no genitals of its own) is stealing them from the individual and that he or she will die as a result. Although it has occasionally been described among Westerners, koro is much more commonly found among inhabitants of South China and among Chinese residents of Singapore and Malaysia.

Thriving in communities in which anxiety is high, koro has at times occurred in epidemics, spreading through "social contagion" to involve as many as 2,000 individuals (see the later chapter on mass hysteria). Desperate men with koro may attempt to prevent retraction of the penis by tying strings or applying clamps to it. Unlike rootwork, spells, and zar, koro is viewed as delusional, and it is even included as a formal psychiatric diagnosis in the classification system for mental illnesses used by the Chinese.

A recent study comparing the frequency of delusions in two very different cultures, those of Germany and Japan, confirms the interaction between culture and beliefs. Delusions of guilt or sin are more common in Germany, a largely Christian society that emphasizes individual expression and personal responsibility. In contrast, delusions of reference—thoughts of being harassed or slandered by others, or uncomfortable feelings of "being known"—are more common in Japan, a society that promotes conformity and a group orientation.

Our own American society has quite properly been viewed as a land of sociocultural and religious diversity. That diversity affords a rich learning opportunity for the psychiatrist, but it also presents a conundrum. In caring for our patients, we must simultaneously adopt a broad view that allows us to determine whether their odd beliefs exemplify delusions or are instead appropriate to their unique subcultures. It is not our place to wrench loose their grasp on traditional beliefs or faith but to supplement it with a strong human connection.

▌ Delusions or Legitimate Fears?

In addition to paying attention to the sociocultural context in which unusual beliefs have arisen, clinicians need to try to learn the particular facts of the patient's life.

Statements from patients that sound outlandish, implausible, and entirely consistent with a psychotic disorder such as schizophrenia usually are delusional. But sometimes we're astounded to find that the patient has been speaking the truth all along; that, for example, the delusions of persecution we've diagnosed actually reflect startling truths.

Some patients claim that they are victims of government conspiracies. They assert that they had access to top-secret information during their military service, adding that now they are being hounded by the government "since what I know would be explosive if I ever revealed it. But if I look 'crazy,' no one will believe what I say. This way, the government doesn't have to worry that I'll be able to 'blow the lid off.' They've got me where they want me: on a psychiatric ward." When the staff's efforts to obtain confirmation of the patient's military or government service lead to dead ends, the patient may insist, "Of course they claim I've never served. Of course they've destroyed the records. It's because of what I know. They want me to lose all credibility. And it looks like you're being led like sheep, just as they had planned."

In cases such as these, discussions with relatives and a diligent search for records can often clarify the truth. At other times, we never do find out for sure whether the patient is delusional. Faced with this dilemma, we try to fulfill the principle within the Hippocratic oath that states, "First, do no harm." We offer the patient treatment for the symptoms of anxiety or depression, the surface problems that have made it difficult for him or her to carry on. But we frequently wonder whether the claims of conspiracies have any real basis.

The dilemma is epitomized by a 1992 Canadian case. "Mr. A," who acknowledged years of treatment in the United States for schizophrenia, said that, after making an idle remark about presidential assassination, he had been arrested for threatening the president and served a sentence in federal prison. After release, he had come to Canada to escape Secret Service "persecution." The doctors hospitalized him briefly, treating him with antipsychotic medication. Shortly after his discharge, however, he reappeared at the hospital. He claimed now that Secret Service agents had located him and were following him and had even snapped a picture of him from behind a parked car. In his distraught state, he had considered drowning himself. He was diagnosed with paranoid schizophrenia and readmitted right away.

Soon after Mr. A's admission, the hospital received a call from a Canadian immigration official. He identified Mr. A by name and asked whether he was receiving psychiatric care. The official indicated that U.S. government agents were interested in Mr. A's whereabouts and needed to keep track of him at all times. Faced with this confirmation of at least part of the patient's story, the ward staff changed their approach and they made arrangements for Mr. A to seek political asylum in Canada.

In a similar case of presumed paranoia, Phil Ochs, the singer/songwriter of the 1960s who was both a friend and a rival of Bob Dylan, insisted that he was being followed by the FBI. His assertions were dismissed even by his closest friends as "crazy." Yet some time after Ochs hanged himself at age 35, it was uncovered that the FBI had indeed compiled a file on him. And it was as thick as a phone book.

The obvious moral here is that sometimes people who appear paranoid have a fear of persecutors who are all too real.

▌ Philosophical Dilemmas

The work of psychiatry will always be accomplished with the broad brush strokes of art as well as the formulas of science. Our diagnoses and treatments sometimes arise less from medical certainties than from informed hunches, and our hunches have served the patient well if we see a stabilizing effect. When the cacophony of psychosis fades to more muted tones—when our patients no longer clash with their environment—we consider our immediate work done. We then move to reintegrate them into society. It is a paradox of our profession that even as we genuinely honor and celebrate the uniqueness of each human being, we strive with a single-minded devotion to contain our patients' behavior within the parameters of social norms.

Generally our patients and their families reach out to us for this very reason, and we are reassured that what we do is kind, humanizing, and even life preserving. But occasionally we struggle with a nagging awareness that our patients' cures come at a cost: that, as healers of delusional patients, we are primarily in the business not of building but rather of dismantling our patients' carefully crafted creations of themselves and their world.

In Peter Schaffer's play *Equus*, it is this misgiving that plagues psychiatrist Martin Dysart, finally escalating to a point of personal crisis. Dysart knows that in curing the delusions of young Alan Strang and returning him to a "normal" life, he will be stripping him of the extraordinary passion for which Dysart himself longs. The doctor, whose books on ancient Greece provide him with his only connection to the "primitive," contrasts his intellectual understanding of the word with Alan's total experience of it:

> Such a fantastic surrender to the primitive. And I use that word endlessly: "primitive." "Oh the primitive world," I say. "What instinctual truths were lost with it!" And while I sit there, baiting a poor unimaginative woman with the word, that freaky boy tries to conjure the reality! I sit looking at pages of cen-

taurs trampling the soil of Argos—and outside my window he is trying to *become one*, in a Hampshire field!

The same theme made an appearance in the Hollywood film *Don Juan De-Marco*. Marlon Brando portrays the psychiatrist who is charged with curing his young patient (Johnny Depp). The lad insists that he is the legendary Don Juan, the greatest lover who ever lived, and he will prove it through the stories he tells. In listening to and learning from his patient's captivating stories, the doctor's marriage eventually is revitalized, his passion for living is reinstated, and his views of psychiatry are fundamentally changed.

The vital and thought-provoking questions raised by these fictional accounts are carried even further in the highly regarded autobiography of Kay Redfield Jamison. In *The Unquiet Mind* (1995), Jamison—who is both a professor of psychiatry and a psychiatric patient—challenges her colleagues to consider the positive aspects of bipolar disorder. If properly monitored, she claims, mental illness can confer unique advantages. Jamison writes movingly about the joys she has experienced during her manic phases and attributes to her illness many of the accomplishments of her early life. She concludes that if it were possible for her to choose a life with or without bipolar disorder, she would choose without hesitation to have it.

For a culture that has stigmatized the mentally ill at every turn, Jamison offers new ways of thinking about mental illness. Her provocative comments mirror the dilemma faced by Dr. Dysart, who agonizes over "curing" Alan at so great a cost. Nevertheless, when we, as clinicians, are confronted with a delusional patient who is obviously agitated and anguished, our perplexities evaporate as the clamor of the patient grows ever louder. When Dr. Dysart reveals his tormented heart to Hesther, his friend and colleague, she responds with a simple reminder about his healing role: "The boy's in pain, Martin. That's all I see."

As psychiatrists and therapists, when we see our patients in misery, there is no philosophical debate and no moral dilemma. Relieving our patients' suffering is the first priority.

HALLUCINATIONS

Seeing Is Believing

The mind is a city like London,
Smoky and populous.

—Delmore Schwartz (1913–1966),
"The Mind Is an Ancient and Famous Capital"

SEEING IS BELIEVING." Until recently, that aphorism served us well. But increasingly such conventional wisdom is being put to the test. Technology allows us to manipulate images in photographs and films, creating flawless visual depictions of the impossible. In the movie *Forrest Gump*, Tom Hanks, a masterful actor, appears to be an even more masterful Ping-Pong player, swatting balls back with a consistency and ferocity that would astonish any world champion. Gary Sinise, portraying Lieutenant Dan, was undoubtedly committed to handling his part convincingly. However, the lure of an Oscar would probably not have been enough for him to allow his legs to be amputated, though this very fate befalls his character in the film. The computer-created image of the legless lieutenant is utterly believable.

The book *Metamorphoses: Photography in the Electronic Age* provides another example. The book is a compendium of electronically altered images: turn-of-the-century figures are meshed with modern landscapes to form a seamless collage; a representation of Jesus appears amidst a scene from everyday Mexican life. Thus, we are beginning to realize through advances in a variety of media that we cannot always trust our eyes.

Or our ears. During the golden age of radio, simulated sounds lent realism to the stories of *The Shadow*. When the sound technician crumpled sheets of cellophane in front of the microphone, listeners were certain that a fire was crackling away. Today, a single electronic synthesizer can reproduce a full orchestral arrangement of Beethoven's Fifth Symphony. Violins, trumpets, and piccolos are all encased in the same computerized keyboard from which flow the more novel simulations of popcorn popping, machine guns rat-a-tat-tatting, ghosts wooooing, and pigs grunting—all in the key of your choice.

At times, these marvels of technology strike us as exquisite and moving, at times ghastly and unnerving. But the task of wrestling with the authenticity of visual and auditory images—as well as sensations involving touch, taste, and smell—has eternally challenged people who experience genuine *hallucinations*.

Hallucinations have always been one of the most fascinating aspects of clinical psychiatry. They are formally defined as perceptions that occur in the absence of corresponding external stimuli. Put more simply, one sees, hears, feels, tastes, or smells something that is not really there; in fact, some patients experience hallucinations involving multiple senses. In contrast, *delusions* are thoughts or beliefs—not perceptual experiences at all.

Whereas the public often dismisses hallucinatory phenomena as virtually synonymous with "madness," each of us has experienced a cousin of the hallucination called the *illusion*. In the darkness of our bedrooms, for example, we momentarily mistake the winding edge of the sheets for a slithering snake. Or the wind from an open window rustling against the curtains has us convinced for a few seconds that we have heard an intruder come in. New mothers have often reported that they have responded to the sound of their newborn's crying only to discover, upon reaching the crib, that the baby is—and obviously has been—sound asleep. This last phenomenon is quite commonplace and seems to stem from the mother's natural concern for her baby's welfare and her heightened vigilance to stray sounds in the environment.

Illusions are also commonly experienced following a significant loss, when the bereaved person's longing overwhelms every other thought and desire. The following recollection illustrates this phenomenon:

> When I was six, my constant companion, my dog Rex, was struck and killed by a car. My grandparents lovingly spared me the sight of Rex's mangled

body, so that when I returned from school I discovered only a headstone marked with his name. With no other evidence of his death than a painted rock and a fresh mound of earth, I could not believe that Rex was gone.

Several days later, while walking home from school, I noticed a woman some distance ahead of me walking a dog on a leash. At the sight of them, my heart stopped. I was right all along! Rex had only been lost, and I was filled with joy. I dropped my books and ran toward them, shouting Rex's name. When they turned to see what all the commotion was about, my heart sank. I could see that the dog on the leash looked nothing at all like my Rex.

Like hallucinations, illusions are false perceptions; unlike hallucinations, however, they are based on *real images or sensations* that we have simply misinterpreted. A commonly used term for illusions that acknowledges both the similarities and differences is *pseudohallucinations*.

▌ The Senses in Context

The term *pseudohallucinations* can also refer to nonpathological sensory experiences other than illusions. In some cultures, "visions," "trance" states, or "possession" are regular components of religion and ritual. They may be not only culturally sanctioned but actively induced. Such societies often do not distinguish between reality and imagination as Western cultures do; indeed, hallucinations and altered states of consciousness may be described as fully "real." Among the Mitsogh tribe in Gabon, West Africa, for example, hallucinogenic drugs are ingested to permit members to unravel the "reality" behind everyday appearances. Even frightening or phantasmagoric perceptual experiences may be well within the norms of those cultures.

Western societies have generally remained more skeptical of claims involving purely subjective perceptual experience, and certainly they do not support the use of drugs to achieve heightened experiential states. People who dabbled in hallucinogenic substances during the 1960s, for instance, were viewed as members of the "counterculture." Their subsequent experiences—religious or otherwise—were understood simply to be due to the direct effects on the brain of artificial chemicals.

But, even in the West, religious visions not associated with drug use have been accorded a somewhat different reception at times. Joan of Arc, for example, was both revered and reviled for the great military power she amassed in 15th-century France due to her supernatural experiences, which incorporated both visual and auditory elements. A contemporary clinician, one well versed in the diagnostic criteria for schizophrenia, might have leaned toward a more medical explanation—and remedy—for her hallucinations. Instead, at the age of 19, Joan was branded a heretic and burned alive at the stake. Exemplifying the public's complex and evolving response to her novel sensory perceptions, Joan was canonized 500 years after her death.

Within the Catholic tradition, occasional sightings of the Virgin Mary have produced a rich folklore surrounding the communities in which the purported visions occurred. Lourdes, France, continues to draws thousands of people every year to the spot where young Bernadette, in 1858, claimed to have seen and received messages from the "beautiful lady" in a cave above the riverbank. In 1917, three children of Fatima, Portugal, also saw a beautiful lady dressed in a white gown and veil who appeared to them as they tended their sheep. The children's claims of repeated visions drew the attention of the townspeople, who eventually built a shrine to honor "Our Lady of Fatima."

Whether these phenomena were pseudohallucinations, pathological hallucinations, or genuine visitations may never be agreed upon. Some psychiatrists have noted that Joan of Arc, Bernadette, and the children of Fatima experienced their first religious visions in adolescence, the time during which schizophrenia commonly begins to manifest itself. For true believers, however, such interesting facts are mere coincidences and do nothing to explain these sacred mysteries. The question of authenticity remains a compelling—and unresolved—one.

There is no dispute, however, about the bases of other unusual perceptual experiences. It is neither uncommon nor necessarily worrisome, for example, that some children speak of their "imaginary playmates." These youngsters may excitedly describe the appearance and characteristics of these pretend people or animals. They may even talk to them, seeming to experience Betty or Sammy or Spot even though they can acknowledge (regretfully) that their compatriots do not really exist.

We know too that normal people subjected to prolonged isolation can have pseudohallucinations. The famous 19th-century captain, Joshua Slocum, documented them as he traveled around the world in his tiny boat, the *Spray*. Sleep deprivation, fatigue, monotony, and extreme hunger and thirst can all have the same effect. Mountaineer Ed Webster wrote of the false images before his eyes as he tried to scale Mount Everest—without bottled oxygen:

> Each breath strained my lungs to their capacity. I couldn't seem to force in enough air. As soon as I began to move, I was exhausted—I needed to rest after every second step—yet I had to climb still higher, where the air was even thinner. Time, like willpower, seemed to slip away. My already tenuous grasp of reality was rapidly weakening. . . .
>
> Looking up, I saw flashes of color and the movement of fluttering objects.

> Then I noticed that several people, apparently Buddhist monks, had gath-
> ered. Nothing about this felt unusual or out of place. The rocky ridge above
> me was ornately carved and brightly painted. Colorful prayer flags were
> strung between the outcroppings, and the purple-robed monks paced back
> and forth, chanting. . . . Only later did I realize that the scene had been a hal-
> lucination.

Although Webster managed to dodge them, barely, comas and near-death experiences can affect the brain physiologically to induce other kinds of vivid visual perceptions. Patients rescued from the very brink of death have described a "world of
colors," "a lovely, dazzling light," or "a brilliant radiance." A few have interpreted
these sensations as mystical or divine signs from God. They may be convinced, for
instance, that angels visited them at their almost final moment or that they saw and
heard Jesus. Following a critical illness that had left him in a coma for a month, Nobel prize–winning writer Saul Bellow spoke in more prosaic terms of his own mental
pictures during that time. As he put it, "I was playing hopscotch with death and had
some marvelous hallucinations that I hope to write about sometime."

In contrast to most of these situations, psychiatrists become involved only when
the false perception experienced by an individual is absolutely convincing to him or
her, is not willed or readily controlled, and— perhaps most importantly—interferes
with day-to-day functioning. In such cases, the perception is indeed a hallucination,
a cardinal sign of a biological or emotional problem. These patients have lost insight,
believing and behaving as though the perceptions are not just compelling but real.

▌ Auditory Hallucinations

As we will see, auditory hallucinations can stem from a variety of causes. For that
reason, some detective work is necessary whenever a psychiatrist is asked to evaluate
a person with hallucinations they hear. A thorough assessment will help reveal
whether the hallucinations are caused by a physical problem, such as a brain tumor
or a medication side effect. Most commonly, however, psychiatrists observe auditory
hallucinations in people with schizophrenia.

Occasionally, patients with schizophrenia cherish their hallucinations because
the voices are encouraging or flattering, but much more often they hear statements
that are threatening, insulting, accusatory, or obscene. A single voice may be present
continually, or two or more voices may carry on their own conversation, possibly
commenting on everything the patient does. Even if the voices mutter or drone unintelligibly, patients almost always perceive them as omnipotent or omniscient forces

in their lives. We have found that when our patients with schizophrenia are able to describe the hallucinatory comments in detail, the content is often strikingly disparaging—perhaps mirroring society's condemnation of people, such as the seriously and persistently mentally ill, who are generally of lower socioeconomic status and achievement.

In rare cases, severely psychotic individuals hear voices from animals. This bizarre conviction has been dubbed the *Dolittle phenomenon,* after the doctor who could "talk to the animals." But in the majority of cases, the voices are reported to come from people. They may be anonymous people, or they may be individuals the patients recognize (even though they may not know them personally). Here, for instance, is a segment from an interview with a 30-year-old woman, Peggy, who had been preoccupied with former President Gerald Ford. She recognized that the hallucinated voice was his and felt that he belittled her:

Marc: "How long have you been thinking about President Ford?"
Patient: "Ever since he became president in 1974."
Marc: "We know that sometimes you've had visual hallucinations where you feel like you *see* him. Have you ever *heard* him talk to you?"
Patient: "Oh, yes. He just tells me that he's got more than me, that he can do 'this' and I can't do 'that.' And he said he's going to live a good long life. He said he's going to outlive me."
Marc: "What do you think about that?"
Patient: "He said he might live to be a hundred. And sometimes I see visions of Ford. He's almost 80 years old but he doesn't look it."
Marc: "What about your medicines? Do the medicines help?"
Patient: "Yes, but Ford still talks to my mind."

Curiously, although Peggy felt that the voice taunted her at times, as the interview proceeded she made it clear that her dream would be to play golf with the former president—a simple game of golf "would leave me fulfilled," she said. In the years since that conversation, she has continued to state that President Ford is the man she most admires.

Mr. Charles (as told by Jackie)

At one of his routine visits, a long-term patient of mine, Mr. Charles, seemed to respond only reluctantly when I called his name. He moved slowly from a secluded corner of the waiting room. For a time, I had watched him as he stood there, looking out a window and rocking back and forth. He wore sunglasses though it was raining furiously outside, and he sported a frayed "Durham Bulls" baseball cap.

As he ambled toward me, it was evident that something was very different this time. He took a circuitous route, avoiding the north wall of the waiting room and casting frequent glances out the windows. Then someone coughed and he jumped. A two-month-old infant with her mother started to cry. He picked up the pace, scurrying toward me. He grabbed my hand, shaking it vigorously while half dragging me from the waiting room to my office.

I have always gotten along well with Mr. Charles. We talk about his symptoms, of course, and the medication side effects he sometimes has, but we spend more time talking about his life, how he's doing, how he keeps busy. A 43-year-old college-educated man from the land Southerners call "Up North," Mr. Charles suffered his first psychotic episode when he was 24 and serving in the Navy. Mental illness struck his life with a ruthlessness that cost him his commission, his job, and his marriage. Since then, he had drifted south to live with some cousins. Although he had attempted to work, his symptoms did not always respond well to the medications and other interventions, and he was hospitalized repeatedly at state institutions.

By the time I first met him three years ago, Mr. Charles was on disability (hardly a comfortable stipend) and living in a boarding home. He had made a few acquaintances there, a chum with whom to play cards, or watch sports, or walk to the corner store for cigarettes. The course of his illness had been fairly static since then. Although he was always wary, he had come to trust me, at least a little. But I always found him difficult to read because his face displayed so little emotion. Only when we spoke about basketball did he perk up.

As even a transplanted Midwesterner knows, Alabama is COLLEGE FOOTBALL land. A bouncing round ball carries very little status in the region. But Mr. Charles was a North Carolina basketball fan, and he knew that I had completed my psychiatric residency at Duke. We had delightful conversations about the merits of each team.

And this was March, a month with unique significance to basketball fans: "March Madness" is well named. It is college basketball's three-week ascent into heaven (or descent into hell, depending upon your team allegiances), and it was upon us. I wondered if Mr. Charles's interest was as keen as always, but first someone needed to open up the conversation, and Mr. Charles was unusually quiet.

"Mr. Charles, how ya' doin'?"

No answer. Hunched in a chair that he had moved as far into the corner as possible, he hunkered down, wringing his hands slightly. I knew that occasionally I would have to draw him out, but, again, this was different.

"Can you take off your shades for a minute, Mr. Charles? I'd like to see your eyes when we talk."

He shook his head and pulled his jacket closer to him. That was peculiar too. His appearance. Usually his attire, though casual, was clean. Today his clothes were mismatched, his shirt dirty. He hadn't shaved. And I could swear that I saw a sparkle—could it be aluminum foil?—in his baseball cap.

I leaned in a bit closer and softened my voice.

"Mr. Charles, what's the matter?"

With that, he stood up abruptly, paced briefly, then sat down again and grabbed his head.

"Mr. Charles, what are the voices saying?"

He looked up, surprised. "You can hear them too?" he said hopefully.

"Well, no."

He was disappointed, and a mixture of frustration and fear crossed his face. "Then you can't help me get rid of them," he said.

"Get rid of the voices?"

"No, the transmitters. They're what's causing the voices."

Transmitters? I paused and quickly flipped through his chart. Nope, no mention of transmitters, or even auditory hallucinations since our clinic had started treating him. Instead, his problems had always centered around paranoia, social isolation, and difficulty sustaining relationships.

As if divining what I was thinking, he said, "You won't find anything there. I have never told anyone about these transmitters. They were put in my head when I was in the Navy. The voices, they had gone away, but now they're back. It's that VA, that goddam fucking VA."

I must have looked every bit as taken aback as I really was, because he added, "Oh, sorry about my language." I had never heard Mr. Charles swear before. Four-letter words were absolutely incongruous with the gentle, soft-spoken soul he had always seemed to be.

"Can you tell me what the transmitters are saying?" I asked, tentatively. I needed to know more but, at the same time, he was obviously very upset about their resurgence.

"They tell me that I'm no good, that I'm a faggot. That the CIA and FBI are going to come and use me to help them spy on some of my friends. There are two voices. One is a man, the other's a woman. The woman is mean to me."

He glanced up over his sunglasses and whispered, "She makes fun of me. The man takes care of me, but he tells me to watch out for the VA." He started tugging at his hat. "Why don't they go away? I've tried everything. I lined my hat with foil to keep the beams away."

He pulled off his hat to show me. Sure enough, it was thickly lined with several layers of aluminum foil.

"And I called the VA and went to see them yesterday. No one will listen." He clenched his hands, pounded his knees, and started to cry. "I can't stand them anymore. *You've got to remove the transmitters!* No one else will. I tried to get the ER docs to do it."

This explained a jumbled message I had received that morning. The Emergency Department had called to say that they had seen a "Mr. Carlos," who came in complaining of voices and metal receivers and who demanded a CT scan and removal of the machinery in his head. They had asked him to sit in the waiting room but it proved too much for him. He fled.

"Do you think a change in your medication would help?" I asked. In the past, Mr. Charles had often retained enough insight into his own symptoms to let me know whether the doses were too high, too low, or just right.

"How, how can it help? This isn't my *nerves*, this is *real!* You don't believe me, do you? You think I'm just being crazy. I don't know, maybe I am." He slumped in his chair, looking disconsolate.

Some psychiatrists would insist that it is *never* proper to appear to endorse a patient's mistaken thinking. Based on years of experience with the seriously mentally ill, I disagree. Often the only way to reach a patient in the depths of psychosis is to operate within the system of the patient's thinking. That means using the patient's beliefs—distorted or not—to facilitate his or her receiving the right treatment. I applied this same flexibility to my treatment of Harold (see Chapter 5 of this book), the man who was convinced that he was Moses, and it has allowed me to help countless others. "How about this, Mr. Charles," I said. "I'd like to do two things. Let's adjust your medicine somewhat, because your nerves are just shot over this, aren't they? A change in the dosage might help you better deal with the transmitters. But you *know* I'm not a surgeon and can't remove things from your head. How about if I call the VA and ask them to stop broadcasting? Would that help?"

He looked buoyant. "Will you do that for me? Will you do it now?"

What could I say but "sure"? Under Mr. Charles's expectant gaze, I called one of my more tolerant colleagues and asked him to please see to it that the VA stopped these transmissions as soon as possible. I then wrote out a letter addressed to the VA and gave a copy to Mr. Charles. Greatly soothed, he also let me call the boarding home to explain that he was having some troubles and the staff needed to keep a closer eye on him. By the end of our talk, he was clearly heartened, though he quickly put the cap back on "to keep the voices quiet."

I checked in with Mr. Charles the following week. This time, his appearance was a touch better and he wasn't wearing sunglasses. But his hat was still lined with foil. He reported on his progress:

"I think your letter is doing some good. The voices are softer, and that lady, she's not so mean after all. Now the voices are helping me with my card games." A grin slowly crossed his face. "They even tell me who's gonna win the NCAA. And you *know* it's gonna be North Carolina."

Over time, the voices and the paranoid delusion of transmitters receded. But, at two visits out of every three, Mr. Charles still wears his foiled-lined hat. He explains that he does it "just in case the voices start up again," and, unfortunately, the tenacity of his schizophrenia means that they very well might. My goal is to keep the volume dial turned as low as possible.

▌ Trying to Tune Out

We all know that a Broadway show is likely to be a hit if theatergoers leave humming the tunes. A good song is "catchy." Couples have "their" song, and certain lullabies, like heirlooms, are passed down within families.

We know too that music can be an irritant. Teens delight in the raucous heavy metal their parents detest. The hard-driving beat booming out of the convertible that pulls up behind us rattles the instrument panels of our cars and rattles us as well. Some people adore rap, others can't abide it. And most of us have had the experience of a certain song we liked at first but now we simply can't get out of our heads. To protect the culpable family member, neither Jackie nor Marc will identify which of them is the source of this reminiscence:

> An annual tradition in my family was watching the Miss America pageant. We enjoyed selecting our own Miss America and guessing who would be the judges' favorite. But what a price to pay! When Bert Parks sang the parting song, "There she is . . . Miss America . . . ," my Dad was hooked for another year. For weeks following the broadcast, he went about the house humming and whistling the tune, driving my mother to near distraction even as he lamented his own inability to "get the tune out of my head." We kids thought this pattern was hysterical and waited patiently until we noticed that the "Miss America" tune was beginning to disappear from his whistling repertoire. Then we would deviously slip up behind Dad and, in feigned innocence, begin softly singing the song until he was off and humming once again.

But the annoyance of a cloying tune, however maddening, pales in comparison to the *musical hallucination*. For patients with true musical hallucinations, tunes like "Waltzing Matilda" and "The Yellow Rose of Texas" are like elevator Muzak that escaped when the doors opened, now following them wherever they go.

In one such case, a 70-year-old woman saw her neurologist after hearing nonstop music for three weeks. At first, she thought it must be coming from another apartment, but friends assured her that they couldn't hear it. She had her hearing aids checked, thinking that they were somehow picking up an itinerant radio broadcast, but the circuitry was fine. Even when her doctor put her in a soundproof room, the songs (mostly ditties from the 1930s and 1940s) played on without interruption. After listening to "When Irish Eyes Are Smiling" 50 times, she had had enough. Her doctor was finally able to unmask the culprit: the high dose of aspirin she took every day for her arthritis. When she reduced her dosage, the music finally stopped. And it has never come back.

Medications, such as aspirin or the benzodiazepines (lorazepam [Ativan] and triazolam [Halcion] are two examples), have been implicated in a few cases of musical hallucinations. In others, a brain abnormality, such as a tumor or stroke, is to blame. Tinnitus, a fairly common problem in older age that produces a buzzing or ringing in the ears, can sometimes be remedied when medications are changed or impacted earwax is removed. But when the subjective sounds are the result of ear pathology, such as nerve damage, the most that can be offered is reassurance and the manipulation of background sound with white-noise machines.

Usually, afflicted patients are not mentally ill at all, even if they complain that the music is "driving me crazy." For example, one 19-year-old woman with new-onset musical hallucinations was convinced that she had become psychotic, but a physical examination revealed that the cause was simply a perforated eardrum. Other patients may be relatively unconcerned—or even pleased about their hallucinations. In a case involving an 87-year-old widow, for instance, her family was much more worried than she. The elderly woman admitted that she had been hearing songs for three years—mainly old Scottish tunes from her childhood that seemed to drift up the staircase—and that she relished them, even singing along when the mood struck. She declined any efforts at treatment.

▌ Command Hallucinations

Whereas the musical variant can be irritating but otherwise benign, another subtype of auditory hallucination can cause concern not just for clinicians, patients, and their families, but for the public as well. *Command hallucinations* are voices that demand that the patient carry out a particular act. Close to a third of patients who hear voices perceive command hallucinations, but only a small—obviously consequential—minority proceeds to act on them. Examples of command hallucinations with dire consequences are those mandating self-mutilation or suicide.

In rare cases, harm to others, including homicide, is the outcome. For instance, psychologist Daniel Martell and psychiatrist Park Dietz scrutinized 16 years' worth of the appalling New York City cases in which individuals pushed—or attempted to push—other people onto subway tracks. Of the perpetrators who acted alone, none had known their victims, and the majority of them were experiencing psychotic symptoms at the time of the offense—such as hearing voices exhorting them to commit the crime.

One factor that determines whether a command hallucination will be obeyed is the severity of the perceived consequences for disobedience. The patient may believe that the destructive behavior compelled by the faceless voices is still a lesser evil than the violence or death that would surely result if they were ignored. Another factor is the patient's interpretation of the content of a command auditory hallucination. For example, three researchers described an Ontario man with a history of command hallucinations spanning 17 years. None of these voices had ever led to violence until the man believed he heard the voice of his deceased grandmother, who was "serving as an oracle of God." With total clarity and absolute authority, she ordered him to "save your mother" and "do it now." Whereas others might have viewed these statements as ambiguous, they were perceived by the patient as divine instructions to save his mother from the forces of evil—and to do so, he needed to kill her. After his arrest, he said that he heard his mother calling his name affectionately and knew unquestionably that she was with God and grateful for his actions.

Like so many other psychiatric phenomena we have described in this book, command hallucinations too can be misused by criminals in an effort to deny culpability for violence. The legal system has become increasingly wary of those who might be faking psychotic symptoms to obviate responsibility for criminal actions. The perpetrator typically seeks to be adjudicated "not guilty by reason of insanity"—a hapless victim of command hallucinations or other symptoms that compelled violent acts. To arrive at the truth, prosecutors and forensic experts need to establish whether the defendant has a history of other criminal behavior, a history of treatment for a mental disorder, and a motive for violence.

Sometimes the defendant's efforts to mislead the court can be almost absurd. In the 1993 murder trial of Richard Lucio DeHoyos in Santa Ana, California, the defense attorney was faced with an imposing task: to save DeHoyos from the gas chamber by convincing the jury that DeHoyos was not guilty by reason of insanity.

The facts were clear. Nine-year-old Nadia Puente was walking home from school on March 20, 1989, when DeHoyos, a drifter, lured her into his car by posing as a teacher. DeHoyos acknowledged that he had then driven the girl to a motel, where he raped and asphyxiated her. Later on, he wrapped her body in a blanket and dumped it into a trash bin at a Los Angeles park.

His attorney pleaded with jurors to decide that DeHoyos was insane at the time of the crime. His reasoning? That no one in his right mind would have committed such a heinous crime.

The jury recognized this perfectly circular argument for what it was. It didn't help that some of the expert witnesses called by the defense contradicted each other, one testifying that DeHoyos was indeed faking his hallucinations and other symptoms. DeHoyos's courtroom antics in trying to appear psychotic were pitiable characterizations of how he must have believed mentally ill people behave: he frequently barked and growled like a dog, for instance.

All to no avail. Four and a half years after Nadia Puente died, Richard DeHoyos was sentenced to death row. His case reminds us of two points sometimes overlooked in discussions of violence in America, especially by those who would further stigmatize the mentally ill: first, most people with mental disorders—even severe ones—do not commit violent crimes; and second, most violent crimes are committed by people who do not have severe mental disorders.

▌ Visual Hallucinations

Hallucinations that involve the sense of sight are called *visual hallucinations*. Like their aural counterparts, these sensations—sometimes pleasant but more often disturbing—can occur for myriad reasons, schizophrenia among them. The complexity of visual hallucinations ranges from brief *photopsias* (sparks or flashes of light) to elaborate, colorful, and riveting spectacles.

Like imaginary playmates, *dreams* and *daydreams* are mental creations with visual elements that do not typically indicate any type of physical or emotional pathology. Another benign example is the *hypnagogic hallucination*, a phenomenon in which, shortly after relaxing in bed, a person's dreams begin even before he or she is fully asleep.

But many other false visual images do indicate a serious problem. For example, patients who are suffering from *delirium tremens* (or DTs) due to alcohol withdrawal may report seeing insects, bugs, or snakes on the ceilings or walls—or even on their own bodies. They may furiously pick at themselves or the air as a futile remedy. Seizures that involve particular parts of the brain can cause sudden intrusions of scenes that are violent, even horrifying. Hallucinations can develop as a neurologic consequence of HIV infection. And in the case of a 69-year-old man who had had a bullet lodged in his head for 45 years, scar tissue and the leaching of metal from the bullet caused visual hallucinations for the first time in his life.

Sheer stress itself can lead to hallucinations as well. One new recruit into the Israeli army, overwhelmed with anxiety about his capacity to serve, suddenly saw human-sized ants approaching and then climbing all over him. Remarkably enough, allowing him to ventilate his fears about military service was all that was needed to alleviate the problem.

Sometimes visual hallucinations can be traced to medications. Some prescription drugs, such as digoxin (for heart ailments) and levodopa (for Parkinson's disease), have been implicated. Even medications that fall short of inducing actual hallucinations, such as streptomycin (an antibiotic) and thiazides (widely used for hypertension), can create disturbances in how colors are perceived. Over-the-counter medications taken to excess can result in visual hallucinations as well. Patients who consume large amounts of antihistamines or antidiarrheal compounds, for instance, may experience this unsettling side effect.

Although medications can present a problem for some patients, particularly the elderly, drug-induced hallucinations are much more commonly observed among those who use illegal substances. Clinicians—and despairing families—know all too well that some individuals exploit illegal drugs precisely because they can provoke visual hallucinations. In the 1950s, Aldous Huxley wrote in *The Doors of Perception* and *Heaven and Hell* about his drug-induced visionary states, which allowed him to escape the "spiritual bankruptcy" of the modern world. Whereas amphetamines ("speed") occasionally have this effect, psychedelic drugs such as LSD and mescaline are mainstays. The perceptions they elicit involve riotous colors, wild distortions of shape and size, and reverberating intersecting lines—like Mondrians gone berserk. Drugs may also spawn *synesthetic* visual hallucinations, in which, for example, a loud noise is transmogrified into a vibrant color.

Synesthesia, one of the strangest sensory experiences imaginable, warrants an aside. Synesthesia is the subject of the 1993 book *The Man Who Tasted Shapes*. Studying the history of this neurologic phenomenon, Dr. Richard Cytowic discovered that numerous artists, poets, and composers have used their art to express their synesthesia. Russian composer Alexander Scriabin "composed" a display of light and shapes to accompany his symphony *Prometheus, The Poem of Fire*. He coded each color and shape to a specific note and assigned hues to musical keys. Thus, the audience is treated to a "sensory fusion" probably not unlike Scriabin's personal synesthetic experience with the "look" of music.

In the same way, certain poets, using what seem to be highly imaginative metaphors, appear to have been expressing their synesthesia. French symbolist poet

Arthur Rimbaud, for example, assigned unusual sensory value to the sounds of vowels. In his poem *Le Sonnet des Voyelles*, "A" is compared to a "hairy corset of clacking black flies" and "I" to "purple red spittle." The poem reflects Rimbaud's poetic principle that the exploration of self through poetry can be achieved only through "a systematic derangement of all the senses." But Cytowic suggests that there is nothing systematic accounting for Rimbaud's odd metaphors. He believes these are very likely created out of Rimbaud's living experience with synesthesia.

A Visual Roster

The ubiquity of visual symptoms in medical practice has led to the creation of a virtual dictionary of new terms. *Phantom vision* can result when the ability to see is lost or sharply diminished, perhaps due to an injury to the eyes. Involving continuous visual hallucinations, phantom vision is the ocular correlate to *phantom limb syndrome*, in which people "feel" a limb even after it has been lost through an accident or amputation. Elderly individuals plagued by a drastic decrease in visual acuity may report the *Charles Bonnet syndrome:* although these patients are cognitively and emotionally normal, failing vision leads to paradoxically vivid sights, such as fully formed faces that the patients know aren't really there. People with *palinopsia* continue to see an image even after the object has been removed. And in *autoscopy*, often associated with seizures or migraines, the person "sees" his or her own body as though it were projected like a searchlight beam into space—a literal "out-of-body experience." However unnerving these visual hallucinations, they are not linked to mental disorders, they do not interfere with normal functioning, and they rarely require significant medical or psychiatric intervention.

A contrasting picture, however, is presented by hallucinating individuals who see things smaller than they really are. This strange variant is found in two distinct syndromes. The *"Alice in Wonderland" syndrome*—in which both size and color are altered—is illustrated by the case of a seven-year-old Japanese girl. She reported that her mother's head was green and way too small for her body. In her case, Epstein-Barr virus infection seemed to be the cause. Smallness also characterizes *lilliputian hallucinations*, named after the little people in Jonathan Swift's 1726 tale *Gulliver's Travels*. In a representative case, a 78-year-old woman complained that dressed-up dwarfs were dancing away on her abdomen; they even cooked up some food for the party. On another day, tiny fishermen staged a battle scene. Later, she witnessed a Japanese feudal lord surrounded by his samurai warriors. It was finally determined by her doctors that these hallucinations were a rare manifestation of senile dementia. Although the dementia was irreversible, treatment for its symptoms could still be offered. In another illustrative case, a 19-year-old female soldier groused that a little man who dressed as she did would intermittently appear on her forehead. Fortunately, after only 10 days of a psychiatric hospitalization focused on providing support and empathy, the soldier's psychological strain eased enough for the little man to disappear.

In 1932, Dr. J. Lhermitte was the first to describe lilliputian hallucinations, which, as we've seen, can be amazingly detailed. He wrote,

> These little persons, or these animals in miniature . . . appear to be strange not only in their small size in contrast to all things around them, but also in their colors, gestures, attitude and performance. Indeed, they often form an ordered troop of little gentlemen as big as thumbs, dressed elegantly, sometimes dressed with richly embroidered fabrics, with precise clothes as if they were from the era of Louis XV. The little gentlemen bend and smile at each other.

Ms. Janey (as told by Jackie)

Ms. Janey was a large woman from a tiny hamlet who rarely came to the clinic. In fact, we generally saw her only when her symptoms worsened and she was eager for a shot to, as she put it, "calm my nerves." But the entire staff had taken particular notice of Ms. Janey, for she often talked about the "movie stars" who inhabited her legs. She could see them beneath her skin, she said, and sometimes they danced about.

Surprisingly enough, this symptom, in and of itself, usually was not terribly troublesome to her. During some visits, she knew her hallucinations were just that, and she felt able to ignore them or simply live with them. During other visits, she never mentioned them at all; she just wanted to chat about her granddaughter in college, of whom she was justifiably proud. But we knew that when the stress in Ms. Janey's life had gotten out of hand, the little movie stars became an immense irritant to her. And they had persisted despite the large number of medications we had tried. Part of the problem was that the dosages always had to remain small; at higher doses, Ms. Janey experienced side effects such as stiffness or tremors.

What a picture she presented on a bright August day as she stormed into the clinic, hair flying, shirt unbuttoned, ample bosom spilling out! Always gregarious, she usually displayed a warm, rich sense of humor, but not today.

"Oh, Doctor Jackie. I need your help," she implored. "They be marchin', marchin' out of me!" She gestured toward her legs, then flung her arm out to show me that "they" were leaving her body and heading out the door.

"Who? Who is leaving?" I asked.

"My stars, my movie stars. Comin' out of my legs and leavin'." She burst into tears.

"But Ms. Janey, what's the matter? I thought you'd be happy if they left. Does it pain you for them to be leaving? I mean, does it *hurt* for them to be leaving your legs?"

"Lordy, no, it ain't hurting, not like knife pain. But why would they want to leave me? Marilyn [Monroe] has been with me for years and Mr. Clark [Gable] has been my friend, kept me company!"

She seemed to be panicking. She rocked in her seat, tears streaming down her face. I moved my chair very close to hers and asked if I could hold her hands. She nodded and then flung her arms around my neck and sobbed.

After a few moments, her tears subsided and she seemed less shaky.

"Let me turn you loose," she said. She flashed a weak smile. "No need to be bawlin' like a baby without a teat."

I patted her hand and asked her to tell me about everything else that was going on. It emerged that her daughter had stopped by earlier in the day and had casually mentioned that she was going on vacation for a week. She wanted Momma to come along.

"But I knowed she really didn't want me to go. She saves and saves her money and spends too much on me. And I knows she needs some time with her new husband. She's very good to me, checks on me every day and says I can come live with her if I wants to. She makes sure I get my hair done just right and takes me to church, even on Wednesday night. She hasn't gone away for a long time."

She smiled ruefully, shook her head, and took a deep breath. "You thinks maybe I got scared, and that's why my movie stars left?"

"I don't know, Ms. Janey, maybe. Haven't they left before? Seems to me that they have."

"Oh, Lordy, yes. And you know what? They come back every time. Maybe I should let them take a vacation, too, just like I need to turn my little girl loose." I nodded, amazed at her ability to state her own conflict so succinctly.

She stood up, straightened her clothes, patted down her hair, and blew her nose. She tucked the messy handkerchief into her sleeve.

"I feel better. How about you give me my shot, and I'll be on my way."

We negotiated a dosage, and she got her shot. And we planned to have the clinic nurses check on her frequently while her daughter was away.

Three weeks later, I met with Ms. Janey again. Marilyn and Clark were back in her legs. And it just so happened that her daughter was back from vacation too.

Flashbacks

In the movie *Born on the Fourth of July*, wounded war veteran Ron Kovic (Tom Cruise) ascends the platform to deliver a patriotic speech to the townspeople. It is the Fourth of July—his birthday—and his first public appearance following a long and harrowing recovery from the war injury that left him paralyzed. His carefully pre-pared speech is interrupted when he becomes aware of an approaching helicopter. The sound of the chopping blades becomes an auditory cue that reconnects him with vivid scenes from an Asian village. Unable to grasp what is happening, his face regis-ters profound anxiety and confusion. In an emotionally wrenching scene, Kovic struggles for the words to continue but cannot complete his speech. He is assisted off the stage to polite scattered applause.

Kovic's visual phenomenon is extremely well known to clinicians in veterans' hospitals and clinics and arises in many other treatment centers as well. Patients who have experienced overwhelming trauma—such as combat, rape, or natural disas-ters—can develop *posttraumatic stress disorder*, or PTSD. In addition to symptoms such as crippling anxiety and intrusive, distressing recollections, PTSD patients of-ten report *flashbacks* in which they suddenly visualize and reexperience the original trauma.

Mr. Curtis (as told by Jackie)

A flashback was vividly described by a patient I treated at the euphemistically named "Mental Hygiene" Clinic within a Veterans Administration Hospital. Mr. Curtis, a 40-year-old Vietnam vet dressed in a gray sweatsuit, was work-ing hard to avoid interacting with the other veterans in the waiting area. This was the first appointment he had kept; he had failed to show up for two oth-ers. He walked into my office and brightened when he saw the window.

"Thank God, a window. There's never any windows in VA clinics. All the offices are like tight little boxes."

He shivered, then pressed on. "Doc, I need help. I thought this would get better but it hasn't. My wife is ready to leave me. This morning, I swear, I woke up with my hands around the bedpost. I coulda sworn it was a Charlie. It's happening more and more. Last week, I was playing with my kid in the yard, and I heard a helicopter, and the whole landscape changed for just a minute. My kid was gone, I was looking at a swamp. It was hot and steaming and it stunk, just like 'Nam. I heard the choppers, and the men hollering for help, and I couldn't move, I couldn't go back in to save Kenny."

At the mention of "Kenny," Mr. Curtis struggled to maintain a steady voice, but telling this story brought a rush of emotion that he could not contain. As he turned away from me and walked back toward the window, I couldn't help but notice the darkened streak of sweat that marked the back of his shirt. His anxiety was threatening to overwhelm him.

Over the ensuing weeks, I learned more about the many ways in which his ordinary environment become a temporary war zone. He told me of his mortification when he found himself diving for cover at the sound of a backfiring car. Not understanding his disturbed state of mind, the people around him took this as a hilarious joke. To save face, he had pretended that his action was indeed intentional—an attempt at slapstick humor. And at a recent family picnic, someone had set off fireworks—grenades to him—and, just as in Vietnam, he found himself running for cover toward the dense surrounding woods. Mr. Curtis described all these experiences as terrifying and, at the time, fully "real."

As I sat with him during our fourth visit, it seemed to me that these attacks were now occurring with greater frequency and were brought on by ever-milder provocation.

"I can't read about war, or Vietnam," he told me. "I can't even see something related to it—even a TV ad with too much hoopla—without it happening again."

He described the harrowing "escapes" that accompanied these seemingly innocuous events, and each narration brought initial anxiety, followed by relief as the story was over and he was reminded that he was safe. At the end of the hour, completely spent, Mr. Curtis slumped in his seat, but his gaze remained on the light streaming through the window. He was no longer visibly perspiring. His face appeared more relaxed. I pushed back my chair a bit to give him more space, feeling that nothing should intrude on this brief moment of peace.

Mr. Curtis knew all too well that flashbacks—like PTSD as a whole—can be extremely hard to treat. But we had just launched a research study, one that entailed combining a particular antidepressant with behavior therapy. As the antidepressant helped patients brighten, the behavioral work would desensitize them to provocative cues in the environment—such as the sounds and sights that can precipitate flashbacks. Once these stimuli lost their power to control the PTSD patient, it was our hope that the flashbacks would become much less frequent.

Over several months, with a firm commitment by Mr. Curtis to consistent attendance, his symptoms diminished dramatically. Reminders of Vietnam no longer seemed to lurk around every corner, and his sleep became a peaceful haven once again. His avoidance of others—as I had noticed that first day in the clinic waiting room—eased enormously. His flashbacks, when they occurred at all, were no longer all-consuming. He could recognize that they were transient and that he had the psychological strength and resilience to tolerate them.

Eleven months after we had first met, Mr. Curtis pronounced himself cured. I must have looked a bit skeptical at his choice of so definitive a word, because he laughed, then offered a quick compromise: "Okay, maybe I'm not 'cured,' " he said. "But I *am* 1,000% better."

That was good enough for both of us.

Tactile Hallucinations

Lamar (as told by Jackie)

Lamar is a funny-looking man. I try not to talk pejoratively about patients, but, well, he is. He's tall and skinny, has long, wild whiskers, and he combs his red hair over his bald spot when he remembers to comb his hair at all.

He's also one of the sweetest men I have ever met. Lamar is unfailingly polite, even in the throes of an exacerbation of his mental illness. Even when he is accusing us of trying to kill him. Even when he is disrobing in the waiting room because of the "bugs" in his clothes.

And he also has one of the most dire cases of treatment-resistant schizophrenia I have ever encountered. No medication has ever seemed to help much.

Lamar tells us he is a thanatologist, an expert in death and dying, and he has filled notebook after notebook with philosophical ramblings that propose to explain the road to death. I understand them as a metaphor, because I believe that Lamar views his schizophrenia as causing *his* "death"—the death of his dreams. In a real sense, it has done exactly that.

Lamar was pursuing graduate studies in geology when the illness first struck. In spite of numerous hospitalizations, supportive psychotherapy, behavioral and cognitive therapies, patient and family education, and housing in therapeutic group residences, Lamar has drifted downhill to where he is today.

His troubles vary from visit to visit. Whereas sometimes he focuses on the voices that plague him, more often he reports that bugs are attacking him—he can feel them crawling all over him, burrowing into his heart to destroy him. One week, he will shower twice a day and dress immaculately to "keep the bugs away." The next week, he will give up and arrive at the clinic grimy and smelly, carrying his laundry and despairing that "the bugs are back." He brings his clothes in to have Audrey wash them. Because Audrey is his favorite nurse, he hopes that her special touch will rid him of this curse.

Audrey is diligent about bringing back pristine clothes, but it never helps. A few days later, Lamar will be arrested yet again for walking naked down the road. He will be angry and thrashing as he rants about thanatology. A brief stay in our hospital will bring him little relief; instead, he will ask to go to the state hospital, where the voices say that the laundry is done with a unique kind of soap.

Lamar was last taken there six months ago, and it is there that he remains. I call the doctor to see how he is faring and get the usual report: he is only slightly better. Our hope for any lasting improvement hinges on the prospects for expansion of the pharmacologic options against schizophrenia—and the prospects do seem bright. But for now, we wait, and Lamar tries to take it one day at a time.

False Feelings

Tactile hallucinations involve the false perception of being touched. Among the most common of the subtypes is *formication*, the feeling that something is creeping or crawling on or under the skin. Although we all loved the kindly spider Charlotte in the children's story *Charlotte's Web*, most of us still have a touch of *acarophobia*, or the fear of crawly things. Some patients, such as Lamar, go much further, becoming convinced that their bodies are actually overcome with bugs. Their remedies can be nearly as dramatic as the disorder itself: one afflicted man spent $1,000 a month on pesticides, and another patient regularly squirted an insect killer into her ears.

We have long been aware that the conviction that one is beset by insects or parasites can be either a delusion (if one has the belief but doesn't claim to feel the crawling) or a hallucination (if the movements are actually experienced). But it is the latter that has interested us in particular. Prescient to our discussion of *folie à deux* in Chapter 7 of this book, in one case in five, the patient's ghastly reports of infestation actually induce parallel delusions or hallucinations in another person—usually a close relative. In essence, the pseudoinfestation is so compelling that it becomes "contagious."

Along with schizophrenia and other psychotic disorders, illicit substances figure in as prominently here as they did in the section on visual hallucinations. Amphetamines and DTs have long been associated with tactile hallucinations. The phenomenon also occurs in up to a third of cocaine users; indeed, during the time Sigmund Freud was extolling it as a valuable medication, one of the patients to whom he prescribed cocaine developed formication. In cases involving such "cocaine bugs," the sensations can be so intense that patients pierce their skin with needles, trying to extract the insects. In these and other cases of hallucinatory parasitosis, patients may also scratch, rub, pick at, and dig at their skin, leaving telltale wounds.

Joey (as told by Marc)

We also know that some cases of pseudoinfestation can be attributed to dysfunction in the brain. Tumors, insufficient blood flow, and direct injuries have all been implicated, but generally we can't figure out exactly how the abnormality in the brain leads to this peculiar outcome.

Joey was certainly a memorable patient. A handsome man in his 20s, he had lived a rebel life, putting off an education and a steady job to see America from the seat of his Harley-Davidson motorcycle. On admission to our ward, he spoke passionately with the staff about his adventures, although his speech was somewhat garbled: an accident during his travels had caused a severe head injury.

After over a year of physical rehabilitation, Joey was able to walk, albeit with a cane. As I learned more from his parents about the horrific accident, I realized that his physical recovery had been astonishing. Watching him mingle with the other patients, I concluded that emotionally, too, he seemed to be doing extremely well—he appeared affable and outgoing, having a smile for everyone.

However, I observed firsthand the reason for the psychiatric hospitalization within moments of my meeting him. Joey carried with him a Styrofoam cup into which he loudly spit several times a minute. Each expectoration was preceded by a lengthy, guttural buildup that repeatedly ground the interview to a halt.

I pointed it out. It is often the case that patients are delighted when the doctor openly addresses an issue that is obviously making him or her uncomfortable. Joey showed me not only the contents of the cup but a backup supply he kept in his duffel bag.

"I've got bugs in my throat. My parents said if I checked myself in here today, you'd be able to help."

Interspersing his story with gargling and coughing, Joey explained that "bugs" must have gotten into his throat when, following the accident, he was intubated to support his breathing. "Maybe the tube wasn't clean," he suggested. "Maybe they had it on the floor."

As his physical impairments had lessened, this residual problem—the conviction of real, live insects in his throat—only became more conspicuous. His parents had had quite enough, and yet they knew it would be impossible to arrange boarding-home placement for Joey if he disturbed other residents all night long with the noise.

Joey explained that while it was obvious that his Styrofoam spittoons put people off, the scratching, crawling sensation in his throat was intolerable. Ear-nose-and-throat doctors had told him that his symptoms might remit if he gave himself a rest from his continual cleansing efforts—that he was further irritating already-irritated membranes. But to Joey, to stop was unthinkable.

Joey's was the first case involving a tactile hallucination that I had ever encountered. I searched through the research literature but found only anecdotal reports with few solid treatment recommendations.

Meanwhile, Joey was extremely helpful and engaging around the ward despite his problem. Theorizing that the bugs were lodged in his windpipe, he tried furiously smoking cigarettes to flush them out. He only coughed more. He then figured that they had taken refuge in his esophagus, and so he drank copious amounts of hot liquids—also without success. As the spitting continued, there were indeed complaints from other patients that they couldn't sleep because of it.

Every once in a while, Joey had me paged to the ward so he could show me a "bug." He would triumphantly hold up a soggy shred of paper towel, on which a dot—perhaps an imperfection in the towel itself—could be seen. Another time he showed me a speck that just about had me convinced until I realized that it was a poppy seed from that morning's bagel. I began to worry that if the gruesome straining and expectorating didn't stop, he'd soon be coughing up blood.

I had to assume that the brain injury had, through some unknown mechanism, resulted in this overwhelming sensation of infestation. Joey simply had no other features of a mental disorder. And no amount of education and explanation helped him. It was obvious with each attempt that the immediacy of the discomfort of the phantom movements in his throat would win out.

I evolved a new plan, thinking that if I made spitting more difficult for Joey, he might give up. I naively underestimated his persistence. A medication that reduces the secretion of saliva led Joey simply to redouble his efforts at expunging his body of the creatures. The notion of a housing arrangement separate from his parents—one that would encourage greater independence—seemed even less attainable.

Finally, I prescribed a medication called haloperidol, which is used in a variety of disorders in which psychotic symptoms occur. Before we started it, the staff kept a baseline tally of the spitting over the course of an hour. After the haloperidol was begun, initial improvement encouraged all of us, but our ability to increase the dose was constrained by the emergence of side effects.

We had to settle for a compromise dose, one that certainly didn't cure Joey but nevertheless led to a better result than we had anticipated at the start of treatment. The frequency of Joey's coughing went down to only a few times per hour, and eventually he started sheepishly to imply that the bugs, while still there, might be dead. It has always intrigued me that, even as patients' symptoms begin to improve, they often maintain a loyalty to their core convictions, seeking to make sense of them in light of new evidence:

"Now I know," he said, "that when I finally cough them out, they'll really be gone once and for all. If the critters are dead, they can't reproduce!" Fortunately, the boarding home accepted that kind of logic.

Shortly after treating Joey, I met a young woman, a taxi dispatcher, who told me that she had started feeling "these little things" under her skin. Apprehensive about encountering another patient with tactile hallucinations so soon, I touched her skin at a spot she pointed to. To my surprise, I could discern a tiny, hard knot. She pointed out several others, each of which I could verify. A referral to an internist confirmed the diagnosis of a physical disease called sarcoidosis, which was ultimately managed with medication. As has been the case many times throughout my career, I was reminded to keep my mind open to all of the diagnostic possibilities!

▌ Olfactory and Gustatory Hallucinations

Among the rarest of the hallucinations are those that involve the sense of smell or taste. *Olfactory hallucinations* involve the perception of odor, such as burning rubber or decaying fish. *Gustatory hallucinations* involve the perception of taste and are usually highly unpleasant as well.

Both gustatory and olfactory hallucinations are more common in medical than psychiatric practice. Either hallucination can occur in seizure disorders, for example; when present, these powerful sensations are described by patients as the single most prominent and consistent feature of their seizures. "Bad," "rotten," "sickening," and "like burning food" are descriptors seizure patients often apply to the hallucinated smells. Their gustatory sensations are typically strikingly "bitter," "sweet," "salty," or "strange."

Similar adjectives dot the language of some patients with migraines or various kinds of brain injury. The composer George Gershwin complained to his doctor of sensing a terrible odor and, in 1937, died from the cause: a brain tumor.

But, as we've intimated, patients with schizophrenia or other mental disorders do occasionally have hallucinations involving taste or smell. They may claim, for instance, that foul odors have been forced upon them, and—in a vain attempt to prevent their entry—the patients block up the chimney. Or they may describe a noxious odor that they believe emanates from their own bodies. As in hallucinatory parasitosis, these patients may wash themselves excessively, constantly change their clothes, and steadfastly avoid other people for fear of repulsing them.

Leona (as told by Marc)

Leona came across as remarkably shy and discomfited. It was obvious that she would have liked nothing more than to vanish—or have *me* vanish. Yet, as the resident physician assigned to her case, I needed to understand the reasons for her admission. She looked to her husband to answer each question, and ultimately I found myself succumbing to her avoidance, directing all of my inquiries to him. Sitting on the bed, Leona shimmied farther and farther away, as if this exercise would make her seem smaller, less conspicuous.

Leona's husband, Mark, also seemed anxious, but he was still determined to explain the situation. Between his euphemisms, embarrassed silences, and fleeting gestures toward Leona, it became clear that the problem was an intensely personal one.

"She just been saying it smell 'down there,' " he said, hesitantly. He incriminated the relevant anatomy with a glance toward his wife's lap. "Been a good wife and mother, but seem like that's the only thing she talk about anymore. Tell me it smell but that I just won't admit it." Leona hung her head and scrunched her nose, probably wishing that, as in a *Star Trek* plot, one of us would be beamed off the planet.

Mark and I left Leona to unpack. We talked privately, and I was impressed with what a devoted and loving husband he seemed to be. A seamstress and the mother of two little boys, Leona had been "down" since the birth of their second child, and she had not reported to work for months. Although always on the quiet side, she had enjoyed visits with the next-door neighbor, but now even that element of sociability was gone. She confined herself to the house, ate and slept little, cried for no reason, and, most recently, asserted that she had a repugnant odor that rendered her unfit to be with others.

Subsumed by this thought, Leona's child care had suffered such that Mark was worried about the kids. And clean bills of health from three different gynecologists had done nothing to assuage her feelings. Instead, these spirited efforts at reassurance merely confirmed for her that even experienced doctors had nothing to offer and that they were too disgusted to admit the truth.

Although the treatment team's working diagnosis was major depression with psychotic features (in this case, olfactory hallucinations), we all agreed that we needed to exclude a medical explanation. Although Leona was pleased that she was being given so many tests, she appeared defeated each time one came back as normal.

Psychological testing was more illuminating. Analysis of Leona's personality and intelligence helped confirm that she was severely depressed. I suspected that she suffered from a postpartum depression that had never been recognized; rather, it had smoldered, then flared, resulting in the disabling psychotic symptom of an unremitting, abhorrent odor. The testing also established that she was mildly mentally retarded, further constraining her coping resources.

Efforts to engage Leona in group activities were entirely unsuccessful. She predicted ostracism and refused even to try. It was clear that, had the nurses not brought her the meal trays, she would have starved rather than venture out to get them herself.

Whereas insurance companies these days routinely intercede when doctors recommend such lengthy stays, back then Leona was able to remain in the hospital for eight weeks. And it was time well spent. Too infrequently do psychiatrists get to see their patients grasp the brass ring of complete recovery. Yet, in Leona's case, the combination of the support of the staff and both antidepressant and antipsychotic medications gradually abolished her hallucinations. Although she still believed that an odor had plagued her in the past, she acknowledged gleefully that this was no longer a problem. She looked forward to resuming a lifestyle free of this obstacle.

As we noted in the case of Joey, Leona did not take the abatement of her symptoms to mean that she had ever imagined them. Indeed, she could not have accepted that her life had been completely controlled by her hallucination, and with such damaging consequences. At the discharge conference, Leona asked Mark to admit that, although she was now symptom free, she did emit an odious smell in the past. In a statement brimming with diplomacy, he weakly said, "Well, maybe there was one time." She smiled, finally vindicated.

Research into the treatment of olfactory and gustatory hallucinations is constrained by their relative rarity. But recently, a Harvard study reported on four elderly psychiatric patients who experienced unpleasant smells or tastes. One complained of a fecal taste and odor; the second reported that water and food tasted "bad" and "foul"; and the third and fourth noted intolerable "metallic" tastes in their mouths. The unpleasant sensations of the first two patients were attributed to their mental illnesses. Those of the last two were the consequence of a particular antidepressant medication that was otherwise uniquely effective for them. The use of zinc supplements—long known to help correct the disordered perceptions of taste or smell that occur in some medical conditions—essentially cured the olfactory and gustatory symptoms in all the patients. The precise action of the zinc in reversing the problem is uncertain, but perhaps it's moot because it so clearly improved the quality of life of each of the patients.

▌ Reality and Replica

As our opening discussion of *Forrest Gump* suggests, the fusing of reality and fantasy has a formidable history in film. *Forrest Gump* flirts with this theme in the service of telling a lighthearted story. But writer-director David Cronenberg's 1982 film *Videodrome* may have taken it the furthest—ultimately down a very sordid road.

The main character in *Videodrome*, Max Renn, embarks on a journey into a realm in which external reality, hallucinations, and video images "programmed" into him become indistinguishable. The line between reality and representation vanishes. In a commentary on the daily saturation of our lives with manufactured imagery, *Videodrome*'s Professor Brian O'Blivion declares, "Television is reality: reality is less than television. Your reality is already half video hallucination. . . ." Cronenberg's film offers a sinister prediction about the increasing interdependence between technology and perception and about the temptation we face as new media encourage us to peek at the other side of the looking glass.

Our modern world provides us with ever more sophisticated ways of supplanting our reality, of suspending our belief and engaging our minds—and bodies—in simulated experiences. At Epcot Center in Orlando, Florida, a ride through the "human body" alters the senses as the rider's capsule dips and jerks in perfect unison with a stunning visual display. Utterly engaged, participants feel as though they are actually traveling through the human bloodstream. The effect of this combined sensory experience—visual, auditory, and tactile— is remarkably riveting and all-encompassing. But, moving far beyond such circumscribed amusements, we are left to wonder whether the ongoing explosion in cybertechnology will cause the virtual increasingly to supplant the real. Will the future fuse the objective and the illusory, the true and the false?

For the patient with hallucinations, this dilemma is less an engaging theoretical possibility than a pragmatic, daily struggle of life.

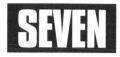

MASS HYSTERIA

Witch Hunts and Social Contagion

A statement once gets loose
cannot be caught by four horses.

—Japanese proverb

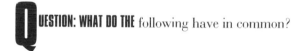UESTION: WHAT DO THE following have in common?

1. The American banking industry in 1990
2. Massachusetts school children at a school assembly in 1979
3. Cotton mill workers in Lancashire, England, in 1787
4. Twenty-nine schoolgirls in Malaysia in 1962
5. Nine hundred people in the West Bank of Jordan in 1983
6. Europe during the Middle Ages

Answer: At first glance, absolutely nothing. But if we were to add to the list "Salem, Massachusetts, in 1692," the picture might become a little bit clearer.

Salem is synonymous with "witch hunts"; in fact, its thriving tourist trade depends upon that immediate association. The witch hunts occurred when a false belief ran amok, forming a *collective delusion*. Sparked by the accusations of four young girls, a community already preoccupied with the risk of eternal damnation became panicked into believing that witches were among them. The lengths to which the rumor went were impressive. "Tests" were devised to identify who was a witch and who was not. Possible witches were thrown into rivers and weighted down, the townspeople knowing that a witch would save herself and emerge unscathed. Only the innocent would drown, and their families could breathe a sigh of relief that, although dead, their loved ones were *definitely not witches*.

By the time this travesty had ended, more than 20 people had been convicted even without the water test. Nineteen were hanged, one was pressed to death under the weight of huge stones, and four others died in prison. Ultimately, however, the Salem jury realized that innocent blood had been shed and that it was actually they who had sinned. In repentance, each juror signed a statement known as The Salem Jury's Rule. It reads in part,

> We confess that we ourselves were not capable to understand . . . but were for want of knowledge in ourselves and better information from others, prevailed with to take up with such evidence against the accused as on further consideration and better information we justly fear was insufficient for touching the lives of any. . . . We do therefore hereby signify to all in general (and to the surviving sufferers in especial) our deep sense of and sorrow for our error in acting on such evidence to the condemning of any person, and do hereby declare that we justly fear we were sadly deluded and mistaken. . . . And we also pray that we may be considered candidly and aright by the living sufferers as being then under the power of a strong and general delusion, utterly unacquainted with and not experienced in matters of that nature.

In 1697, the Massachusetts Day of Repentances for these egregious murders was established. Even as late as 1957, the small Massachusetts community was paying restitution to the families of those who had become the victims of the Puritan witch hysteria.

Like the residents of colonial Salem and other settings (including Sweden, Spain, England, Iceland, and South Africa) in which outbreaks of "witch hysteria" have occurred, the individuals in the six groups on our list have fallen prey to *mass hysteria*—if not nearly so famously.

Elsewhere in this book, we have examined the cases of individuals who harbor beliefs and experience perceptions that are simply not valid. The delusional person may think he is God. The hallucinating person may see demons coming to get her. But how does an ostensibly normal person, or a small group of people, or even an entire community, get swept up into a frenzied conviction that the shakiest of rumors is a terrifying reality? And how can a mistaken idea, like a disabling virus, make so many people so dreadfully sick that in short order an entire town's ambulances are scarcely enough to rush them all to hospitals?

▐ Mass Hysteria: What Qualifies?

As with the other phenomena we have discussed, mass hysteria has its nonpathological counterparts with which nearly everyone can identify. Virtually all of us have lived through—and probably participated in—a fad or craze. "Disco fever," which took the 1970s by storm and made John Travolta a role model, is an example of a period fad that became a national obsession. As more and more people "caught the fever," disco clubs sprang up overnight. The movie *Saturday Night Fever,* which propelled the BeeGees to stardom, rocked America as a rush of new musicians jumped on the bandwagon. It seemed at the time that our devotion to disco was here to stay.

Viewed from the perspective of the 1990s, disco, with its requisite male attire of screen-printed polyester, seems rather quaint—but only because we are now engaged in more fitting pursuits. Disco clubs have been replaced by health clubs, to which we race with equal zeal. Each day, millions of us, stylishly outfitted in fashionable aerobic attire, pay for the privilege of sweating and groaning on NordicTracks and Lifecycles. In our faddish fervor for exercise, we have created a lucrative new industry.

Are fads, then, a form of mass hysteria? We believe that that's an overstatement, but we note too that there's no universally accepted definition of mass hysteria. An assortment of opinions surrounds the issue. We side with those who insist that to qualify for the label of mass hysteria, there must first be a baseless belief from which behaviors spring absolutely spontaneously. Although fads do seem to arise spontaneously, in reality people decide whether to join in. As a result, they are really nothing more than collective behaviors—often whimsical in nature—that, like Nehru jackets, are appealing for a time but later seem embarrassing. By this same school of thought, riots at musical and sporting events, which occasionally have led attendees to be trampled or suffocated, are not altogether spontaneous either. The fans have specifically come together to hear the Rolling Stones perform or see their national soccer team play, and their zeal is deliberately whipped up with enough sound, action, and flashing lights to put any video game to shame. In such overstimulating settings, fainting teenage concertgoers—from the days of Elvis and the Beatles through today—collapse either from emotion-sparked hyperventilation or the legitimate panic of being trapped in the middle of an unruly crowd. In a similar—but safe—way, Grateful Dead concerts were known to trigger "movement epidemics" that were not wholly spontaneous: during certain songs, Deadheads would suddenly fill concert aisles with a spinning, whirling, trancelike dance that was simultaneously mysterious and magnetic.

Finally, we remove from the list cult movements, such as those driven by the fanatical leaders Jim Jones (the People's Temple), David Koresh (the Branch Davidians), Marshall Applewhite (Heaven's Gate), and Luc Jouret (Order of the Solar Temple). These charismatic leaders had formed tightly knit relationships with susceptible individuals and deliberately misled them into believing in their own special abilities and divine knowledge. Many would say that the outcomes of murder and suicide were almost inevitable in these cases.

At the same time that we exclude these particular cases, however, we need to point out that mass hysteria—like most human behavior—exists on a continuum. At one end are behaviors elicited within a specific, even carefully crafted context, such as the cult examples we've just cited. At the other are those that arise purely *de novo*, such as the remarkable cases of *mass sociogenic illness* and *mass anxiety* we will describe later in this chapter.

▌ "Limited" Hysteria

Somewhere in the middle of the continuum is a variant termed *induced psychotic disorder*. Here, one individual's false ideas spread to one or more people with whom he or she is close. The French phrase *folie à deux*, literally "double delusion," applies when the unfounded convictions stretch to just one other person. *Folie à trois/quatre/cinq* . . . applies when the false idea is transmitted within a circle of three/four/five or more. The following example of *folie à deux* illustrates this peculiar phenomenon.

Marion (as told by Jackie)

Marion was a stout woman with a large billowy frame and penetrating eyes. She was new to our clinic, and her records from another mental health center had not yet arrived. Because she wouldn't tell us whether she had any family we could call, my initial diagnosis was based strictly upon her vague answers and nonverbal behaviors. Certainly, she was distant and guarded—not irritable and hostile, but she put off the staff nonetheless. I had to work hard over several visits to establish any connection with her, but I had finally started to feel that a relationship of trust was developing. I found out that she could laugh gaily when something struck her fancy, although I could never predict exactly what would tickle her.

On this day, she circled the waiting room, her back always to a wall, checking over her left shoulder for something or someone. Her few remaining teeth were in obvious disrepair and her tongue and gums were stained from chaw.

I called her in, and she shook my hand in a diffident manner. She had called and asked us to see her soon, and we had obliged.

"So, Marion, how can I help?"

"My sister is dead."

I sat bolt upright. I had been working with her for only a couple of months, but this was the first I had heard of a sister, and Marion's startling disclosure was quite a distressing introduction to the subject.

"Well, a half sister. My ol' man got married again after my momma died."

"Where's your sister's . . . body?"

"She's at home. She's been with me for a while." She looked blankly out the window, then jerked around as though I might have caught her in something. "But she surely is dead." Marion cackled.

"How did she die?"

"He got her. He got into her body like he got into mine and now she's dead."

With that she stood up, then started to sway, holding herself and humming something mournful. I wondered how fast I could get the police out to her place. Just how *old* was this corpse?

"Do you want to meet her?" she asked.

"Who? Your sister? I thought she was dead!"

"She is, he got her, just like he's been trying to get me. She might as *well* be dead."

So she *wasn't* dead. "Yes, I'd like to meet her," I sighed. "When can she come in?"

"Well, actually, she's downstairs smoking a cigarette. I'll get her."

Quite off balance, I waited alone in the exam room, looking frantically through the chart but relieved that the sister was at least alive. There were no details about her family in the records, but then Marion had never been forthcoming. She had always been a loner, often depressed, but nonetheless assertive and loud. She was also not given to taking her medicines. She had never been convinced that she had a mental illness, and her noncompliance with the "unnecessary" medications meant that she continued to suffer with symptoms that included an elaborate system of delusions. In the past, she had said that a man was in her stomach, eating away at her, sometimes trying to kill her, sometimes trying to make love to her and impregnate her. He came and went unpredictably.

Marion arrived back at the room and brought her sister in; rather, she *pushed* her into the room.

"See, I told you, she's dead. Dr. Feldman, this is Myra. Myra, this is MY doctor."

Myra was a tiny, bland, mousey woman, stoop shouldered and clothed in a worn gray dress. Her pink slip straps showed, her shoes were scuffed, her stockings were in tatters. Myra refused to shake my hand and instead clasped her stomach. She closed her eyes and shuddered. I thought she was going to faint.

"Please, Myra, sit down," I said. "Can I get you something? You look like you're in terrible pain. What's the matter?"

Myra opened her eyes and looked toward Marion. She seemed to be looking for her sister's permission to respond to my questions. But I needed to hear *her* story. I turned to Marion: "Marion, why don't you wait for us in the TV room so that I can talk to Myra alone?"

Without a word, however, Myra grabbed for her sister. Marion wasn't going anywhere. The interview progressed as Marion supplied the details whenever Myra hesitated, even for a moment.

The story emerged that Myra had never married and had not worked outside the home for almost two decades. Over many years, she had nursed first her grandmother, then her father until he died the year before. She continued to receive a check from a trust fund but had no other resources. She also had no known psychiatric history: no hallucinations, no delusions, no emotional problems of any kind. She denied ever having seen a psychiatrist or counselor. Instead, it seemed as though she had always been a very isolated, slightly depressed lady who nonetheless managed to take care of herself and others.

Myra had moved in with Marion six months earlier. In that short period, Marion's stronger personality, and her delusion of the little man in her body, had spread like Alabama kudzu into Myra's life as well. If the situation weren't so obviously uncomfortable for Myra, I would have pointed out that her symptoms were blatantly cloned from Marion's.

Myra twisted and turned, complaining bitterly that the man inhabiting her ate at her stomach. He was killing her; maybe she was already dead. No, he had never wanted to make love to her, but she'd be glad for that to happen and to have his baby. Yes, maybe it would be best if she *were* dead. She had considered killing herself, but she couldn't leave her sister alone in this world.

The suicidal references prompted me to act with some urgency. Although there are many approaches to treating *folie à deux*, the one I chose was to try to separate the two afflicted individuals and prescribe antipsychotic medicine—to at least one of them—on a short-term basis.

How could I possibly separate these two enmeshed sisters? Although it took a while to convince them, I finally won their shared consent to admit Myra to the hospital. And the staff there was made well aware of the fact that Marion had agreed to follow my strict orders not to communicate with her sister.

At first, both sisters challenged that directive quite a few times. On the third day, however, as Myra became more at ease with the staff, she agreed to the plan—and to my recommendation of a low-dose antipsychotic medication. She started politely to decline to take the phone when Marion called. Instead, she spoke with the staff—particularly about how empty and lonely her life had felt after her father had died. She had sought to strengthen her relationship with Marion, she said, but over time she found herself overwhelmed by her domineering and persuasive sister. She began to accept—and experience—Marion's convoluted assertions.

At discharge, the results were gratifying for Myra and for me. Therapy and the brief medication use had loosened the grip of the delusions. Myra, the sister without psychiatric problems up until now, was able to give up the shared delusional thinking. And, although Marion resisted it, Myra decided to live elsewhere in town.

I continue to see both of them—Myra, much less frequently. Although Marion retains her unusual beliefs, Myra has been able to maintain her gains and expand her social network. She appears happy. The key to her success has been her maintaining a more distant, although still supportive and caring, relationship with her less-healthy sister.

■ Mass Hysteria: A Different Kind of Outbreak

As we have mentioned, there is no consensus about the definition of mass hysteria. Still, there are commonly accepted clinical features that can guide us. We generally think of mass hysteria as producing ill effects on the mind and/or body. Symptoms can be psychological in nature, such as acute anxiety. Or they can be physical, such as nausea and vomiting. Unlike *folie à deux*, the symptoms sweep through groups of people that can number into the thousands and who do not necessarily have any personal relationship with one another. The victims are people who have usually had their emotions under adequate control and who generally feel perfectly well.

Author Charles Mackay was a pioneer in the description of mass hysteria. Published in 1841, his book, *Extraordinary Popular Delusions and the Madness of*

Crowds, detailed the amazing power of the phenomenon. One of the zaniest chapters details so-called tulipomania. In the early 1600s, tulips were all the rage. Novel and in demand, a single tulip bulb cost a fortune—more than many people would earn in a lifetime. A fellow who naively ate a tulip bulb, blinded by his hunger into thinking it was a lowly onion, was criminally charged for the act. Mackay makes the point that, among its effects, mass hysteria can drive people to become irrational, imbuing the tulip (or anything else, including a belief) with a value out of proportion to its actual worth.

▌ Thought Control? Or Out-of-Control Thoughts?

The cause of the outbreak is often a baseless belief, a misimpression, or a rumor that begins small but, like a hurricane, travels and becomes more devastating as it picks up speed. Orson Welles's "War of the Worlds" radio broadcast in 1938 is an infamous example of the power of a false idea gone berserk. Although the play was announced as fictional several times, panic still spread throughout the country as millions became convinced that the Martians had landed and were taking over the Earth.

Similar anxieties were unleashed, albeit on a much smaller scale, in response to a Pittsburgh disc jockey's April Fools' Day hoax. The deejay's 1988 on-air account of an unidentified flying object brought a flurry of calls to the station from listeners ready to confirm that they had witnessed the UFO's rumbles and flashes of light. Frantic citizens also flooded the switchboard at the Allegheny County police department. But fans of the station should have expected that the invasion of foes was itself false. On April Fools' Day a year earlier, the same deejay had announced on the air that an alligator was lurking in Pittsburgh's sewer system. To solve the problem, he asked listeners to flush their toilets at the same time: three, two, one, *now!* A lot of people obliged, although at least *this* time the police didn't receive panicked calls about it.

From a perch distant in time or geography, it is tempting to view these cases as rather quaint. Perceiving ourselves as more aware and enlightened, we're likely to bristle at any suggestion that, in fact, we too are pitifully gullible. Yet, our very sophistication spawns tensions from which misguided passions can arise. Dazzlingly complex technology, for example, allows us not only to spread information as fast as it is generated but to transmit it even before it has been verified, creating a climate ripe for runaway rumors. These same technological achievements, which confound our minds and imaginations, do more than fascinate us; they also frighten us with their mysterious and powerful capabilities. In this context, it is easy to see how rumors about subliminal messages have become such a potent force in American culture.

Concern over subliminal "thought control" arose decades ago when movie theater operators were said to have used subliminal advertising to boost concession sales. Some department stores were accused of using intercom subliminals to influence shoppers. In the 1970s, the notion was promulgated that some companies were using subliminal sexual messages to sell their products: for instance, the ice cubes in a beverage company's magazine ad would supposedly be transformed into an image of writhing naked bodies if the viewer chose to stare at it long enough. As interest in the subliminal theory grew, some companies suffered heavy financial losses from the rumors that had taken hold. Procter & Gamble lost an enormous number of sales when its moon and stars logo came under attack as having satanic implications.

Eventually, the public's intense interest in subliminal advertising waned, only to reemerge in the music industry. In the 1980s, heavy-metal musicians became the new targets of the subliminal fixation, and satanic messages were purported to be ensconced within the hard-driving beat. The metal genre, which became known for its violent sexual themes, was indeed offensive and alarming to many, yet there was no basis for the accusations that the music masked subliminal missives. In fact, its overt iconoclasm and openly offensive material seemed to run counter to the idea of subliminal content. *why hide it when the very basis of the music was to shock?* Yet, the myth persists that certain music, especially when played backwards, yields alarming messages.

▌ An American Tale

The sexual-sublimination angst persists to this day as new targets have been discovered. In a recent example, a localized rumor eventually spread from coast to coast, casting nasty aspersions on three of America's unlikeliest villains. At first, the rumors of subliminal sexual messages in several of Disney's animated movies seemed to be a joke. But Jim Stratton, a reporter for the *Daily Press* in Newport News, Virginia, was tipped off to the credence some people gave these rumors as he thumbed through a newsletter published by an antiabortion group. An article in the newsletter informed parents that the popular Disney film *The Lion King* contained subversive material. The article cited the scene in which the adorable Simba kicks up a cloud of dust: "Watch closely as the cloud floats off the screen and you can see the letters 'S-E-X,' " the article warned (and invited) readers. Incredulous and somewhat amused, Stratton called the newsletter's publisher, where a spokeswoman informed him of clandestine messages hidden in two other Disney features. According to her, there is a scene in *Aladdin* in which the title character murmurs, "All good teenagers take off your clothes." And the claim was made that, in *The Little Mermaid*, during the course of a wedding ceremony, the presiding bishop becomes "noticeably aroused."

Not satisfied, Stratton gathered together a dozen reporters to view *The Lion King* scene to see for themselves whether the supposed message was actually there. No one was convinced. Stratton decided to write a story covering the three incidents in a tongue-in-cheek manner. This story was picked up by the Associated Press, which then printed a version of its own, announcing that a Christian group had identified subliminal sexual scenes in popular Disney movies. That widely published story brought the alleged subliminal messages to the attention of millions who otherwise would never have read the *Daily Press*, let alone the antiabortion newsletter.

The circuitous origins of the rumor were eventually teased apart. The antiabortion group had gotten its information from a reader of *The Movie Guide*, a Christian entertainment magazine. *The Movie Guide* was prompted to do the story by concerned citizens, such as a woman who heard about the "take off your clothes" message from her daughter, who heard about it through a grapevine that was ultimately traced back to a rather excitable college student. Disney vigorously denied the allegations, pointing out that the line is "Scat, good tiger, take off and go." *The Movie Guide* ran a retraction—only after having had the video analyzed by a digital recording studio.

But the matter still is not settled. Although this was by no means the first case in which accusations of subliminal tampering were made against Disney, it remains one of the most widespread, and it has changed many viewers' opinions of the company's animated films. Never mind that the furious allegations have been weakened by retractions, contradictions, and even confessions by some of the most vehement accusers that they have not actually seen the films they have so firmly denounced. Once rumor takes root in fertile soil, truth and logic are difficult to recapture. As of this writing, the Disney rumor continues to thrive.

▌ Contagion: Literal and Figurative

Group therapists who use the term *contagion* mean it in a technical way. In this context, it applies to an empathic process in which one group member expresses a particular emotion and then another member becomes aware of a similar emotion in himself or herself. But a warpage of this subtle, usually helpful dynamic fuels the social contagion that can lead not simply to pervasive rumors but to actual mass hysteria. Such an event is especially likely when a group or community is unsettled to begin with—in other words, when the emotional climate is already highly charged.

During the Black Death of the Middle Ages, millions of people were terrified and bewildered. An unknown force had descended, eventually killing an incredible 75 million citizens in Europe alone. We now know that the bacterium *Yersinia pestis*—transmitted by fleas and rodents and propagated by poor sanitation—was the cause of the devastating illness and death. At the time, however, townspeople commonly believed that the plague had befallen them because of a malignant energy from the stars or as a divine punishment for their sins. In some cities, such as Florence, Italy, fully half of the population died. As writer James Fenton has noted, "This is why the plague is not one of many epidemic diseases, but the disease of all diseases, the disease that could destroy a city, its rituals, its morality—every measure by which it reckoned its own worth."

In this fiercely unsettled atmosphere, *Yersinia* prompted some epidemics not due to the bacterium per se. Among these were the so-called psychic epidemics. A phenomenon called "dancing mania" propelled itself through Europe as a result of the intolerable tension built up by the unpredictability of the Black Death. The citizens were desperate for salvation from the peril. Yet, surrounded as they were by ever-expanding death, salvation seemed impossible to achieve. Those overcome by the dancing mania are thought to have been seeking a state of ecstatic release and redemptive visionary experience. Unfortunately, their efforts were in vain, and the exhaustion brought on by the medieval dancing mania itself even killed some of the participants.

Some would say that our modern age has produced its own expression of dancing mania. In our anxiety over maintaining the competitive edge, staying current, keeping up with technology, and, ultimately, holding onto our jobs, we are "dancing" ever faster to a tune that is harsh, dissonant, and continually changing keys. Unlike our European forebears, our dancing mania is merely metaphorical—but in these anxiety-ridden times, it is driven by the same frantic need for self-preservation.

◼ The Movement Is the Message

Other dramatic movement epidemics like the dancing mania of the Middle Ages have dotted more recent history. In the 19th century, for instance, the famous French neurologist Jean-Martin Charcot needed to maintain a special ward at Salpêtrière Hospital in Paris just to house the many "hysteroepileptics" referred to him—patients with convulsions that were purely hysterical.

In the United States, during both the 19th and early 20th centuries, there was an unusually strong association between religious groups and epidemics of movements that have been irreverently dubbed the "jerks." The jerks were physical displays of religious fervor that typically occurred during revival meetings. They could be of a variety of types, evoking descriptions such as the "falling exercise," the "dancing exercise," and the "barking exercise." In one variant, supplicants' heads would zip from side to side so fast that their faces could scarcely be seen. As their zeal took even greater hold, their whole bodies would snap forward and back, their heads nearly touching the floor in front and behind. Another subtype melded sudden jerking and loud grunting; another still consisted of frenzied dancing. Like additional variations that involved excessive singing or running, these odd spectacles stemmed from religious fanaticism and unbridled excitement.

Even as we approach the 21st century, wild displays of religious ecstasy emerge again when the conditions that created the jerks reappear. A reporter who attended a modern-day revival meeting in Melbourne, Florida, described it as follows:

> A woman named Sandy is the next to go down. She lies on her back, her head twitching as though jerked by a puppeteer. Then she begins doing what appear to be tiny sit-ups: her stomach muscles tighten and her head lurches convulsively off the floor. Then [an old man] keels over and twitches. More people collapse. Some emit little moans and mumbles and yips. Soon, Sandy explodes in wild, loopy, liquid laughter. After several more minutes, everyone gets up.

Sometimes, communal "giggles" (termed "holy laughter") have surfaced in religious settings. Since 1994, parishioners at the Toronto Airport Vineyard Christian Fellowship have been getting together six nights a week for group laugh-ins called "the Toronto Blessing." The phenomenon of uncontrollable group hilarity has been spread by pastors to Anglican churches around the world. They see it as a manifestation of the Holy Spirit, though other observers suggest that the sight of a whooping congregation is frightening, even reminding them of demonic possession. They don't see the slogan "I'd bust a gut for the Lord" catching on anytime soon.

As with all forms of mass hysteria, movement epidemics know no geographic borders. The "mysterious madness of Mwinilunga," for example, led Zambian schoolgirls to twitch uncontrollably. In another epidemic, Malay athletes were seized by bouts of spasms. And "running manias" and "laughing epidemics" have struck Tanzania, Uganda, and other African countries, often in the face of forced closures of beloved missionary schools.

▌ Cultural Context

As we evaluate such incidents in other societies, the sociocultural context in which patients' beliefs and behaviors arise is as important as the role of particular events or individuals. We have emphasized in every chapter that it is vital to consider the social, political, ritualistic, and institutional forces that propel a behavior. Failure to do so can convert culturally appropriate rituals and roles into pathology. Do we really want to recommend psychiatric consultation for little kids who insist they've seen Santa coming down the chimney?

Therefore, before deciding on the meaning of an odd belief or behavior, even one that seems to be sweeping through large groups of people, we need to ask a series of questions: What is its meaning in relation to the prevailing norms? Even if the belief or behavior itself is fairly common, is it far too extreme in the cases at hand? How do the members of the culture explain it?

For example, one patient revealed to Marc a curious religious custom she remembered practicing as a child. She was taught that if she followed a precise ritual on a particular feast day, she could release a suffering soul from purgatory, where it awaited entry into heaven. The ritual involved a set series of prayers that, in order to work, had to be spoken in church. If she wanted to pray for more than one soul, she had to exit the church after each complete series and then reenter once again. In her childlike enthusiasm to release as many souls as possible from their suffering, she found herself springing up and down like a windup toy as she went out the big doors and came right back in again. Her friends, equally inspired, were doing the same thing. An outsider would have found these behaviors laughable or bizarre—but to these tender and well-meaning children, their behaviors made perfect sense.

Adding to the complexity, we also have to bear in mind that the fact that a cultural interpretation can be offered does not necessarily mean that mass hysteria *has not* occurred. Although a traditional healer, a *bomoh*, was able to cure 29 Malay schoolgirls who claimed in 1962 to have seen a spirit near a fruit tree, their screaming and fainting spells were not a part of any ritual. They were abnormal even within the context of that unique culture.

Another example has occurred in locales ranging from Puerto Rico to Papua New Guinea. When it spreads, *amok* (the origin of the English phrase "running amok") is an authentic example of mass hysteria. In amok, a male phenomenon, a period of brooding is followed by an outburst in which victims direct violence toward people and objects. Exhaustion ensues, ultimately leading to a return to normal behavior. *Piblokto* is yet another culturally based but authentic example. In this Arctic hysteria, Eskimos begin to scream, tear off their clothing, and throw themselves on the snow or ice. Once the attack passes, the patient appears fine and often does not remember the episode.

Mass Sociogenic Illness

In the common variant of mass hysteria called *mass sociogenic illness*, a number of people almost simultaneously develop physical complaints that certainly suggest a real illness but in fact have a purely psychological cause. It is as though mere sight and sound make them terribly ill. Usually beginning when the air is already crackling with anticipation or stress, mass sociogenic illness has a number of defining characteristics.

First, even though the individuals involved appear and feel ill, all the lab tests and physical exams are normal. Second, hyperventilation, dizziness, and fainting are almost invariable. Third, the symptoms spread through the group with blazing speed. Fourth, the people affected strongly resist a psychological explanation for their sudden afflictions, even when the evidence is incontrovertible. And fifth, though relapses can occur if the same malignant factors all conspire again, the long-term outcome (as in the culture-specific examples cited above) is good.

Consider this example from a summer outreach program in Florida for disadvantaged kids. One hundred fifty children, ages 4 to 14, were enrolled in the program, which provided educational and recreational activities. Every day at noon, the children assembled in a large dining hall where they were served prepackaged meals. The same meals were among 3,800 prepared by a single Florida plant and distributed to 68 additional sites throughout the state.

The ham-and-cheese sandwiches, diced pears, apple juice, and chocolate milk looked good enough. But as lunch began, one 12-year-old girl complained that her sandwich didn't taste right. She said she felt nauseated and came back from the rest room reporting that she had thrown up. Other girls began to complain that their stomachs hurt too and that the sandwiches really did taste funny. A number of them began to report headaches, tingling in their hands and feet, abdominal cramping . . . and fear. The supervisor, obviously worried about all the complaints, announced to the children that the food might be poisoned. The horrified children were told to stop eating immediately.

Within 40 minutes, 63 children were sick. More than 25 of them had vomited. Ambulances were called, and the 63 kids had to be divided among three different hospitals.

But an hour later, it was all over.

Every examination and every test performed on the children were normal. At considerable expense, meal samples were analyzed, but no bacteria or pesticides were detected. Food processing and storage techniques were reviewed in detail and found to be adequate, with no possible contamination source. Most convincingly, no one had become ill at any of the other 68 sites at which the very same food was served.

These children were unmistakable victims of mass sociogenic illness. But how did this social wildfire get started? What led to the mobilization of such immense expenditures of time and money?

Looking back, it was recognized that the statement of the first girl had precipitated a small chorus of complaints. Her reason for the remark, perhaps as coincidental as the momentary feeling of light-headedness that many of us get from time to time, nonetheless proved to be very powerful. The number of victims, all suggestible children, expanded exponentially as an authority figure, the supervisor, announced that the food might indeed be tainted. Typical of settings ripe for mass hysteria, the program itself was already an unsettled environment; two days earlier, a newspaper article had reported on management and financial problems within the youth center. The children, being attuned to their emotional shifts, seemed to have registered the pervasive anxiety of the staff.

That same year, Santa Monica, California, was the site for our second example of mass sociogenic illness, this time involving even more people. Nearly 600 budding musicians from junior and senior high schools had come together for the annual Stairway of the Stars concert. Instead, it proved to be a stairway to the emergency room. Complaining of headaches, dizziness, weakness, belly pains, and nausea, the performers—like stacked dominoes—toppled one by one. The soprano section was decimated when 16 girls fainted. The auditorium had to be evacuated and ambulances sped to the site of the concert.

Two hundred forty-seven of the student performers ultimately succumbed. And, as in the Florida case, all proved to be perfectly normal. Mass hysteria emerged as the culpable communicable disease here too. The students' anxiety about their scheduled performance—an unhealthy dose of stage fright—created a tense situation in which mass illness was able to fester.

▊ Unsettling Influences

In these examples, the symptoms were passed from person to person within the group. Although many people were afflicted, the hysteria nonetheless remained

John Dewey Library
Johnson State College
Johnson, Vermont 05656

within the confines of the group. But news travels quickly these days, and both word of mouth and the media can play a significant role in spreading the ailments from town to town.

In 1979, for instance, the presumed illness of one boy at a school assembly in Norwood, Massachusetts, rapidly spread to others. Alarmed teachers dismissed the group while staffers called the fire department. Blaring sirens from approaching emergency vehicles only exacerbated the panic, and soon the whole building was evacuated. Some kids were whisked to the hospital. Doctors arrived on the scene to examine the ones who were left.

Within four hours, Norwood's phantom epidemic was over, only to emerge four days later at a junior high school in the neighboring town of Hopkinton. Rumors of the mystery illness had found new hosts nearly 15 miles away.

Psychiatrists Gary Small and Jonathan Borus scrutinized the cases in Norwood and Hopkinton. They discovered that anxiety relating to the impending loss of the principal was a likely precipitant in the Norwood school and that media coverage, although well intended, had nonetheless fueled the mayhem: Norwood newspapers published photos of the sick, tearful children—riveting visual images that seem to have facilitated the spread to Hopkinton. The newspapers also dutifully reported on inconsequential faults in the ventilation and heating systems at the Norwood school, thereby heightening the anxiety and the itinerant rumors. It is extremely doubtful that Hopkinton would have felt the sting of mass sociogenic illness if not for the media coverage of the Norwood episode.

Like the misleading findings about the Norwood building, evaluations of the victims can result in deceptive "false-positive" findings as well—illusory explanations for the symptoms that serve only to fan the flames. Almost exactly two years after the Norwood episode, for example, the Massachusetts town of Templeton became the latest site of mass hysteria. A choir performance (again) was marred by serial fainting among the members. And within an hour, just about everyone was fine.

That is, until the lab results came in two days later. Some of the urine tests disclosed trace levels of a chemical compound found in plastics and other products. How had such a substance found its way into our children's bodies? aghast parents wanted to know. It was feared that public health was in jeopardy. Agents ranging from gas to moth spray were proposed as the villains, and distressing uncertainty reigned—that is, until it was shown that the chemical compound was a contaminant in the urine collection bottles themselves. Drs. Small and Borus postulated that existing concerns in Templeton about pollution contributed to this overinterpretation of an incidental, and ultimately irrelevant, lab finding.

■ New Age Illness

"Fashions in illness change," wrote British researcher Simon Wessely, "but will always reflect the preoccupations of the age." Indeed, the hysteroepileptics who freely populated Charcot's hospital in the 1800s have all but vanished, only to be replaced by people with symptoms more in vogue. As we saw in Chapters 3 and 4 of this book, an epidemic of multiple personality disorder has emerged in part from sustained media coverage.

Like mental disorders, physical symptoms have arisen out of popular thinking. From radon and asbestos, to silicone in breast implants, to the drugs Bendectin and diethylstibestrol (DES), the world appears to be fraught with chemical dangers. But, as argued by Dr. Marcia Angell in her 1996 book *Science on Trial*, a cautious public cannot always discern which hazards are real (such as DES), which are overstated (asbestos and radon), and which are spurious (Bendectin and, surprisingly enough, almost certainly silicone). We are not automatically trusting of what authorities tell us. When there is a "momentary" malfunction of a nuclear reactor or when chemical spills have leached into our groundwater, we are not necessarily comforted by the government's official assurance that all is well. We remember Love Canal and the Woburn wells.

Clearly, environmental pollutants have been responsible for all manner of disease, from respiratory failure to leukemia. Who could doubt the devastating evidence from Chernobyl? And yet, even this very real nuclear accident—one that undeniably caused acute radiation poisoning in some people—has also produced benign sociogenic illness. When UCLA pediatrician E. Richard Stiehm visited Kiev in the early 1990s, he found concerned doctors and anguished parents trying to explain the sudden onset of illness in a staggering number of children. The "elusive epidemic" reported by Dr. Stiehm was characterized by symptoms of pallor, lethargy, and fatigue. But when Stiehm conducted tests on hospitalized children, not one was found to be suffering from radiation poisoning. Instead, Stiehm reasoned that the immense anxiety of the parents had induced a vicarious "illness" in their offspring: unconsciously, the children were compelled to experience the very symptoms that parents and doctors feared would be caused by radiation exposure. Because we know from Hiroshima's survivors that radiation effects peak only after 15 to 20 years have passed, the magnitude of the long-term health consequences of the Chernobyl accident is yet to be known. But to this point, it has been the psychological fallout from Chernobyl that has been most instrumental in leading the children to have such intensive inpatient physical evaluations and treatment.

▮ The Environment as Culprit

In the case of Chernobyl, it is easy to understand how legitimate fears could produce a sociogenic epidemic. But far less dramatic environmental concerns have seeded equally pronounced epidemics. In 1995, after studying many classic cases, Drs. Carl-Johan Göthe, Carl Molin, and Carl Gustaf Nilsson of Stockholm coined the term *environmental somatization syndrome* (ESS). Individuals who exhibit ESS have no physiologic basis for their symptoms and yet become convinced that their health disturbances are caused either by environmental contaminants or by work-related ergonomic stress (repetitive movements or uncomfortable postures). One of the main characteristics of ESS is its tendency to precipitate fearsome epidemics of mass sociogenic illness.

The Swedish researchers provide numerous illustrations of ESS. They recount, for example, the outbreak of *chronic carbon monoxide poisoning* (CCMP) that swept through the Nordic countries in the 1940s and 1950s. During the World War II blockade of international transports, solid fuels had to be used in certain regions for heating and for driving motor vehicles. An increase in cases of actual carbon monoxide poisoning ensued and, with it, the fear of carbon monoxide in general. Solicitous clinic staff members evolved a new theory to explain their patients' vague symptoms, even those unaccompanied by any physical or laboratory abnormalities: perhaps they had been exposed to carbon monoxide at levels too low to cause acute illness. The health services soon found themselves flooded by patients who believed that the diagnosis of CCMP would explain their aches and pains.

But even after the war had ended and the petroleum fuel supply had finally been restored, the influx of patients with symptoms of CCMP did not stop. It took the passage of many more years for change to occur. The erosion of interest in CCMP as an explanation came only after it was demonstrated that the classic symptoms of CCMP (such as fatigue and subjective heart troubles) were found every bit as often in unexposed groups as in groups exposed to heavy doses of carbon monoxide.

Recently in selected areas in the United States, a debate surrounding the mandated use of reformulated gas precipitated a similar epidemic. In an initial trickle of protest, some citizens in southeastern Wisconsin claimed that the gas, which contains additives that make it burn more cleanly, caused them to suffer headaches, nausea, and respiratory problems. Heavy media coverage followed, turning the trickle into a groundswell of public fury. Thousands of residents began registering their discontent with legislators and local officials. However, after interviewing 1,339 Wisconsin residents and thoroughly investigating the complaints, health officials were able to confirm that the fears were baseless. They pointed out, for instance, that there had been no outbreaks of symptoms in the other states selling the very same reformulated gas. In short, reformulated gas has only one effect: reducing air pollution.

Our preoccupations with environmental "diseases" are often transient in just this way. In the 1970s and 1980s, *oral galvanism, micromercurialism,* and *metal syndrome* became popular explanations, both in the United States and Europe, for whatever ailed you. The first theory underlying these neologistic terms was that symptoms such as anxiety, mild dysphoria, and poor sleep could be explained by tiny currents from the metals in dental work. Eventually, that theory gave way to the belief that the leaching of mercury from amalgam fillings was the cause. The resulting media frenzy was staggering. Göthe and his colleagues note, for example, that the largest daily newspaper in Sweden emblazoned a 1989 article with the headline "The Amalgam Must Be Forbidden! The Dental Profession Mass Produces Autoimmune Diseases!" In the story, the reporter shrilly leveled erroneous accusations that mercury from fillings was the cause of a motley assortment of maladies, including multiple sclerosis, myasthenia gravis, allergic disorders, and asthma.

Like CCMP, this explanation gradually lost its popularity. A large number of careful studies refuted the notion that amalgam restorations present any kind of health risk, and even alarmists found it difficult to argue with solid data. In fact, a 1992 study indicated that children with amalgam fillings actually had a *lower* prevalence of allergies and asthma than children without them.

The list that opens this chapter includes one item that further establishes that mass ESS is by no means confined to Western countries. The fifth item, the case from the West Bank of Jordan, refers to an epidemic of abdominal pain and other symptoms that started when a 17-year-old schoolgirl reported that the sulfur smell from a lavatory had made her sick. Within three hours, 62 other students had developed pain and nausea. Over the next three days, 727 schoolgirls and 222 other people (both Arabs and Israelis) were struck. In this case, unbridled media coverage and the tense emotional climate in Djenin Hospital clearly exacerbated the situation. In essence, a disagreeable odor was transformed through word of mouth into a dangerous airborne toxin.

According to the Swedish study, a variant of ESS is at the root of the U.S. epidemic of "repetitive strain injuries" (from typing, for instance), which now account for 60% of all workplace illnesses. Undeniably, repetitive strain injuries are a real physical problem for some people, but factors such as boredom, constant pressure to produce, poor labor-management relations, and the challenge of rapidly changing technology ("technostress") seem to have helped carry them to epidemic proportions.

▌ Sick Buildings and Sick People

Sick building syndrome—in which masses of employees become ill due to "toxins" in the workplace—is yet another new subtype of ESS. Sick building syndrome has certainly spread far beyond the workplace, however. In its most extreme form, people with this puzzling disorder (sometimes saddled with the rubrics *multiple chemical sensitivity; environmental illness, 20th-century disease*, or *total allergy syndrome*) claim to have become temporarily paralyzed from just a whiff of perfume; in response, some churches have asked congregants to leave their Chanel No. 5 at home. Being near electrical appliances can ostensibly disable victims as well or cause what appears to be a drunken stupor *(electric allergy)*. Terms such as *carbonless copy paper syndrome* have been coined in an effort to attribute dizziness, palpitations, and headaches to specific chemical substances.

Todd Haynes's 1995 film *Safe*, which has been dubbed an "environmental horror movie," tells the story of homemaker Carol White, a victim of 20th-century disease. Fatigued and prone to frightening coughing jags, Carol treks from her luxury home in L.A. to a chemically free safe haven in New Mexico. She seeks relief from the "poisons" of her shampoo, her husband's cologne, even her new sofa ("totally toxic," she calls it). Carol finds a network of similarly afflicted people, many of whom wear face masks and oxygen tanks as naturally as jeans. Ultimately, though, Carol's quandary emerges as an indistinct and complex one: is her illness *really* a toxic reaction to the environment? Or is it her only route of escape from a life of numbing complacency, deference, and predictability?

In the rush to isolate the disease-causing agents, the potential role of such intricate psychosocial factors in propagating the symptoms is routinely ignored. ESS patients and their supporters often establish pressure groups to influence the media and lobby authorities, as though they should be the arbiters of what constitutes "real" disease. These steps result in what Göthe and colleagues describe as

> expensive, medically senseless, and potentially dangerous countermeasures of a quasiscientific nature. . . . This not only intensifies [the patients'] complaints and prevents rational therapy founded on scientific principles and reliable experience, but also further propagates the disorder in the community.

Self-labeled victims and their advocates, including their attorneys, may also beg the question of the authenticity of the toxic threat. Far too often, their polemical response is, Whether or not any toxic exposure has ever been proved, we *believe* there's a problem. That should be enough. We expect the requisite modifications to be implemented—regardless of cost. If the modifications are not made, lawsuits are predictably filed against architects, office building owners, manufacturers, and contractors.

A new type of specialist called the "clinical ecologist" has cropped up to deal with the alleged environmental culprits. No longer are "spirits" to blame for the symptoms; now formaldehyde fumes from particleboard or electromagnetic fields are the standard explanations offered. As a result, the specialist typically recommends widespread, even drastic structural modifications—such as high-powered ventilation systems, uncarpeted floors, metal kitchen cabinets, sophisticated water filtration equipment, and nonfluorescent lights—of which the therapeutic effects are dubious. For example, even after moving into one thoroughly outfitted "sterile" apartment complex called Ecology House, sufferers continued to have headaches, pain, and insomnia. Rather than acknowledge the likely psychological underpinnings to their symptoms, the residents came up with a new explanation: the unsealed concrete walls. *Why not just seal them up?* Not so fast—for, as one consultant on the project put it, "Not everybody tolerates sealers." Some residents have taken to sleeping on balconies or in bathtubs to escape the "fumes."

▌ Mass Anxiety

As we've pointed out in our discussion of mass sociogenic illness, mass hysteria as a whole has always been more likely to arise when people are dissatisfied with existing conditions or feel on edge. And these tribulations, such as those caused by the gust of modernization that has swept through parts of Africa, may be far outside the control of any one person. Another example is the constant strife in Guatemala that has resulted from extreme poverty, political and judicial corruption, and unchecked street crime. The result has been a child-snatching hysteria: unknown numbers of panicked Guatemalan parents harbor the unfounded belief that their children—often their only precious belongings—are being abducted by foreigners as forced organ donors. Innocent Americans visiting the country have sometimes been attacked and almost killed by angry mobs certain that the foreigners were trafficking in human organs.

A "stress-and-strain" model, then, can apply to cases of mass hysteria, including those in which severe anxiety bubbles over even though physical complaints per se do not arise. An American example of this mass anxiety is the "Seattle windshield-pitting epidemic" in the 1950s that stemmed from the tensions that had built up over hydrogen bomb tests. A few residents thought they had noted pitting marks in the windshields of their automobiles, and anxiety over the apparent nuclear fallout reigned until they could be reassured. The same climate of unease gave rise to the McCarthyism that overtook the United States during this period. Arthur Miller's 1953 play *The Crucible*, based on the Salem witch hunts, was simultaneously a cautionary tale for a country then gripped by an anticommunist frenzy.

Conflicts between governments have had similar results elsewhere. The widespread reports of a phantom slasher in Taipei arose from the insecurities of the Taiwanese, who faced a tense confrontation between their government and that of Communist China. Indeed, such baseless mass sightings have emerged around the world as among the most common manifestations of mass anxiety.

For five months in 1946, for example, UFOs were sighted all across Scandinavia, especially Sweden. A theory arose among inhabitants that remote-controlled German rockets, confiscated by the Soviets at the end of World War II, were being test-fired over the hapless countries. Newspapers reinforced this misimpression of "blue-white ghost rockets" and "radio-controlled bombs," contorting rumor into published fact. Because the war had ended only a year earlier, residents were all too ready to interpret these celestial signs as ominous. Swedish military defense personnel launched an official investigation in which they encouraged residents to report sightings; they then explored the "crash sites." "Bomb fragments" were analyzed and coincidental fires blamed on the rockets. A lake was drained to look for clues. Even the deaths of three cows were attributed to poisonous material carried by a projectile.

But the cows died because cows die. The bomb fragments were old antennae or other refuse. And the rockets turned out to have resulted from a confluence of astronomical and meteorological circumstances: solar and comet activity had produced the ghost rockets.

These sightings represented a particularly large and diffuse outbreak of mass anxiety. Although obviously disruptive, the mass hysteria in this case also paradoxically helped the Swedes and others. The citizens were able to turn their amorphous fears of potential Soviet domination into a series of concrete events—the rocket sightings. Their anxiety could then be contained by being directed toward a specific, tangible threat.

There have been many other sightings that have later emerged as dubious at best. Great groups of people thought, for a time, that they had spotted a "phantom" Virgin Mary in Egypt. Such unconfirmed group apparitions of Mary have been reported over the centuries in locations ranging from Mexico, France, and Belgium to Conyers, Georgia, and Hollywood, Florida. In other examples of sightings, a "phantom monoplane" appeared over South Africa and a "phantom anesthetist" struck Matoon, Illinois.

▌ An Equal Opportunity Affliction?

In the examples we've discussed throughout this chapter, many people were drawn into the whirlwind of hysteria, but not everyone in the same place at the same time was. *Why not?*

Adding to the complexity of mass hysteria is the fact that our age and sex affect our susceptibility. Because they are generally more responsive to social cues, for example, females are affected more commonly than males. Impressionable children and adolescents, less resilient than adults, have also emerged as the likelier victims of mass sociogenic illness.

Another factor, differences in personal suggestibility and susceptibility, becomes especially notable when mass hysteria strikes a group in which all the members are of the same age and sex. When 34 Thai girls suffered a sudden bout of screaming, shaking, and hallucinating, for instance, 34 classmates who did not develop any symptoms were examined by psychiatrists as well. It turned out that those consumed by the hysteria were more anxious and fearful to begin with and some had had "trances" at other times in the past or had witnessed spirit-possession ceremonies. In other words, this subgroup of girls was more vulnerable to mass hysteria before they all came together on that fateful day.

The same dynamic applies in other cases: who is affected and who is not isn't random. In the case of mass sociogenic illness in Norwood, Massachusetts, the children who became sick were already at higher risk. They were shown by researchers to have been much more likely to have experienced loss through parental divorce or the death of a family member and thus their backgrounds were viewed as more unsettled.

People contending with acute demands are predisposed to mass hysteria as well. Consider the following case. In 1994, a local resident named Gloria Ramirez was brought to Riverside General Hospital in Los Angeles nearly in cardiac arrest. As a nurse drew blood, an overwhelming ammonia smell seemed to rise from Ramirez's body. Seven ER staffers were overcome, falling to the floor as they approached. Others experienced muscles spasms and had trouble breathing.

Had Ms. Ramirez been the victim of a bizarre medical malady or of a tainted street drug? She died before anyone could question her. Like technicians in a "hot zone," doctors donned space suits to perform the autopsy. The findings were that Ramirez had died from kidney failure brought on by cervical cancer . . . which did not explain the incapacitating odor.

Ms. Ramirez's family sued over the defamation of the deceased as theories multiplied about the cause of the fumes. What sort of lifestyle had she lived? What kind of sordid chemical agents might she have put into her body?

Six months later, the State Department of Health Services reviewed the medical records of five of the staff members who had had to be hospitalized after exposure to the ghastly smell, as well as 34 other workers at Riverside. They pored over the investigations performed by others, including scientists at the Lawrence Livermore Laboratories.

The state investigators discovered that the batteries of tests were all negative. They also found that the factor that most strongly predicted the development of symptoms was not exposure to Ms. Ramirez's body. Rather, the most highly correlated features of the victims were being a female paraprofessional and working in an acutely stressful environment. The investigators also noted that the paramedics who treated Ms. Ramirez in an ambulance for 14 minutes prior to her arrival at Riverside, and who drew and even spilled her blood, detected no odor and experienced no unusual symptoms. The state concluded that mass sociogenic illness was to blame.

Case closed? Not entirely. The county coroner later released an amended report claiming that an odd chain of chemical reactions in Ramirez's blood had produced a deadly nerve gas. Victims eagerly pointed to this medical explanation as their vindication, but others have bitterly disputed it as a transparent effort to appease riled workers—including one who had filed a $6 million lawsuit. The final, decisive chapter may never be written in the strange saga of Gloria Ramirez.

▌ You Can't Bank on It

As we pointed out in our list at the beginning of the chapter, even an impersonal entity—the American banking system—has fallen prey to mass hysteria.

How? As Richard X. Bove points out in an article in *American Banker,* the prices of U.S. bank stocks in 1990 went wild. The seeds of panic were sown by the fact that the thrift industry was virtually bankrupt. Although this problem was real, it was magnified out of all proportion by worried investors. Congress issued reports claiming that the whole banking system was in jeopardy, and the alarm was sounded: *the U.S. banking system was no longer safe!*

Millions of people were swept up. Frantic depositors withdrew tens of billions of dollars from their accounts. Regulators audited the banks according to rigid and unrealistic standards, and, in response to their gloomy decrees, Congress demanded that more reserves be tied up in bank coffers to protect against predicted losses. One Wall Street brokerage firm after another assailed the management of the banks, and the cost of bank funding swelled inexorably.

In the melee, bank stock prices plunged. Loans to small and medium-sized businesses had to be yanked, and real estate projects could no longer be funded. Highly leveraged firms were forced to fire millions of workers.

That finally grabbed the president's attention. He pressured regulators to ease up, and aggressive steps were taken to inspire renewed confidence in the banking system. Interest rates were cut, and incentives to lend were supplied.

The scare had come and gone. But the episode proved that witch hunts and tulipomania are always poised to descend once again.

FINAL THOUGHTS— TREATMENT FOR LIES OF THE MIND

Learning From the Past, Catapulting Into the Future

Hope is the feeling you have
that the feeling you have isn't permanent.

—Jean Kerr (1923–)
Finishing Touches

▌ A Brief History of Treatment

In the distant past, many people who had the psychological problems we've discussed in this book were dealt with in an unfortunate, albeit decisive way: they were literally removed from society, often by being institutionalized, at times even by being put to death. In fact, it wasn't until 1792 that a move toward moral treatment was initiated in Europe, eventually crossing the Atlantic to the United States.

The term *moral treatment* meant just that: ethical principles had finally wormed their way into the care of patients with mental disorders. Patients were respected as individuals who were suffering from faulty rearing or from an illness, not transgressors who were wicked and being justly punished by God. They were housed in small institutional settings that deliberately mimicked a large family. There they were fed, clothed, and encouraged to engage in gentle exercise and recreation. Physical restraint was always the last resort.

Meanwhile, U.S. psychiatry officially came into being. In 1844, 13 physicians who directed "insane asylums" formed the forerunner of what is now the American Psychiatric Association. Termed *alienists*, these physicians promoted the belief that the mentally ill belonged in specialized treatment settings. Public enthusiasm for institutional treatment was furthered by moral treatment's impressive cure rates (which its advocates sometimes inflated). By 1887, every state had established at least one public hospital to serve the mentally ill.

But these facilities expanded too slowly to handle the massive influx of patients. People desperately in need of care simply overwhelmed the meager system. Adding to the turmoil, public institutions often housed immigrants and the impoverished in addition to those considered insane. At first, towns and cities paid for the care of their citizens but, to cut costs, some began to relegate patients to local almshouses. To stop this practice, officials declared mental patients wards of the state, entitling them once again to state hospital care. But communities seized this opportunity to shift to state coffers the cost of caring for people who were elderly, physically disabled, or demented.

Inundated as they were, over the next several decades these state facilities evolved into impersonal institutions housing over 1,000 patients each. Lengths of stay increased from a few months to many years. The pendulum had swung back. In 1895, for example, a hard-hearted editorial in the *Journal of the American Medical Association* decried "the sentimental tendency to demanding all possible freedom and lack of restraint for the insane." So much for empathic moral treatment.

Few truly useful medications were available during the 1800s. Instead, primitive tranquilizers or narcotics were sometimes employed to blunt the "madness." Morphine, various tonics, aromatics such as ether, and even hemlock derivatives and wine were among the pharmacologic options. Sometimes these agents were combined. Brigham's Mixture, for example, was a concoction that included conium from the poison hemlock, ferric carbonate, wine, molasses, and sassafras oil. A physician who self-experimented by swallowing an extract from fresh conium seeds experienced partial leg paralysis for two days.

If these substances were either unavailable or insufficient to control the symptoms, physical restraint or outright physical abuse were other mechanisms employed in the name of treatment. Bloodletting and mechanical devices such as the spinning "tranquilizer chair" were used in some cases, though by the mid-19th century they were falling out of favor with doctors. *Phrenology* (touching and interpreting the shape of a patient's head) was also losing its luster.

In 1994, Drs. Jeffrey Geller and Maxine Harris published *Women of the Asylum*, a book filled with the actual writings of women who spent time in the early asylums. They quote a woman named Tirzah F. Shedd, who, in 1865, wrote about the horrors of institutional treatment:

> I once saw Miss Conkling held under the water, until almost dead, and I feared she would never get her breath again.
>
> I saw Mrs. Comb held by the hair of her head under a streaming faucet, and handfuls of hair were pulled from her head, by their rough handling, simply because she would not eat when she was not hungry.
>
> I have seen the attendants strike the hands of the patients with their keys, so as to leave black and blue spots for days.
>
> I have seen them pinch their ears and arms and shoulders and shake them, when they felt that they could not eat; and were thus forced to eat when their stomachs were so rejecting it as to be retching at the time.
>
> There is one married woman there who has been imprisoned seven times by her husband, and yet she is intelligent and entirely sane.
>
> When will married women be safe from her husband's power?
>
> And yet, she must assert her own rights, for the government does not protect her rights, as it does her husband's, and then run the risk of being called insane for so doing! I do not think the men who make the laws for us, would be willing to exchange places with us.
>
> This house seems to me to be more a place of punishment, than a place of cure. I have often heard the patients say:
>
> "This is a wholesale slaughter-house!"

In the early and mid-1900s, a few psychiatric procedures were developed that were sometimes surprisingly effective, particularly with those who suffered from psychosis or depression. One of these procedures, still in vogue in some Eastern European countries, was *insulin coma therapy*. Also called "insulin shock," it involved administering insulin to a patient to lower his or her blood sugar so far that seizures or coma resulted. Patients with schizophrenia or other psychotic disorders sometimes showed considerable improvement with this technique—but it carried with it a 1% mortality rate. *Frontal leukotomy*, and even more extensive brain surgery called *frontal lobotomy*, emerged in the 1930s. These procedures would reliably reduce patients' violent outbursts, but at a high price: they also rendered them listless and apathetic, seeming to destroy their souls. Nonetheless, the early enthusiasm for such "psychosurgery" won Portugese neurologist Egas Moniz the 1949 Nobel prize, and a highly refined brain operation called *cingulotomy* is still performed in the United States in rare cases. *Convulsive therapy*, introduced for psychiatric illness in 1938, involved administering seizure-inducing agents such as camphor and pentylenetetrazol and was often helpful in the short-term for reasons that were unclear. It was later supplanted by the use of huge boluses of electricity in early *electroconvulsive therapy*, or ECT. This primitive ECT was administered without the sedatives and muscle relaxants that are standard today. Although they bear no relation to the way ECT is now practiced, these archaic techniques continue to alarm potential candidates for the treatment who have seen the movie *One Flew Over the Cuckoo's Nest*.

Medications that were dramatically more effective than those previously available began to arrive on the scene in the 1950s. With the discoveries of chlorpromazine (an antipsychotic medication) and amitriptyline (an antidepressant), the mushrooming population of the state asylums finally began to plateau and then decline from its high of 558,000.

The early to mid-1960s was an especially prominent time of change—not always beneficial, however—for those with serious mental disorders. The trend of the nation was toward enhancing civil liberties, and this helping hand reached out to those housed in institutions. The nation was also seized with the initiative to enable and ensure community treatment. Patients were to be treated in their own towns, around familiar places and faces. As excitement over this new ideal grew, many patients, including those whose severe mental illnesses had led to years of institutional confinement, were suddenly discharged from state hospitals—a phenomenon called *deinstitutionalization*.

But although hearts were in the right place, dollars were not. Fewer than half of the projected community mental health centers were actually established. Those that were opened were charged with expanding their services to the waves of the newly discharged, but state and federal legislatures failed to provide enough money. The result? In many states, so-called *transinstitutionalization* occurred and continues to occur. Patients are rarely in state mental hospitals; instead, they've ended up in meager substitutes such as nursing homes, boarding homes, jails, or homeless shelters. Those with milder lies of the mind can retain their jobs and insurance; those with the worst forms typically cannot. With the spotlight continuing to shine on the financing of health care, mental health clinicians continually try to juggle the demands of ensuring high-quality care and ready availability as the rottweiler of cost controls nips at their heels.

Our hopes for the present and future stem from the progress being made on many fronts. The advances in psychiatry have accelerated as psychiatrists have become better able to identify the mental illnesses that afflict their patients. The American Psychiatric Association's *Diagnostic and Statistical Manual of Mental Disorders*, now in its fourth edition (and abbreviated as DSM-IV), compiles mental illnesses into logical groups and subgroups and lists objective criteria for the diagnosis of each. Thus, clinicians can diagnose their patient's maladies with accuracy and consistency. At the same time, our understanding of the reasons our minds betray us is expanding. The long-held societal view that mental illness is a collection of "uns"—undefinable, untreatable, unpredictable, and uninsurable—is gradually changing. Technologies are being invented and refined, and new medications and different forms of therapy are being tested every day. Importantly, mental health professionals are talking—and honestly thinking—in terms of recovery for patients, not just maintenance.

All of these favorable developments are being fueled by the emergence of the consumer movement among patients and the advocacy organizations that have developed among family members and other concerned individuals. They point out that, at any given time, 25% of the hospital beds in the United States are filled by patients with mental disorders—more than the combined total for cancer, heart disease, and respiratory illness.

The numbers are impressive, to say the least. Shouldn't our response be as well?

■ Evaluation Is a Powerful Tool: Assessing Lies of the Mind

Throughout this book, we have offered examples of psychological conditions that range in severity from occasional nuisances to extreme intrusions. Some appear out of the blue. Others are insidious but relentless in their development. Regardless of the precise features, all of these maladaptive ways of thinking, feeling, and behaving have to be assessed and treated in a consistent and logical way. Sensible treatment always originates from a careful evaluation.

The evaluation can be as simple as an interview or as complex as a battery of brain tests that includes *neuropsychiatric testing*, *magnetic resonance imaging* (MRI), and *cerebrospinal fluid analysis* (through a spinal tap). Techniques such as *functional MRI*, *positron emission tomography* (PET), and *single photon emission computed tomography* (SPECT) can literally illustrate the malfunctioning brain. As Kay Redfield Jamison writes in her 1995 memoir *The Unquiet Mind*,

> a depressed brain [in manic depression] will show up in cold, brain-inactive
> deep blues, dark purples, and hunter greens; the same brain when hypo-

manic, however, is lit up like a Christmas tree, with vivid patches of bright reds and yellows and oranges. Never has the color and structure of science so completely captured the cold inward deadness of depression or the vibrant, active engagement of mania.

Often, however, the style and sensitivity of the examiner are more important than the technologies brought into play. Without an alliance between the doctor and patient, assessment and treatment efforts are shackled.

The individuals whom mental health care providers see have a rainbow of attitudes about the whole affair. Some patients come enthusiastically, eager to conquer a distressing problem and sure that, with a little help, they can do so. Others are defensive and distrustful, feeling coerced into a form of treatment still highly stigmatized in our society. We have found that the social pleasantries that come naturally with the cooperative patient—a calm demeanor, the introduction of oneself, a handshake—can be even more important with the angry individual. These social rituals depathologize the setting, announcing that "though I'm the 'psychiatrist' and you're the 'patient,' above all we're just two people who hopefully will be working together toward common goals." All of us respond best when we know that we are being respected and truly listened to. Initial questions will be open ended and will concern the feelings and events that have been causing trouble. Gentle follow-up questions that communicate caring allow patients to express what is important to *them*.

We have also discovered that we can learn a lot from pregnant pauses and halfhearted answers. Patients sometimes tell doctors only what they think they want to hear. Following up on hesitant replies ("Oh, I'm all right, I guess"), weak endorsements ("The medication's probably working, but I'm really not sure"), and circumlocutions ("My marriage? Could be better, could be worse") has allowed us to tap into reservoirs of emotion and worry that the patient would otherwise have left concealed.

Patients use much more than their voices to tell their stories. Their manner of interacting, their style of dress, the movements of their bodies—all contribute vital pieces to the diagnostic puzzle. Brief "snapshots" from actual cases will be provided throughout this chapter to illustrate specific points.

Kyra (as told by Jackie)

Kyra is so familiar to us that we know exactly what to watch for when she's becoming ill. Sometimes it isn't subtle. She pranced into the clinic one morning dressed from head to toe in green, like an avocado with legs. On her head was a hat of crushed jade-green velvet with a green plume fluttering from it, and she was clad in a tight green silk dress, green fishnet stockings, and green sequined shoes. Her makeup was vivid as well, with glaring eye shadow and luscious red lipstick adorning her face. She had applied stick-on nails and painted them a rainbow of colors, pasting green "sparklies" (as she called them) onto six of them. Each finger was adorned with a large rhinestone ring.

Kyra snapped her fingers at the secretary, pointed to my office, and proceeded in without knocking. She almost dragged her father in behind her. She leaned over my desk, fists tightly clenched on her hips, and looked around in a conspiratorial fashion.

"Are we alone?" she whispered. "Where are the bugs? Can we talk?" She then let loose with the ear-scorching collection of curses she always produces when her mental disorder flares.

Green is Kyra's manic color. We use her flamboyant appearance as a guide to assess the degree to which she is ill. When she is feeling fine, she is pleasant and easygoing, and she dresses neatly in casual clothes. Through the radical alteration in her manner of dressing, speaking, and interacting, she lets us know—unmistakably—when she is getting sick, even before any of us has asked a single question.

As Kyra's occasional fashion statements illustrate, clinicians need to notice nonverbal clues. Are the patient's clothing and hairstyle appropriate (even given hefty allowances for taste)? Is the patient easy or difficult to engage in conversation? If easy, is he or she in fact so loquacious you can't get a word in edgewise? Is the patient's thinking clear, or is it much like a bunch of superimposed road maps, so convoluted that you can't possibly begin to follow it? As we've seen in every chapter, lies of the mind can be glaring (such as violence sparked by command hallucinations) or so subtle that they are unearthed only with careful observation and detailed questioning (such as quiet, singular delusions or specific phobias).

In evaluating a patient, *collateral* information is, paradoxically enough, central. Collateral information is that obtained from family members and others knowledgeable about the patient's life. We need to make every attempt to speak with a relative or someone else who can comment on how the patient is and has been functioning.

Determining the Cause

The source of the trouble.   Certainly, there are many reasons for psychological ailments. We have talked about some of them already. In any kind of medical care, the patient and practitioner must try to understand what is causing the symptoms before a full plan of treatment can intelligently be devised. To treat the symptom alone (the Band-Aid approach) may well mean that we are missing a looming underlying problem. A few staples and some glue will not repair a bridge on the verge of collapse.

The best approach is the broad approach. The list of physical conditions that can cause emotional symptoms, for instance, is stupefying. Those who zealously embark on treatment without attention to these factors will often find that they have performed a serious disservice. A number of examples will illustrate the point.

1. Alcohol and other substances can wreak havoc on one's psyche.   Heavy, long-term abuse can lead to disturbing phenomena such as protracted delusions or hallucinations. Perhaps the most dramatic mental disorder due to years of alcohol abuse is *Wernicke-Korsakoff syndrome*. People with Wernicke-Korsakoff syndrome have a severe impairment of memory, especially for recent events, that stems from a thiamine deficiency due to their alcohol use. They try to compensate for their defective memories through *confabulation*, giving ready, fluent, but inaccurate answers to fill in their memory gaps.

Scott (as told by Jackie)

I recently interviewed Scott, a patient with no prior psychiatric problems. He appeared very energetic and upbeat but nevertheless reported hearing frightening, castigating voices. Baffled, I arranged to continue the evaluation, and he returned two days later, now complaining not of hallucinations but of depression of suicidal proportions. This wildly shifting presentation led to a bit of detective work, and a conversation with the young man's girlfriend confirmed our suspicions. He had been abusing cocaine and was experiencing the fallout of the mood swings and occasional psychoses that can develop with cocaine addiction. Our focus moved away from considerations of possible schizophrenia or psychotic depression to the treatment of his substance abuse.

Gwendolyn (as told by Marc)

Years ago, I evaluated a woman named Gwendolyn, who had been brought to our hospital's emergency room after she was found cowering in a corner at work, trembling and terrified. Only very reluctantly did she reveal that she hadn't slept for days, was having persistent diarrhea, and was seeing flashes of light. The cause of these symptoms seemed to be stress: her mother had recently died and her daughter had been arrested three days earlier on charges of prostitution.

But further inquiry led to another disclosure: though she had always been a moderate coffee drinker, Gwendolyn had recently increased her coffee consumption to *50 cups a day* in order to "stay productive"! Despite the magnitude of the stressors in her life, we recognized that her extreme, disabling anxiety and other symptoms had been caused primarily by caffeine intoxication *(caffeinism)*.

When a mental disorder is precipitated by a substance, the obvious intervention is to assist the patient in reducing or eliminating its use. The clinician, family, and patient must thoroughly understand the nature of the addiction, however, because it is unsafe to stop certain substances abruptly.

2. Prescription and over-the-counter medications can also induce serious problems. For example, reserpine (a blood pressure medication), steroids, and birth control pills have all been associated with depression. Steroids have also been linked to episodes of psychosis. And many popular cold remedies, asthma preparations, and sleep medications have *anticholinergic* side effects. For susceptible individuals such as children, the elderly, or those with preexisting brain disease, these anticholinergic effects can cause emotional and behavioral symptoms as well.

Bert (as told by Jackie)

Bert was a 72-year-old man in fairly good health, although his memory was far from razor-sharp. After he had caught a cold, his wife gave him an over-the-counter medication that combined a decongestant and an antihistamine. Having forgotten that he had already taken a dose, Bert took two more capsules in the middle of the night. The next morning, his wife gave him some cough syrup and two 12-hour timed-release tablets (figuring that if one works, two will work twice as well).

By mid-morning, Bert was hauled to the doctor's office by his wife, who said, "He's talkin' out of his head. He's crazy. His face is all red and he can't stop talkin' or walkin'." The doctor discovered that Bert had a fever and a sharply elevated pulse rate and blood pressure. His pupils were dilated, he was breathing rapidly, and his mouth was very dry. It was apparent that Bert was experiencing toxicity from having taken too many medications with anticholinergic side effects. After a cardiac monitor was placed, Bert was treated with an antidote called physostigmine. Improvement was rapid, and after two days of hospitalization, he was discharged.

Anyone with troubled thoughts or behaviors should be examined and questioned thoroughly. Bert's case makes it clear that the practitioner must ascertain what medications, including over-the-counter preparations, patients are taking.

3. Diseases of the brain can sometimes masquerade as primary psychological distur-bances.   However, patterns in symptomatology can provide essential clues. Pa-tients with Alzheimer's disease and other forms of dementia, for example, may become anxious and paranoid toward dusk, a phenomenon called *sundowning.* The reason for this predictable deterioration is that as darkness falls, the visual stimuli that help keep demented patients alert and aware become less apparent. At the same time, particularly on hospital wards and in nursing homes, the bustle of the daytime hours is being replaced by a less active, ostensibly more relaxing routine. For the pa-tient with dementia, the reduction in stimulation can trigger disorientation.

Although physicians often reflexively use medications to calm such patients, simple changes in the environment to enhance stimulation might do the trick. Ex-amples are having the patient remain in the TV/recreation room during the evening and leaving a few lights on at night.

4. Excesses or deficiencies in body chemicals can cause lies of the mind as well.   For instance, having too little or too much sodium or calcium in one's system can cause symptoms spanning the spectrum from lethargy, somnolence, and depression to agi-tation and even psychosis. Patients with too much thyroid hormone can be jittery, impulsive, and confused. Deficiencies of vitamins such as B_{12} or folate can cause pa-tients to appear psychotic, depressed, or amnestic. In a famous example, England's King George III suffered from spells of "madness" due to his body's improper me-tabolism of yet another chemical, delta-aminolevulinic acid.

Vanessa (as told by Jackie)

Vanessa was a skinny, mildly mentally retarded 22-year-old woman with schizophrenia. She came to our clinic one day looking and acting fearful and suspicious. Although she and her mother both insisted that she had been tak-ing her psychiatric medications conscientiously, I was sufficiently concerned about relapse that I admitted her to the hospital. While waiting for the paper-work to clear, I quickly performed a "review of systems" check, asking the pa-tient and her mother detailed questions to see whether she were having symptoms in any part of her body. Vanessa replied only that she had had a cold for over a week; her nose had been runny and she coughed now and then. I thought little of it.

Once Vanessa was admitted to the ward, however, the nurses noted that her heart rate was high, she was breathing fast but shallowly, and she had a temperature of 101.5 degrees. The resident listened to her lungs and thought that she detected congestion on one side. Follow-up tests revealed that Vanessa was suffering from pneumonia, and, as a result, that the level of oxygen circulating in her blood was far too low. We had discovered that her precarious state—her confused thinking and agitated behavior—was attributable not to a worsening of her schizophrenia but to her physical illness: there simply wasn't enough oxygen traveling via her blood to her brain.

We continually remind ourselves that everyone has the potential to become physically ill, including patients who have preexisting mental illnesses. Clinicians, patients, and families should remember that mental deterioration can and often does have a medical cause.

5. Vascular difficulties, such as atherosclerotic changes in the brain that reduce blood flow, can cause impressive transformations in personality. As early as 1812, Dr. Benjamin Rush (the "Father of American Psychiatry") suggested that poor blood supply to the brain was the cause of serious mental disorders. *Strokes* are among the vascular problems that frequently cause psychiatric symptoms, either by directly damaging brain tissue or by inducing *poststroke depressions* that are often responsive to antidepressants.

Edward (as told by Jackie)

Edward's wife brought him to me because he constantly accused her of having an affair, although he acknowledged that he could "never catch the culprit." His personality had changed radically from cheerful to venomous. A computed tomography (CT) scan of Edward's brain showed that he had recently suffered a small stroke. With time and a reduction in the swelling in the area of the stroke, Edward reverted back to his sunnier disposition.

Other types of vascular abnormalities can create immense mood, personality, and cognitive changes as well. For example, *collagen vascular diseases* such as systemic lupus erythematosus can induce serious mental changes; patients with brain involvement can become deeply confused and psychotic, even delirious. Treatment with medications can often restore more normal thinking by addressing the underlying inflammation of the brain.

6. Localized or widespread infections can cause people to look and act very strangely. Patients with AIDS, for instance, can experience effects on the central nervous system that induce mania, depression, or psychosis. Infections should be ruled out as possible causes of psychiatric symptoms. If detected, they must be treated with the appropriate antimicrobial medications.

Pamela (as told by Jackie)

When I was in medical school, our team evaluated Pamela, a 38-year-old professional woman who offered a rather unusual story. She reported a rapid worsening in her memory such that she was losing her way around the city (in which she was born and raised) and forgetting appointments despite carrying around an appointment book. She finally came to the emergency room when she started to experience paranoid feelings and hear denigrating voices. Her work was suffering terribly, as were her relationships with family members.

We hospitalized Pamela and performed a complete physical workup, including CT scan, spinal tap, and dozens of blood tests. Every result was normal except for one: the presence of white blood cells in the spinal fluid was a very worrisome finding, because usually there are none. Unable to find the cause through the usual studies, the treatment team finally had to recommend a radical approach: a brain biopsy. Pamela and her exasperated family agreed. The initial biopsy results were normal and, after six weeks of intensive evaluation, Pamela was discharged on an antipsychotic drug, having obtained little relief from her symptoms.

Within two weeks of her discharge, however, a culture of the brain biopsy tissue had grown out a bacterium called *Brucella*. We recognized it to be the elusive cause of her cognitive problems. Pamela was treated with antibiotics and responded beautifully. After a period of convalescence, she was able to resume her excellent functioning.

7. Neoplasms or tumors, benign or malignant, can also initially manifest themselves through psychiatric symptoms.

Millie (as told by Jackie)

Millie's family had brought her to the emergency department because she had apparently experienced a hallucination of sorts while driving. During the episode, she seemed sure that someone else had gotten into the car with her, spoken to her, and then gotten out. A daughter who witnessed the scene said that her mother had turned to the unoccupied right front seat and spoken as though someone were there.

Millie's physical examination was normal, and her neurologic exam   to which I had paid particular attention—seemed just fine. But I still felt uncomfortable. Erring on the side of caution, I requested a formal neurologic consultation.

Unfortunately, the neurologist who was assigned to Millie didn't care much for "psychiatric" patients. After a cursory exam, he wrote in the patient's chart, "Nonfocal [i.e., normal] exam on this 47-year-old white female." I was worried about the superficiality of his exam, and went ahead and ordered a CT scan of Millie's brain. Unfortunately, my gut instinct proved correct. Millie had what turned out to be an advanced and inoperable *astrocytoma* (a particularly vicious type of malignant tumor). She died just six months later.

Not all brain tumors are malignant, but they can cause people to behave strangely and should never be ignored as a diagnostic possibility. Many times, removing the tumor restores the patient to a completely normal state.

8. Bizarre behavior and thoughts can be seen in people who have suffered head trauma. The case of Joey in Chapter 6 who, after a motorcycle accident, developed tactile hallucinations of bugs in his throat demonstrates just how powerful the effects of trauma can be.

Peter (as told by Marc)

Like Joey, Peter was a young man who had suffered a serious head injury as a result of a motorcycle accident (neither Joey nor Peter had been wearing safety helmets; at that time, fewer than half of the states required them). Peter's personality had changed radically as a result. Although sometimes placid and agreeable, he was now prone to fits of scathing verbal abuse. His wife had initially tried to trace his outbursts to something she had said or done, but continual walking on eggshells did nothing to appease him. It became starkly evident that his anger was entirely unprovoked, and she accepted a counselor's advice to move out. The finality of the separation, and the impenetrable insulation his wife's family provided around her, led Peter mournfully to seek help, signing himself into our psychiatric hospital.

Unmistakably, it was the dreadful damage to Peter's brain that had created this modern-day Jekyll and Hyde. There simply was no way to resurrect the destroyed tissue. Within several hours, Peter was angry with the staff, throwing away the trial medication he had agreed to take only minutes earlier.

Psychiatrists learn early in their careers to abandon their rescue fantasies:

some patients simply cannot be induced to grab the only lifeline in sight. I did my best to change Peter's mind, but it was apparent that I was neither powerful nor persuasive enough to succeed. It is illegal to force treatment on a patient (barring court intercession or a clinical emergency), so we had no other options. Peter signed himself out of the hospital after less than one day there.

The individual's state of mind. Our review of the organic explanations for "psychological" problems leads to the following moral: given that there are many physical abnormalities and substances—both legal and illegal—that can have overwhelming effects on the brain, each patient must be evaluated thoroughly. It can be disastrous to miss an organic basis to a behavioral change, because all subsequent treatment efforts will be misguided.

At the same time, we do have to accept that some lies of the mind do not involve a physical abnormality. Overzealous, repeated medical testing will only increase the patient's discomfort and drive up the medical bill; simultaneously, actual treatment will be delayed. Some psychiatric problems, for example, stem from the patient's unconscious use of primitive or immature defense mechanisms. Others occur in direct response to overwhelming stressors.

Research is helping us to make distinctions between organic and nonorganic causes. Recent interest has focused on aberrant levels of *neurotransmitters*, natural chemicals in the brain that help it function correctly. For example, depression may be related to reduced levels of the transmitters *serotonin* and *norepinephrine*, whereas schizophrenia is thought to be associated in part with elevated *dopamine* levels.

But no currently available lab test will allow us to pinpoint any of these possibilities as the cause of a given patient's symptoms. Although we always like to trumpet our research successes, we are still at only a basic level of understanding how the brain functions and malfunctions. Psychiatry has made great strides in the identification of mental disorders and the relief of human suffering. Yet, as a relatively young discipline, it has far to go in uncovering the causes of and cures for mental illness.

▋ The Treatment Palette Today

Before discussing the mainstays of psychiatric treatment—namely, the various types of therapy and medications—we need to reinforce some overarching principles that mothers have always advocated. Regardless of the precise causes of a person's mental disorder, he or she needs to adhere to a nutritious diet and engage in at least moderate physical activity. Maintenance of consistent hours for sleep and activity and identification and reduction of sources of stress are vital as well. (And nice friends never hurt.)

This commonsense advice often bears repeating as the doctor discusses his or her findings with the patient and the available family members or friends. The treatment plan is then devised with the participation, understanding, and agreement of everyone present. Expectations for recovery have to be balanced against the current realities of treatment options and prognosis.

We need to assess the patient's ability to comply with the treatment recommendations before he or she ever leaves the clinic or hospital. Advice is easy to offer but sometimes difficult to follow. Does the patient have a way to access essentials such as shelter, food, and clothing? Does he or she have enough money to buy the medications the doctor has prescribed? Does the patient clearly understand the medication regimen? Is an adequate support system in place so that the patient isn't adrift on a day-to-day basis?

For obvious reasons, compliance is massively hindered if the patient cannot accept that he or she has a psychiatric problem. Patients in denial typically refuse treatment. The degree to which medication side effects interfere with the patient's lifestyle—including the ability to get an education or a job—also needs to be addressed aggressively or treatment is doomed. Finally (and once again, mothers would agree), abstinence from abusable substances needs to be stressed continually.

Talking Your Way to Health

Advances in neurochemistry and neurobiology have focused unprecedented attention on the workings of the human brain. But what about the human mind? In our zeal to map out the interlocking networks of nerves and transmitters that comprise the brain, is there the possibility that the soul of psychiatric treatment—the rich relationship between patient and practitioner, the so-called talking cure—will be sacrificed? Will we ignore Henry David Thoreau's advice to "be a Columbus to whole new continents and worlds within you, opening new channels, not of trade, but of thought"?

This is indeed a risk that will only be magnified as difficult decisions are made about the costs of health care. Techniques and treatments that can prove their value—whether they be new generations of medications or of therapists—will prevail in the long run. But, at least for now, the odds seem strong that the human-to-human bond of therapy will remain the best approach for many patients. Even as new technology continually supplants the old, no one has yet developed a substitute for an experienced, empathic person with whom to talk. Computer therapy programs that parrot the patient's statements, or offer up variations on the hackneyed phrase "Tell me more about that" simply aren't quite the same—although enthusiastic software developers promise to surmount the technical, ethical, and human obstacles. And although medications are necessary in many psychiatric conditions, seldom are they sufficient for optimal results.

Over 200 named psychotherapies exist, and most of these share a few basic elements: a unifying theory of how the mind goes awry and how treatment works, positive regard for the patient, empathy for his or her distress, and hope for improvement. Many are structured to involve an individual and a therapist conversing privately on various issues important to the patient, and aim to explore the experience of the patient as a person. Marital (or couples) therapy, family therapy, and group therapy are also venues in which people—this time three or more—discuss a variety of important concerns.

Before we outline the enormous range of psychotherapies that are available, we should also talk about who might profit from therapy. Who are the ideal candidates? Patients who are aware that they are in emotional pain (or are causing others emotional pain), who are motivated to change, and who realize that difficult life problems take time to resolve will probably be best able to handle the hard work of therapy. Although some clinicians believe that patients need to be quite intelligent and highly verbal as well, it has been demonstrated repeatedly that many different kinds of patients can profit from therapy.

A plethora of psychotherapeutic models and techniques exists. Each has its ardent advocates and vehement detractors. The most sensible strategy is to tailor the type of therapy to the needs of the patient, not force him or her into rigid theoretical preconceptions. This approach means that sometimes therapists will need to admit to their own limitations. Sometimes they'll need to say flatly to patients, "I know what you need but I'm not the right person to provide it. Let me refer you to someone who is."

Being open-minded also means attempting to work within the context of the patient's cultural or subcultural beliefs and rituals. For example, the folk healers *(curanderas)* in Mexican American communities are too readily dismissed by physicians as intruders into the curative process. In some cases, a curandera can be incorporated into the treatment team as an informational and spiritual resource.

With these caveats reinforced, we will serve up a smorgasbord of psychotherapeutic techniques:

Psychoanalytic therapy.   *Psychoanalytic therapy* is based on the work of Sigmund Freud and others. The stereotype of the psychoanalytic situation—the triangular relationship of a bearded doctor, a densely neurotic patient, and a couch—is the one most Americans equate with psychiatry as a whole. In practice, however, traditional analysis has a limited role in contemporary psychiatric practice. Best suited to patients with deep-seated conflicts who nonetheless function adequately from day to day, analysis focuses on the role of the unconscious and the persistent influence in the here and now of unresolved psychological conflicts that occurred in childhood. The goals of psychoanalytic therapy are to resolve life problems by enhancing the patient's insight and by facilitating healthier, more adult functioning.

In its loosest form, called *insight-oriented* or *psychodynamic psychotherapy*, therapist and patient meet once or twice a week and, facing each other, discuss both childhood and pragmatic (or "reality") issues. In contrast, meetings occur three to five times a week in formal psychoanalysis, often for many years, and the therapist is out of view of the reclining patient (see a Woody Allen film for more information).

Supportive psychotherapy.   In *supportive psychotherapy*, the therapist actively offers support to the patient instead of encouraging the development of insight per se. The therapist helps the patient understand what behaviors are appropriate and inappropriate, encourages him or her to view problems from other perspectives, provides reassurance, and offers practical advice and assistance to help the patient develop social and other skills. Supportive therapy often incorporates *patient education* about mental disorders as well.

Therapy with a spiritual focus, often performed by *pastoral counselors*, incorporates a religious perspective into supportive therapy and is particularly helpful for patients wrestling with spiritual dilemmas.

Brief therapy.   *Brief therapy* has become a favorite of managed care companies because it involves a smaller financial outlay than most other techniques (in fact, in their applications for provider membership, many managed care organizations ask the clinician to define the term *brief therapy* to be sure they're up to speed). Brief therapy centers on discrete topics or conflicts, and the number of visits is typically etched in stone at the onset. Practitioners of brief therapy are more confrontational and directive in this form of treatment, always keeping the patient "on target." Smaller changes in personality and behavior are anticipated than with therapies that are lengthy and more costly.

Interpersonal psychotherapy.   *Interpersonal psychotherapy* is a standardized form of short-term therapy in which the emphasis is on very active exploration of current interpersonal relationships. Techniques to improve these relationships—to make them more satisfying for everyone involved—are taught and advocated.

Behavior therapy.   Clinicians who practice *behavior therapy* believe that behavior can change in impressive ways without the patient's having to develop insight into its foundations. A variety of behavioral techniques are used to encourage or discourage certain behaviors or to uncouple anxious feelings from provocative situations. This form of therapy is often most effective when the problem behaviors or feelings are quite circumscribed. A few subtypes of behavior therapy follow:

Token economies, sometimes established for entire wards or therapeutic residences, involve the dispensing of rewards for positive, prosocial behaviors. For instance, adolescent inpatients who have complied with the unit schedule might receive tokens that they can redeem for bonuses such as passes and special privileges.

Aversion therapy is just as it sounds. In this variant of behavior therapy, an unpleasant stimulus such as a mild electrical jolt or a noxious smell is coupled with an inappropriate behavior. Severely retarded individuals who incessantly beat or bite themselves have sometimes responded to aversive stimuli as objectively innocuous as a light mist of water sprayed at their faces. In other cases, rather than being directly punished, patients are encouraged to envision an unpleasant event unfolding from an improper behavior. Aversion therapy that goes beyond imagination alone is forbidden in many treatment settings because some feel it legitimizes the potential abuse of patients.

Another behavioral technique, *systematic desensitization*, is described in detail in Chapter 1. Patients with fears of certain stimuli (e.g., snakes) or situations (e.g., eating in public) are asked to conjure up increasingly anxiety-producing situations, tolerating the anxiety until it dissipates on its own or via the use of relaxation exercises. Systematic desensitization can also incorporate real-life exposures (e.g., viewing or handling a snake or going out to a crowded, fast-paced diner).

Flooding, also described in Chapter 1, in a case involving noise phobia, exposes a patient to the very situation of which he or she is most afraid. While enduring this worst-case scenario, the patient's anxiety eventually will start to ebb, and so the patient learns that the devastating consequences he or she expects don't actually occur. In a variation of full-blown flooding, the frightening situation or object is vividly imagined all at once, without intervening progressive desensitization. This technique, perhaps too descriptively, is termed *implosion*.

Cognitive therapy.   Proponents of *cognitive therapy* maintain that our behavior is the result of what we tell ourselves about ourselves and our roles in the world.

By this reasoning, psychological distress is attributable to "cognitive errors," or distortions in thinking. A patient's cognitive error may lead him or her to equate the statement "I've disappointed my mother" with "I'm no good." Or the patient may believe "I must perform perfectly in order to be a worthwhile person." Cognitive therapy works to challenge and correct these distortions. It is usually time limited, uses homework assignments to facilitate the patient's progress outside sessions, and can be highly effective in patients with mild to moderate depression.

Group therapy. *Group therapy* techniques gained popularity after World War II, when there were simply too many psychiatric casualties to be treated one by one. Today, the types of groups are as various as the psychological issues in people's lives. The current offerings in group therapy span a wide spectrum of formats, themes, and leadership styles. Some focus on singular problems and have a homogeneous membership, whereas others are remarkably diverse. Some are loose, with participants coming and going at will, others highly structured. And some are supportive in orientation, others blisteringly confrontive. Still, a common core of therapeutic factors characterizes all groups. These factors include universality and identification (that is, sharing common values and beliefs); acceptance of and altruism toward one another; a forum to test out beliefs and behaviors; and a place to ventilate pent-up emotions.

Group therapy can range from groups of women struggling to understand the dynamics contributing to their eating disorders to individuals with relationship difficulties who use the group format to practice their communication skills. Group therapy can also help victims of sexual abuse and other trauma. People who have been victimized by rape, other crime, or war may gain a measure of relief by sharing their thoughts and feelings with others who have endured the same crises. Groups for perpetrators such as sex offenders exist as well, sometimes inside prisons. They are called *encounter groups* because they typically involve the members' vigorously challenging each other about their attitudes and beliefs.

Consumer and family support groups. *Consumer and family support groups* technically are not group therapies; however, they use group processes to facilitate growth, reintegration, and recovery. These formats aim to provide mutual support rather than to tease apart and resolve psychological conflicts. Consumers or family members look to each other in a compassionate atmosphere that often mixes education with advice and companionship. Gatherings, projects, and discussions offer means by which consumers can interact socially, enjoying nonjudgmental fellowship. One well-known group is *Alcoholics Anonymous* (AA), in which peer-run meetings are devoted to a single goal: the maintenance of sobriety. Although the characteristics, formats, and even rules of individual AA groups vary considerably, AA has transformed the lives of millions.

Families often find that they, like the patients themselves, are stigmatized by society. When the mentally ill are portrayed on television, for instance, they are almost always fallaciously depicted as violent. The general public then leaps to the conclusion that there must have been something terribly wrong within the family itself that caused such an egregious outcome. Support groups for families offer a means of dealing with stigma and coming to terms with the feelings engendered by having a loved one with mental illness. Such groups have been fostered by the National Alliance for the Mentally Ill (NAMI),[1] the National Depressive and Manic Depressive Association (NDMDA),[2] and the National Mental Health Association (NMHA).[3]

Advocacy groups stimulate patients and family members to champion the rights of those with mental illnesses. These groups work to inform their members and the public, encourage—and fund—research, and lobby decision makers. For example, NAMI has instituted a five-year antistigma campaign that entails programs for public enlightenment.

Marital therapy.   In *marital therapy*, the relationship is the patient. This type of therapy involves the identification of marital problems. It also offers the spouses feedback from the therapist and regular opportunities to practice new, healthier ways to solve relationship problems.

Family therapy   *Family therapy* is often based on the central assumption that disturbed families are systems that, paradoxically, work to maintain their dysfunction. Therapy helps each member of the family understand the role he or she plays in keeping the system in turmoil. At times, family therapy (or marital therapy) is used to supplement one person's individual treatment. For example, it may be discovered that the efforts at individual treatment of a depressed patient's emotional

---

[1] NAMI, 200 N. Glebe Road, Suite 1015, Arlington, VA 22203; telephone: (800) 950-NAMI; URL: http://www.nami.org/.

[2] NDMDA, 730 N. Franklin St., Suite 501, Chicago, IL 60610; telephone: (312) 642-0049; URL: http://www.ndmda.org/.

[3] NMHA, 1021 Prince St., Alexandria, VA 22314; telephone: (703) 684-7722; URL: http://www.nmha.org/.

problems are being subtly sabotaged by relatives who unconsciously wish to maintain the status quo.

Family counseling, unlike family therapy, has an explicitly didactic focus. The clinician offers the family members education about their loved one's psychiatric illness and treatment, the likely causes of the problem, and the prognosis. He or she will also correct common misconceptions, such as the discredited idea that parents can induce schizophrenia in their offspring through improper child rearing. Finally, the counselor teaches practical coping strategies and family stress management, emphasizing the need for family members to care for themselves and avoid escaping through drugs or denial.

Hypnotherapy. *Hypnotherapy* has been used as a therapeutic tool in patients who are troubled yet cannot allow the escape of their conflicted thoughts and feelings. Retrieval of early memories through hypnotherapy is extremely unreliable (see Chapter 4) however. Some patients have reported success in using hypnosis to combat problem habits such as smoking or overeating.

Psychosocial rehabilitation. *Psychosocial rehabilitation* is an important adjunct to medications for those with serious mental illnesses. Whereas medications target distressing symptoms, psychosocial rehabilitation helps patients increase their motivation and their opportunities for socialization. For example, "drop-in centers" provide relaxed atmospheres fostering social interactions. Educational, prevocational, and vocational offerings include sheltered workshops, in which clients learn the basic expectations of employment, and vocational rehabilitation, in which training, job placement, and on-the-job counseling services are available.

Choosing A Professional

All human relationships that involve meaningful exchanges possess qualities much like a musical composition. In the interactions that occur, patterns evolve that are harsh or pleasing, discordant or harmonious. The relationship between therapist and patient is no exception. But how do patients and their families know which mental health professional is most likely to stimulate a balanced and satisfying outcome? What factors should guide consumers in choosing a therapist? As we have shown, there are myriad philosophies and approaches in treating mental illness. Having a large range of options brings comfort to some patients, whereas others find such an array taxing and confusing. These choices can be narrowed first by identifying the right category of professional to treat a particular problem and then by asking the right questions about the proposed treatment.

Mental Health Professionals

Many of the disorders described in this book, particularly in more severe forms, require treatment with medications as well as counseling. As a physician, the *psychiatrist* is the only mental health professional specifically trained in both the medical and emotional aspects of mental illness. A psychiatrist can prescribe medication and, if necessary, hospitalize patients. In cases involving severe symptoms, a psychiatrist is often the logical choice. *Clinical psychologists* are master's- or doctoral-level professionals who also have expertise in diagnosing and treating mental disorders, although they cannot prescribe medication. They are often consulted to administer tests (such as the Minnesota Multiphasic Personality Inventory, or MMPI) that help them construct psychological profiles of patients. Like psychiatrists, psychologists generally have training in psychotherapy and may be a good choice for patients who do not need close monitoring of medications. *Counselors* include social workers, psychiatric nurses, and others who are trained in helping patients and families cope with their problems. In addition to providing supportive counseling, these professionals can be an excellent resource for patients needing assistance with housing, social outlets, vocational rehabilitation, and other services involved in mental health rehabilitation. Their services are usually less costly than those offered by psychiatrists or psychologists.

Persons seeking professional help should look for a clinician who is licensed and certified in his or her area of practice. Some states do not offer licensure for particular types of counselors or therapists, making an informed choice more difficult. In the absence of licensing laws, individuals should seek a referral from a trusted professional, such as a family doctor. Caveats and considerations relating to therapy practices can be found at the end of Chapter 4.

Appropriate Questions

How the professional functions will have an enormous impact on the satisfaction of the patient and family as well as the treatment outcome. Asking specific questions up front can assist patients and families in making the best choices. In addition to queries about the clinician's training and experience, the following questions (adapted from Agnes Hatfield's 1991 book *Coping with Mental Illness in the Family*) are examples of those that will guide consumers in making reasonable treatment selections:

■ What are the expected benefits, risks, and alternatives to the proposed treatment?

- How often will the plan of treatment be reviewed and adjusted if necessary?
- For how long is it anticipated that treatment will be needed?
- Will the professional's services be covered by the patient's particular insurance?
- Will information have to be provided to a managed-care or other entity for payment to occur? Will the patient's insurance constrain the treatment options?
- Are there other treatments that might work just as well at less cost?
- What options exist for payment of outstanding balances?
- Will the clinician usually be available if crises arise? Can the family initiate contact during a crisis?
- If the patient consents, will the clinician explain his or her diagnosis and prognosis to the family?
- Will guidelines be provided to the family about how best to respond to the patient at home and in the community?
- Does the clinician welcome the input of family members and friends about the patient's behavior and progress?

The Medication Arsenal

When we first meet them, some of our patients announce that they "just have nerves." We try to disabuse them of the idea that the cure is to be found in "pulling themselves out of it" or "keeping a stiff upper lip." But this pervasive belief—the all-too-common misimpression that lies of the mind are due to a lack of willpower—has rendered the use of psychiatric medications a bit politically incorrect. Many ask, "Why *should* someone need the 'crutch' of a medication? Shouldn't people be able to cope on their own?" or "We *all* have problems—you don't see *me* taking anything, do you?"

Tyrone (as told by Marc)

I constantly have heart-to-heart discussions with patients, such as Tyrone, who can scarcely endure their psychiatric problems any longer, yet refuse to take a medication that would almost certainly help. All too often, any medication I suggest is instantly dismissed as a crutch. The irony is that Tyrone, like so many others, had been using horrific amounts of alcohol to numb his pain, never viewing this uncontrolled form of self-medication as a crutch.

When Tyrone finally relented and agreed to a medication trial, he voiced the deep fear that "the boss will find out. I'll be canned. He won't stand for it." A few sessions later, however, he returned, saying, "You'll never believe it. The boss caught me as I was about to take my pill. Just as I was about to sputter some sort of excuse, *he pulled out his own bottle*. We're on the same thing! He's suffered with depression too!" With more than 21 million people world-wide having taken fluoxetine (Prozac), just one of the many psychiatric medications available, these coincidences are becoming more and more commonplace.

Regardless of the naysayers, the availability of effective medications has proved to be an extraordinary weapon in the arsenal against mental illness. Nonetheless, we admit that medications are both wonderful and terrible: doctors, patients, and family members must understand that the trade-off to the emotional improvement is the potential for side effects and even for life-threatening complications if the medication is misused.

We'll demonstrate the range of available medications by detailing the options for three of the most common psychiatric maladies: depression, bipolar disorder (also called manic-depression), and psychosis. As we have illustrated in our case reports in the preceding chapters, the standard medications for these three conditions may at times have an important place in the treatment of each of the lies of the mind.

Medications for Depression

Patients suffering from depression are continually sad or at least unable to experience pleasure. They may also have to endure poor concentration, marked changes in sleep and appetite, diminished motivation and energy, tearfulness, hopelessness, and/or suicidal thoughts. Fortunately, depression is among the most treatable of all the mental disorders. Studies have shown that antidepressants alone work in up to 80% of the patients who use them, generally by increasing the availability of norepinephrine and/or serotonin. Moreover, because there are several different classes of antidepressants, if one doesn't work, another probably will. Because antidepressants typically take three to six weeks to work, however, patients must not stop taking them even if improvement isn't nearly so prompt as they would have liked. Depression develops over a period of time; reversing it takes time too.

We'll outline the main classes of antidepressants below:

Tricyclic antidepressants.   The *tricyclic antidepressants* (TCAs), such as amitriptyline (Elavil), imipramine (Tofranil), and doxepin (Sinequan), have been on the market for many years. We can measure the blood levels of some of the TCAs, so that we can adjust the dose until it results in a level that we know is highly correlated with improved mood. These guideposts to dosing can be invaluable.

On the other hand, the TCAs influence several different neurotransmitters, and their broad effects are mirrored in a rather extensive list of possible side effects. At times, we can usefully exploit the side effects; for example, their sedating properties are terrific for people who can't sleep. At other times, the side effects, particularly those due to their anticholinergic actions (remember the case of Bert?), can be troublesome. Their tendency to dry people's mouths can result in a telltale clicking sound as people speak. Older individuals may develop *orthostatic hypotension* as a result of TCA use: if they stand up too fast, they feel swimmy-headed and are at risk of falling.

Any of these side effects can be so aversive that patients quietly stop taking the pills. TCAs are also highly dangerous if excessive amounts are consumed, so they're rarely sensible choices for suicidal patients.

Monoamine oxidase inhibitors.   The   *monoamine   oxidase   inhibitors* (MAOIs), introduced in the mid- to late 1950s, are becoming quaint. They attained popularity as antidepressants though actually they were introduced to treat other conditions. As reports of euphoria began to be offered by patients whose tuberculosis was being treated with early MAOIs, the antidepressant properties of this class of drugs were soon recognized.

These pharmacologic senior citizens (which include phenelzine [Nardil] and tranylcypromine [Parnate]) are indeed effective antidepressants. They work to increase the levels of neurotransmitters in the brain by inhibiting the enzymes that would otherwise degrade them. Unfortunately, because of the chemistry of the MAOIs, patients who take them must abstain from, or at least restrict intake of, foods containing the amino acid *tyramine*. Whereas not too many people would mourn the loss of fava beans, lovers of strong cheeses and aged sausages would never be candidates for the MAOIs. Patients who dabble in tyramine while taking MAOI antidepressants are at risk for an enormous rise in blood pressure. Patients on MAOIs must also avoid certain classes of medications, including some cold preparations and painkillers. In a sensational New York case that garnered national attention, an 18-year-old college student named Libby Zion, who had been taking phenelzine for depression, died after doctors gave her an injection of a narcotic called meperidine (Demerol). The medical situation was made even more treacherous by her reportedly having abused cocaine as well.

Even with careful use, side effects from MAOIs can include the orthostatic hypotension noted above, as well as muscle twitching and weight gain. Still, for the patient who has responded well to MAOIs in the past or has failed other medication trials, a selection from this class of antidepressants can make good sense.

Serotonin reuptake inhibitors.   The *serotonin reuptake inhibitors* (SRIs) are among the most widely publicized antidepressants on the market. What other class of antidepressant has graced the cover of *Newsweek*—twice, no less? Since the introduction of the first SRI, fluoxetine (Prozac), they have become enormously popular, even more so with the arrival of variants such as sertraline (Zoloft) and paroxetine (Paxil).

SRIs are reputed to effect changes in personality (turning a Type A person into a Type B), and therefore they've been both lauded and chided as "designer drugs" or "cosmetic pharmacology." But only 10% of those on Prozac will experience the dramatic transformations touted in Dr. Peter Kramer's bestseller *Listening to Prozac*. Similarly, their reputations have been enhanced in some circles and derided in others due to their increasing use in pets—to quell Sparky the dog's compulsive paw licking, perhaps, or Frasier the parrot's overzealous feather grooming.

In humans, and presumably the rest of the animal kingdom, these medications have a fairly selective effect in increasing the availability of the influential brain neurotransmitter serotonin. They generally have mild side effects: the SRIs are every bit as effective as the older antidepressants but not nearly so sedating or anticholinergic. When an SRI's side effects do intrude, they usually involve activation (jitteriness), headaches, stomach upset, or sexual dysfunction. Unlike the TCAs and MAOIs, they are not toxic to the heart, even in overdose; indeed, it is virtually impossible to overdose fatally on these medicines if they're taken by themselves. A joke, probably funny only to psychiatrists and pharmacologists, is that the lone way to kill a laboratory rat with an SRI is to bury it alive in it. However, these medications can never be taken along with MAOIs, and they can sharply hoist the levels of TCAs if they're taken together.

Other antidepressants.   Other effective antidepressants are constantly emerging. Considering the ubiquity of depression, it's no wonder that drug manufacturers are enthusiastically pursuing the development of newer and better antidepressants. One entry, venlafaxine (Effexor), increases the availability of both serotonin and norepinephrine, which has been shown to improve mood. Among the many others that have their proponents are trazodone (Desyrel), nefazodone (Serzone), bupropion (Wellbutrin), and mirtazapine (Remeron).

Electroconvulsive Therapy

Before we highlight the medications useful in other disorders, we need to mention ECT, as we have in several of our case descriptions and elsewhere in this chapter. As currently practiced, ECT is at least as effective as medications in relieving depression, and it usually works a lot faster.[+] In her book *Undercurrents: A Therapist's Reckoning With Depression*, clinical psychologist Martha Manning describes her personal battle with severe depression. Manning, an informed consumer to say the least, reports that ECT succeeded where medications had failed, rescuing her from the very brink of suicide. Testimonials such as hers are helping to eradicate the heedless misinformation and prejudice that greeted former vice presidential candidate Thomas Eagleton's 1972 disclosure that he had received ECT years earlier.

A course of ECT usually consists of six or more treatments over two to four weeks. After the ECT ends, the patient is either placed on an antidepressant to help prevent relapse or given "maintenance ECT" (a single treatment is delivered at intervals ranging from once a week to every six weeks). Side effects from ECT include headaches and memory loss, although any memory loss usually is transient or inconsequential. Still, around one in 200 patients will have long-term memory problems, a risk to which we must alert them during the process of informed consent.

An exciting development on the scientific horizon is *transcranial magnetic stimulation*. This experimental technique applies magnetic force to targeted areas of the brain to alleviate depression, without requiring the anesthesia or electrical impulses involved in ECT.

Luther [as told by Jackie]

Several years ago, a man named Luther was admitted to my service at a VA hospital. Mute and unresponsive, Luther had stopped eating and drinking. He also moved so slowly that, when we removed the pillow from behind his head to complete the physical exam, it took a full 10 seconds for his head to hit the bed.

We had to get the admission information from Luther's family, a charming group from rural North Carolina. "Daddy," as he was called by everyone, had

---

[+] In addition, ECT can be useful in treatment-refractory mania, catatonia, and schizophrenia; in situations in which medication treatment must be avoided; and in other conditions that have not responded to conventional therapies.

been doing fairly well until recently. It then seemed that "Daddy was on the go-down." A man who had had a smile for everyone, he now became increasingly short tempered and highly critical of his two sons, who worked with him on their small tobacco farm. His energy waxed and waned, as did his appetite. His wife would wake to find him prowling the house with a shotgun, whispering that he was sure someone was following him.

The final blow came when he disappeared. The family finally located him in the chicken coop, weeping and wringing his hands, moaning that something was wrong: "God hasn't answered my prayers," he kept repeating. "I want Him to carry me to heaven." His wife and sons had consoled him that night but decided that he needed to see a doctor—even though he looked reasonably fit. They got especially upset when Luther didn't have enough fight to resist their suggestion; in the past, he had ignored their entreaties to get help even when he was terribly ill.

Shortly after his arrival on the ward, it was clear that he was desperately depressed and needed immediate treatment. We didn't feel that he could last the several weeks it would take antidepressant medications to work. We suggested the option of ECT.

The family was outraged. No one wanted to subject Daddy to that. They had all seen *One Flew Over the Cuckoo's Nest*. No, they couldn't allow us to do it. Daddy himself was in no shape to agree or disagree.

Days passed and Luther's only caloric intake was from the dextrose in his IV fluids. His weight was dropping and so were our hopes. Desperate, we called another family conference, and this time everyone showed up: the patient's wife ("Momma"), the two sons, a niece, their "Granny," and all the members of our treatment team. The family asked us to start the conference with a prayer. It proved to be very elaborate, continuing for several minutes with many pronouncements of "Amen!" and "Yes, don't ya know that!"

We explained Daddy's situation again. If we didn't provide some form of treatment quickly, there was a real chance that he would die. Momma offered that maybe it was Daddy's time to die and go to the Lord. I argued that he was suffering from an illness that could be treated. I added, fighting fire with fire, that God had given us the ideal treatment for Daddy, which was ECT.

Again, they prayed for a while, but ultimately Momma still refused. The whole family rose to leave, but then the older son, who had seemed to be harboring a secret throughout the conference, spoke up.

"No, Momma," he said. "We *need* to do this." He looked ashamed. "I hate to say this, but . . . I'm not *ready* to be the man of the house. We need to do this not just for Daddy but for me."

"Do you really feel that way, son?" she asked. "Really and truly?" He nodded. "Well then, I guess we gotta do it." Within seconds, impelled not by medical authority but by the power of the boy's discomfort, she had entirely reversed her position. She immediately signed the formerly taboo consent form.

Fortunately, Luther responded wonderfully. Soon his mood, energy, and thinking were back to normal. We discharged him on the day before Thanksgiving, and he came back to the clinic for follow-up right before Christmas.

This was the Daddy everyone knew. A Santa-like figure with twinkling eyes dressed in a red vest, he gave me a big hug and kiss. But Momma pulled me aside and timidly asked if we could "get him just a little sick again." It turns out that not only had his energy improved, but Daddy's libido—long bridled by depression—was as active as it had ever been. Instead of somehow encouraging him to get depressed again, we were able to offer brief marital counseling and sex education. My contacts back in the Tarheel State tell me they've lived together happily ever since.

Medications for Bipolar Disorder (Manic-Depression)

Lithium is currently the most commonly used treatment for bipolar disorder, having been approved by the Food and Drug Administration back in 1970. Although various hypotheses have been offered to explain the efficacy of lithium, there still is no consensus on just how it works. For the more than two million Americans who suffer from the disorder, however, all that really matters is that it is effective in 70% to 80% of patients who comply with the prescribed regimen.

Because each dose of lithium is eliminated almost entirely by the kidneys, we have to check the patient's renal functioning periodically. Most practitioners will also follow with thyroid function tests and white blood cell counts, because lithium has been known to affect these indices. The doctor will check the level of lithium in the patient's bloodstream frequently at first but only intermittently once the level is stable and appropriate.

Patients and family members will also need to be educated about lithium dos and don'ts (*do* drink plenty of fluids; *don't* abruptly change salt consumption; *do* beware of diuretics or other fluid depleting medications; *don't* routinely use over-the-counter analgesics such as ibuprofen without checking with the doctor). If a patient's lithium level gets too high, he or she may experience slurred speech, hazy thinking, and a staggering gait. In cases in which the lithium level for some reason has gone through the roof, even more serious side effects can result.

Mr. Henry (as told by Marc)

Mr. Henry was a 56-year-old factory worker with a long history of bipolar disorder. His usual daily dose of lithium controlled his mood swings very well—so well, in fact, that he thought that perhaps the diagnosis itself was wrong and that he didn't need to continue the medication. Predictably, he became manic again. Admitted to the hospital, he was quickly restarted on his usual lithium dose.

Unfortunately, the manicky Mr. Henry was so busy racing around the unit that he ate and drank almost nothing. He became dehydrated and, in response, his kidneys essentially shut down like a nuclear reactor trying to abort a meltdown. With nowhere to go, the lithium in his bloodstream shot up. Mr. Henry became delirious, staggering from his bed and shouting obscenities in slurred speech.

We hurriedly transferred Mr. Henry to the intensive care unit, where he was repleted with fluids. With his dehydration reversed, the lithium was gently restarted—obviously with heightened vigilance to his eating and drinking. His wife brought him cherry slushes, his favorite, to encourage him.

Fortunately, Mr. Henry fully recovered. Shortly before his discharge, as we reviewed the events of his hospitalization, we both admitted that we had learned a valuable lesson: lithium is a very effective medicine but, like bipolar disorder itself, it can be very dangerous. We should never be complacent about either of them.

Other medications that are prescribed for some bipolar disorder patients are valproic acid (Depakote) and carbamazepine (Tegretol), although both are more commonly used to treat patients with seizure disorders. Once again, the precise way in which they work is not well understood. Each has its own side effects but can be uniquely effective for some individuals.

Medications for Psychosis

Once the physician is reasonably sure that there isn't a reversible physical cause for a patient's delusions, hallucinations, or bizarre behavior, he or she can select from a growing list of antipsychotic medications. Generally these medications are employed in conjunction with one or more of the psychotherapy techniques mentioned earlier. They can be miraculously helpful in reducing or even abolishing the psychotic symptoms, allowing the patient to work much more effectively in therapy and resume a functional and satisfying life.

There are three fundamental kinds of antipsychotic medications on the market: *low-potency, high-potency,* and *new* antipsychotics. The low-potency medications, so named because a patient needs to take a greater number of milligrams for them to be effective, include such drugs as chlorpromazine (Thorazine). Possible side effects include sedation, dry mouth, and the orthostatic hypotension described earlier.

High-potency antipsychotic medications are plentiful. An example is haloperidol (Haldol). The high-potency drugs sometimes induce side effects such as muscle stiffness or restlessness. Very infrequently, they can cause much more obvious side effects such as *oculogyric crisis* (eyes rolling back) or *torticollis* (twisting of the neck muscles). Although these dramatic problems are almost immediately reversible with a counteracting medication, they can be quite sudden and frightening. For that reason, the doctor will monitor the patient especially closely early on and be ready to offer a different type of antipsychotic if necessary.

Tardive dyskinesia (TD) is a side effect that can occur with both the low- and high-potency antipsychotics, typically if a patient needs to remain on large amounts for many years. TD consists of involuntary actions that range from very subtle motions of the tongue, mouth, or fingers to jerking or rhythmic movements.

The standard antipsychotic medications are of tremendous value in decreasing the so-called *positive* symptoms of psychosis—active symptoms such as hallucinations and delusions. However, many patients experience *negative* symptoms characterized by the absence of energy, motivation, the desire to socialize, and even emotion. Newer antipsychotic medications such as clozapine (Clozaril), risperidone (Risperdal), and olanzapine (Zyprexa) are being touted for being better able to treat the negative symptoms and/or carrying with them a much lower risk of tardive dyskinesia. However, they can have other side effects. Clozapine, for example, carries with it a small chance of suppressing the body's formation of white blood cells. Until we acquire more clinical experience with these medications, we have to view them as new and *probably* improved.

Ezra [as told by Jackie]

Ezra was a 30-year-old man with a long history of schizophrenia. He had been diagnosed at age 17 with symptoms so troublesome that he had been unable to continue high school. By the time I met him, Ezra had been on standard antipsychotic medications for 13 years. These worked well in controlling his positive symptoms but had no impact at all on his negative symptoms. As a result of these symptoms, Ezra passed the days without purpose, watching TV, smoking cigarettes, and occasionally helping his sister around the house.

Clozapine, which could have improved his condition, was not covered by government health plans, and Ezra was unable to afford it on his own. When an even newer antipsychotic, olanzapine, was approved for state funding, Ezra came to see me. Although he was anxious about changing his medication, he wanted to feel better, and with my encouragement he agreed to try olanzapine.

After only two months on the new drug, Ezra returned a changed man.

His positive symptoms of paranoia and hallucinations remained well under control. More importantly, Ezra's symptoms of apathy and lack of energy began subsiding.

I watched as Ezra began stepping out into the world. He enrolled in GED classes and soon took a part-time job in landscaping. He also shyly admitted that he had met an attractive woman with whom he was attending church. At the age of 30, Ezra was just beginning to explore life in a way that most of us take for granted.

Not all patients experience such dramatic turnarounds, but new medications such as olanzapine continue to inspire hope for more fulfilling lives.

Hospitalization

When and why?   Despite our best efforts to forestall it, psychiatric hospitalization becomes indispensable at times. The structure of the hospital can help insulate patients from the stressors impinging upon them, simultaneously providing support and continuous medical and nursing care. Hospitalization usually is reserved for patients whose suicidal wishes, hostile impulses, or other symptoms and behaviors are becoming uncontrolled and for those for whom less intensive forms of treatment are not working well enough.

The inpatient stay can range from a day or two for acute stabilization to many weeks if protracted care is needed to address the patient's difficulties. For example, some patients require evaluation and treatment of concurrent emotional and physical problems, substance abuse, and inadequate housing. In response to the increasing vigor of managed care in the United States, however, hospital stays are decreasing in length, a trend not likely to end anytime soon. Simultaneously, the extent of the progress that can be made during hospitalization itself will diminish, and the emphasis will be on continued outpatient management.

For patients who need close attention but still can function safely in their own home settings, partial hospitalization and day treatment programs can be useful alternatives to an inpatient stay. Patients attend these programs for up to eight hours per day, returning home to practice skills they have learned. Medication adjustment can take place, but not with the continual observation possible in the hospital.

Miriam (as told by Jackie)

I vividly remember Miriam from my days as a resident because she was hospitalized on my service for almost a full year. At the time of admission, Miriam had been overcome by her fears and delusions, most of them focused on her certainty that people were repulsed by her and were going to abandon her. She had become intensely suicidal and was literally starving herself to death.

Even as the staff and I administered constant care to Miriam, we often found ourselves unable to halt her regression. At several points, her refusal to eat escalated into a refusal to drink as well—not even water. She seemed to collapse into herself, eventually refusing to talk and breaking her silence only to write an occasional note.

For the first 10 months, Miriam was so persistently suicidal that staff members, like guards on watch, took turns sitting next to her for 24 hours a day. When the observation was momentarily interrupted on Christmas Day, Miriam grabbed a bottle of Clorox, swigging it in an abortive suicide attempt. As her regression only worsened, she even stopped swallowing her own saliva. In response, we had to place a nasogastric (NG) tube—through her nose, down her esophagus, and into her stomach—so she could be fed. Her mouth had to be suctioned constantly, and she was reduced to wearing diapers due to incontinence.

As time passed, her behavior, incredible already, became even more bizarre. Day by day, she began to drop her head down toward the floor until eventually her chin seemed glued to her chest. I can still see her walking down the hall with a nurse on one side and the IV pole on the other; from the back, she looked headless. We tried everything we could think of to brace her neck and hold her chin up, ultimately settling on a four-post steel brace. But even *that* wasn't enough. The front sides of two of her vertebra eventually fused because of her bowed head.

Although she was no longer communicating, I resolved to provide Miriam with psychotherapy every day. At times, I was essentially talking to myself during the sessions, but I firmly believed that the consistency of my attention would be a decisive factor if she were ever to get well. We also provided therapy to her family at least once a week.

Finally, after so many months of care and exhausting work on everyone's part, Miriam showed a few flickers of improvement. She gained weight, slowly at first, then more quickly. We encouraged her to begin to care for herself and she was able to do so in stages. The NG tube came out. She dressed normally. She began to talk. Even her head came up—as far as it could, given the changes to her bone structure.

At the end of that year of hospitalization, Miriam emerged a different person, much better able to deal in a healthy fashion with life's demands. When I admitted her, I never could have predicted the happy outcome.

I think about Miriam even more in these days of managed care, as the lengths of hospitalizations are inexorably whittled down. Miriam was critically ill and she needed constant care. And that care took time. If we hadn't been able to treat her over such a long period, I would have been able to offer not just a prediction but a virtual guarantee: she would have spent the rest of her days in a nursing home or the back wards of a state hospital—*if* she had lived. The results over time have continued to be immensely gratifying: I know from mutual friends that Miriam got married, attended college, and is now busy rearing her four-year-old daughter.

▌ Conclusion

Prevention is always preferable to cure. But considering the complicated and diverse physiologic, genetic, psychological, and environmental factors continually being identified as bases for mental illnesses, it is doubtful that they can be prevented altogether. Smallpox has been wiped from the face of the earth. Victories over schizophrenia and other serious mental illnesses will not come so swiftly and decisively.

But our ability to address lies of the mind has never been stronger. We have learned from the past. Developments in assessment and treatment are coming faster than ever before. Primary care doctors, such as family practitioners and internists, are learning how to detect and treat some of the more common and mild mental disorders. And the public is starting to lift the veil of stigma and secrecy that has hidden mental symptoms for so long.

We have infused this book with quotations we love, and we conclude with a final one. In 1711, British essayist Joseph Addison wrote, "What sculpture is to a block of marble, education is to a human soul." This book represents our own deeply felt contribution to others about what our patients have taught us. With them, we have explored the secret passageways and hidden alcoves of the mind, tiptoed up its staircases, and proceeded into its shadowy rooms—and we have discovered that the mind is not a haunted house but a resplendent castle.

REFERENCES AND SUGGESTED READINGS

THIS LIST OF REFERENCES and suggested readings is not intended to be conclusive, nor does it embrace every source of information to which we had access while writing this book. It is only a starting point; after all, the last word has not yet been said or written on any of the mental phenomena described in this book. For general information about these or other psychiatric topics, the reader is also referred to the following:

American Psychiatric Association: *Diagnostic and Statistical Manual of Mental Disorders*, 4th Edition. Washington, DC, American Psychiatric Association, 1994

Dunner DL (ed): *Current Psychiatric Therapy*. Philadelphia, PA, W. B. Saunders, 1997

Gabbard GO, Atkinson SD (eds): *Synopsis of Treatments of Psychiatric Disorders*, 2nd Edition. Washington, DC, American Psychiatric Press, 1996

Grohol JM: *The Insider's Guide to Mental Health Resources Online*. New York, Guilford Press, 1997

Kaplan HI, Sadock BJ (eds): *Concise Textbook of Clinical Psychiatry*. Baltimore, MD, Williams & Wilkins, 1996

Perry PJ, Alexander B, Liskow BL: *Psychotropic Drug Handbook*, 7th Edition. Washington, DC, American Psychiatric Press, 1997

▍Introduction

Carrese JA, Rhodes LA: Western bioethics on the Navajo reservation. Benefit or harm? *Journal of the American Medical Association* 274:826–829, 1995

Cui X-J, Vaillant GE: Antecedents and consequences of negative life events in adulthood: a longitudinal study. *American Journal of Psychiatry* 153:21–26, 1996

Doskoch P: The mind of the militias. *Psychology Today*, July-August 1995, p 12

Ely E: The physiology of insight. *Psychiatric Times*, September 1995, pp 29–31

Ford CV: *Lies! Lies!! Lies!!! The Psychology of Deceit*. Washington, DC, American Psychiatric Press, 1996

Ghaemi SN, Pope HG Jr: Lack of insight in psychotic and affective disorders: a review of empirical studies. *Harvard Review of Psychiatry* 2:22–33, 1994

Hutson HR, Anglin D, Kyriacou DN, et al: The epidemic of gang-related homicides in Los Angeles County from 1979 through 1994. *Journal of the American Medical Association* 274:1031–1036, 1995

Kelly C: ASU journalist admits faking story. *Arizona Republic*, November 29, 1994, p A1

Kessler RC, McGonagle KA, Zhao S, et al: Lifetime and 12-month prevalence of DSM-III-R psychiatric disorders in the United States: results from the National Comorbidity Survey. *Archives of General Psychiatry* 51:8–19, 1994

McEnroe C: Amnesia: ah, fragile memory, the linchpin of identity. *Hartford Courant*, October 2, 1995, p E1

Mezzich JE, Kleinman A, Fabrega H Jr, et al: *Culture and Psychiatric Diagnosis: A DSM-IV Perspective*. Washington, DC, American Psychiatric Press, 1996

Murabito JM: Women and cardiovascular disease: contributions from the Framingham Heart Study. *Journal of the American Medical Women's Association* 50:35–39, 55, 1995

Ormel J, VonKorff M, Ustun TB, et al: Common mental disorders and disability across cultures. *Journal of the American Medical Association* 272:1741–1748, 1994

Patel V: Explanatory models of mental illness in sub-Saharan Africa. *Social Science and Medicine* 40:1291–1298, 1995

Roberts G, Owen J: The near-death experience. *British Journal of Psychiatry* 153:607–617, 1988

Schiller L, Bennett A: *The Quiet Room: A Journey Out of the Torment of Madness*. New York, Warner Books, 1995

Shorter E: *A History of Psychiatry: From the Era of the Asylum to the Age of Prozac*. New York, John Wiley & Sons, 1997

Stampp K: *The Peculiar Institution: Slavery in the Ante-Bellum South*. New York, Vintage Books, 1956

Stern KS: *A Force Upon the Plain: The American Militia Movement and the Politics of Hate*. New York, Simon & Schuster, 1996

Storr A: *Feet of Clay: The Power and Charisma of Gurus*. New York, Free Press, 1996

Tseng W-S, Streltzer J (eds): *Culture and Psychopathology: A Guide to Clinical Assessment*. New York, Brunner Mazel Publishers, 1997

Wahl OF: *Media Madness: Public Images of Mental Illness*. New Brunswick, NJ, Rutgers University Press, 1995

Wells KB, Stewart A, Hays RD, et al: The functioning and well-being of depressed patients: results from the Medical Outcomes Study. *Journal of the American Medical Association* 262:914–919, 1989

■ One

Blore DC: Treating a miner with underground phobia. *British Journal of Nursing* 2:1017, 1021, 1993

Davey G (ed): *Phobias: A Handbook of Theory, Research, and Treatment*. New York, John Wiley & Sons, 1997

Davis S: Aliya angst. *Hadassah Magazine*, May 1995, pp 34–36

Flynn TM, Taylor P, Pollard CA: Use of mobile phones in the behavioral treatment of driving phobias. *Journal of Behavior Therapy and Experimental Psychiatry* 23:299–302, 1992

Genova P: The coming polarization of psychotherapy. *Psychiatric Times*, May 1995, pp 18–19

Hayes J: Biblio-maniac. *MPLS-St. Paul Magazine*, November 1994, p 64

Houlihan D, Schwartz C, Miltenberger R, et al: The rapid treatment of a young man's balloon (noise) phobia using *in vivo* flooding. *Journal of Behavior Therapy and Experimental Psychiatry* 24:233–240, 1993

Interview: Dr. Brian Weiss. *Omni*, April 1994, p 85

Jacobsen PB: Treating a man with needle phobia who requires daily injections of medication. *Hospital and Community Psychiatry* 42:877–878, 1991

Juster HR, Heimberg RG, Holt CS: Social phobia: diagnostic issues and review of cognitive behavioral treatment strategies. *Progress in Behavior Modification* 30:74–98, 1996

Kirmayer LJ: The place of culture in psychiatric nosology: taijin kyofusho and DSM-III-R. *Journal of Nervous and Mental Disease* 179:19–28, 1991

Lindemann C: *Handbook of the Treatment of the Anxiety Disorders*. Northvale, NJ, Jason Aronson, 1996

Marshall JR: Integrated treatment of social phobia. *Bulletin of the Menninger Clinic* 59 (suppl A):A27–37, 1995

Nicholson PJ, Vincenti GEP: A case of phobic anxiety related to the inability to smell cyanide. *Occupational Medicine* 44:107–108, 1994

Pam A, Inghilterra K, Munson C, et al: Agoraphobia: the interface between anxiety and personality disorder. *Bulletin of the Menninger Clinic* 58:242–261, 1994

Rapaport MH, Paniccia G, Judd LL: A review of social phobia. *Psychopharmacology Bulletin* 31:125–129, 1995

Ritchie EC: Treatment of gas mask phobia. *Military Medicine* 157:104–106, 1992

Rosenbaum JF, Biederman J, Pollock RA, et al: The etiology of social phobia. *Journal of Clinical Psychiatry* 55 (suppl 6):10–16, 1994

Ross J: Social phobia: the consumer's perspective. *Journal of Clinical Psychiatry* 54 (suppl 12):5–9, 1993

Rothbaum BO, Hodges LF, Kooper R, et al: Effectiveness of computer-generated (virtual reality) graded exposure in the treatment of acrophobia. *American Journal of Psychiatry* 152:626–628, 1995

Singer LT, Ambuel B, Wade S, et al: Cognitive-behavioral treatment of health-impairing food phobias in children. *Journal of the American Academy of Child and Adolescent Psychiatry* 31:847–852, 1992

Stein MB, Walker JR, Forde DR: Public-speaking fears in a community sample: prevalence, impact on functioning, and diagnostic classification. *Archives of General Psychiatry* 53:169–174, 1996

Sved-Williams AE: Phobic reactions of mothers to their own babies. *Australian and New Zealand Journal of Psychiatry* 26:631–638, 1992

When fear takes control. '*Teen*, January 1995, p 24

Whitby P, Allcock K: *Spider Phobia Control* (software). Gwent, Wales, Gwent Psychology Services, 1994

▐ Two

Barsky AJ, Borus JF: Somatization and medicalization in the era of managed care. *Journal of the American Medical Association* 274:1931–1934, 1995

Barsky AJ, Cleary PD, Sarnie MK, et al: The course of transient hypochondriasis. *American Journal of Psychiatry* 150:484–488, 1993

Bohr TW: Fibromyalgia syndrome and myofascial pain syndrome: do they exist? *Neurologic Clinics* 13:365–384, 1995

Bowman ES: Psychodynamics and psychiatric diagnoses of pseudoseizure subjects. *American Journal of Psychiatry* 153:57–63, 1996

Chaturvedi SK, Michael A: Do social and demographic factors influence the nature and localisation of somatic complaints? *Psychopathology* 26:255–260, 1993

The compleat hypochondriac. *The Economist*, May 6, 1989, pp 79–80

Cooke P: They cried until they could not see. *The New York Times Magazine*, June 23, 1991, p 23

Feldman MD, Ford CV: *Patient or Pretender: Inside the Strange World of Factitious Disorders*. New York, John Wiley & Sons, 1995

Fichtner CG, Pechter BM, Jobe TH: Pisa syndrome mistaken for conversion in an adolescent. *British Journal of Psychiatry* 161:849–852, 1992

Hodgman A: I had liposuction. *New York Magazine*, October 10, 1994

Hollander E, Cohen LJ, Simeon D: Body dysmorphic disorder. *Psychiatric Annals* 23:359–364, 1993

Israel B: Disease du jour. *Harper's Bazaar*, March 1994, pp 141–142

Kellner R: Hypochondriasis and somatization. *Journal of the American Medical Association* 258:2718–2722, 1987

Kellner R: *Psychosomatic Syndromes and Somatic Symptoms*. Washington, DC, American Psychiatric Press, 1991

Klinghoffer D: Postscript: a hypochondriac writes. *National Review*, December 13, 1993, p HC15

Lowry D: The curse of hypochondria. *Cosmopolitan*, February 1994, pp 122–123

Micozzi MS (ed): *Fundamentals of Complementary and Alternative Medicine*. New York, Churchill Livingstone, 1996

Noyes R Jr, Holt CS, Kathol RG: Somatization: diagnosis and management. *Archives of Family Medicine* 4:790–795, 1995

Phillips KA, McElroy S: Insight, overvalued ideation, and delusional thinking in body dysmorphic disorder: theoretical and treatment implications. *Journal of Nervous and Mental Disease* 181:699–702, 1993

Phillips KA, McElroy SL, Keck PE, et al: Body dysmorphic disorder: 30 cases of imagined ugliness. *American Journal of Psychiatry* 150:302–308, 1993

Pilowsky I: *Abnormal Illness Behavior*. New York, John Wiley & Sons, 1997

Silver FW: Management of conversion disorder. *American Journal of Physical Medicine and Rehabilitation* 75:134–140, 1996

Spiegel D, Kato PM: Psychosocial influences on cancer incidence and progression. *Harvard Review of Psychiatry* 4:10–26, 1996

Spiegel D, Bloom JR, Kraemer HC, et al: Effect of psychosocial treatment on survival of patients with metastatic breast cancer. *Lancet* 2:888–891, 1989

Stone AB: Treatment of hypochondriasis with clomipramine. *Journal of Clinical Psychiatry* 54:200–201, 1993

Veale D, Boocock A, Gournaky, et al: Body dysmorphic disorder: a survey of fifty cases. *British Journal of Psychiatry* 169:196–201, 1996

Warwick HMC, Marks IM: Behavioural treatment of illness phobia and hypochondriasis: a pilot study of 17 cases. *British Journal of Psychiatry* 152:239–241, 1988

Watson CG, Buranen C: The frequency and identification of false positive conversion reactions. *Journal of Nervous and Mental Disease* 167:243–247, 1979

Wessely S, Chalder T, Hirsch S, et al: Psychological symptoms, somatic symptoms, and psychiatric disorder in chronic fatigue and chronic fatigue syndrome: a prospective study in the primary care setting. *American Journal of Psychiatry* 153:1050–1059, 1996

Wolf M, Birger M, Shoshan J, et al: Conversion deafness. *Annals of Otology, Rhinology and Laryngology* 102:349–352, 1993

Woodbury MM, DeMaso DR, Goldman SJ: An integrated medical and psychiatric approach to conversion symptoms in a four-year-old. *Journal of the American Academy of Child and Adolescent Psychiatry* 31:1095–1097, 1992

Wool CA, Barsky AJ: Do women somatize more than men? Gender difference in somatization. *Psychosomatics* 35:445–452, 1994

▌ Three

Appelbaum PS, Greer A: Who's on trial? Multiple personalities and the insanity defense. *Hospital and Community Psychiatry* 45:965–966, 1994

Associated Press: Rape trial costs $14,732. *Wisconsin State Journal*, January 22, 1991, p 3D

Cohen LM, Berzoff JN, Elin MR (eds): *Dissociative Disorders: Theoretical and Treatment Controversies*. Northvale, NJ, Jason Aronson, 1995

Ganaway GK: Hypnosis, childhood trauma, and dissociative identity disorder: toward an integrative theory. *International Journal of Clinical and Experimental Hypnosis* 43:127–144, 1995

Gorney C: The many faces of S: a question of rape; trial begins in case of woman who claims 18 personalities. *Washington Post*, November 6, 1990, p E1

Kapur N: Amnesia in relation to fugue states—distinguishing a neurological from a psychogenic basis. *British Journal of Psychiatry* 159:872–877, 1991

Keller R, Shaywitz BA: Amnesia or fugue state: a diagnostic dilemma. *Developmental and Behavioral Pediatrics* 7:131–132, 1986

Kluft RP: Clinical presentations of multiple personality disorder. *Psychiatric Clinics of North America* 14:605–629, 1991

Kluft RP: The use of hypnosis with dissociative disorders. *Psychiatric Medicine* 10:31–46, 1992

Merskey H: Multiple personality disorder and false memory syndrome. *British Journal of Psychiatry* 166:281–283, 1995

Ofshe R, Watters E: *Making Monsters: False Memories, Psychotherapy and Sexual Hysteria*. New York, Charles Scribner's Sons, 1994

Patwatikar SD, Holcomb WR, Menninger KA 2d: The detection of malingered amnesia in accused murderers. *Bulletin of the American Academy of Psychiatry and the Law* 13:97–103, 1985

Piper A Jr: *Hoax and Reality: The Bizarre World of Multiple Personality Disorder*. New York, Jason Aronson, 1997

Piper A Jr: Multiple personality disorder. *British Journal of Psychiatry* 164:600–612, 1994

Platte M: Attorney wins $114,800 in assault she can't recollect. *Los Angeles Times*, November 23, 1990, p A41

Putnam FW: Recent research on multiple personality disorder. *Psychiatric Clinics of North America* 14:489–502, 1991

Richeport MM: The interface between multiple personality, spirit mediumship, and hypnosis. *American Journal of Clinical Hypnosis* 34:168–177, 1992

Riether AM, Stoudemire A: Psychogenic fugue states: a review. *Southern Medical Journal* 81:568–571, 1988

Sarbin TR: On the belief that one body may be host to two or more personalities. *International Journal of Clinical and Experimental Hypnosis* 43:163–183, 1995

Shapiro M: Missing adults: painful question for families. *Washington Post*, October 23, 1983, p A1

Smith WH: Incorporating hypnosis into the psychotherapy of patients with multiple personality disorder. *Bulletin of the Menninger Clinic* 57:344–354, 1993

Spanos NP: *Multiple Identities and False Memories: A Sociocognitive Perspective*. Washington, DC, American Psychological Association, 1996

Spiegel D, Cardena E: Disintegrated experience: the dissociative disorders revisited. *Journal of Abnormal Psychology* 100:366–378, 1991

Torem MS: Therapeutic writing as a form of ego state therapy. *American Journal of Clinical Hypnosis* 35:267–276, 1993

∎ Four

Appelbaum PS, Uyehara LA, Elin MR (eds): *Trauma and Memory: Clinical and Legal Controversies*. New York, Oxford University Press, 1997

Appelbaum PS, Zoltek-Jick R: Psychotherapists' duties to third parties: *Ramona* and beyond. *American Journal of Psychiatry* 153:457–465, 1996

Bauer PJ: What do infants recall of their lives? Memory for specific events by one- to two-year-olds. *American Psychologist* 51:29–41, 1996

Bikel O (producer): "Innocence Lost: The Verdict." *Frontline*, PBS, July 20–21, 1993

Bikel O (producer): "Divided Memories." *Frontline*, PBS, April 11 and 18, 1995

Bikel O (producer): "The Search for Satan" (R. Dretzin, coproducer). *Frontline*, PBS, October 24, 1995

Biology enters the repressed memory fray. *Journal of the American Medical Association* 272:1725–1726, 1994

Ceci SJ, Loftus EF, Leichtman MD, et al: The possible role of source misattributions in the creation of false beliefs among preschoolers. *International Journal of Clinical and Experimental Hypnosis* 42:304–320, 1994

Crews F and his critics: *The Memory Wars: Freud's Legacy in Dispute*. New York, New York Review of Books, 1995

Galloway P: Cardinal mourns death of his former accuser. *Chicago Tribune*, September 23, 1995, NEWS section, p 5

Garry M, Loftus EF: Pseudomemories without hypnosis. *International Journal of Clinical and Experimental Hypnosis* 42:363–378, 1994

Godley E: My mother abused me, didn't she? *Modern Woman*, January 1994

Hudak E: Autism communication device was less than it seemed. *Detroit Free Press*, October 31, 1993, p 2G

Loftus E, Ketchum K: *The Myth of Repressed Memory: False Memories and Allegations of Sexual Abuse*. New York, St. Martin's Press, 1994

McHugh P: Psychiatric misadventures. *The American Scholar*, Autumn 1992, pp 497–510

Morain D: Recovered memory murder case unravels. *Los Angeles Times*, December 25, 1995, p A1

Morain D: Father to be retried in recovered memory case. *Los Angeles Times*, January 19, 1996, p A3

Nathan D, Snedeker MR: *Satan's Silence: Ritual Abuse and the Making of a Modern American Witch Hunt*. New York, BasicBooks, 1995

Ofshe RJ, Singer MT: Recovered-memory therapy and robust repression: influence and pseudomemories. *International Journal of Clinical and Experimental Hypnosis* 42:391–410, 1994

Pendergrast M: *Victims of Memory: Incest Accusations and Shattered Lives*. Hinesburg, VT, Upper Access Books, 1996

Rogers ML: Factors to consider in assessing adult litigants' complaints of childhood sexual abuse. *Behavioral Sciences and the Law* 12:279–298, 1994

Rosen M, Podolsky JD: Out of this world: a Harvard psychiatrist believes that alien abductions are real. *People Weekly*, May 23, 1994, p 41

Salem revisited: satanic abuse. *The Economist*, August 31, 1991, p A23

Schacter DL: *Searching for Memory*. New York, BasicBooks, 1996

Shales T: Vicious psyche. "Frontline's" frightening look at regression therapy. *Washington Post*, April 4, 1995, p E1

Shapiro J: See me, hear me, touch me. *U.S. News and World Report*, July 27, 1992, pp 63–64

Smith G: Unspeakable secret: what happened on the night Michael Shea can neither forget nor believe? *Washington Post Magazine*, January 3, 1988, p W12

Taylor J: The lost daughter. *Esquire*, March 1994, pp 74–87

Wakefield J, Underwager R: Recovered memories of alleged sexual abuse: lawsuits against parents. *Behavioral Sciences and the Law* 10:483–507, 1992

[We also wish to acknowledge issues of Psychiatric Times and the False Memory Syndrome Foundation Newsletter too numerous to list. The address and URL for the FMS Foundation can be found in Chapter 4. The address for Psychiatric Times is CME, Inc., 1924 E. Deere Avenue, Santa Ana, CA 92705.]

▮ Five

Abed RT, Fewtrell WD: Delusional misidentification of familiar inanimate objects. *British Journal of Psychiatry* 157:915–917, 1990

Bernstein RL, Gaw AC: Koro: proposed classification for DSM-IV. *American Journal of Psychiatry* 147:1670–1674, 1990

Buchanan A: Acting on delusion: a review. *Psychological Medicine* 23:123–134, 1993

Butler RW, Braff DL: Delusions: a review and integration. *Schizophrenia Bulletin* 17:633–647, 1991

Feldman MD, Davidson ME: The self-mutilating patient: the contribution of psychiatric consultation. *Resident and Staff Physician* 34:69–71, 74, 1988

Fishbain DA, Barsky S, Goldberg M: "Koro" (genital retraction syndrome): psychotherapeutic interventions. *American Journal of Psychotherapy* 43:87–91, 1989

Gaines AD: Culture-specific delusions. Sense and nonsense in cultural context. *Psychiatric Clinics of North America* 18:281–301, 1995

Garety PA, Hemsley DR: *Delusions: Investigations into the Psychology of Delusional Reasoning*. New York, Oxford University Press, 1994

Kourany RFC, Williams BV: Capgras' syndrome with dysmorphic delusion in an adolescent. *Psychosomatics* 25:715–717, 1984

Menuck MN. Differentiating paranoia and legitimate fears. *American Journal of Psychiatry* 149:140–141, 1992

Miller LJ: Psychotic denial of pregnancy: phenomenology and clinical management. *Hospital and Community Psychiatry* 41:1233–1237, 1990

Miller LJ, Forcier K: Situational influence on development of delusions of pregnancy in a man. *American Journal of Psychiatry* 149:140, 1992

Opler LA, Klahr DM, Ramirez PM: Pharmacologic treatment of delusions. *Psychiatric Clinics of North America* 18:379–391, 1995

Rhoads JM, Kamaraju LS, Feldman MD: The unforgivable sin: a theologian's dilemma and a psychiatrist's challenge. *Psychiatric Forum* 14:54–58, 1988

Shengold L: *Delusions of Everyday Life*. New Haven, Yale University Press, 1995

Silva JA, Leong GB: Syndrome of exchanged doubles. *American Journal of Psychiatry* 38:368, 1993

Silva JA, Leong GB, Luong MT: Split body and self: an unusual case of misidentification. *Canadian Journal of Psychiatry* 34:728–730, 1989

Silva JA, Leong GB, Shaner AL, et al: Syndrome of intermetamorphosis: a new perspective. *Comprehensive Psychiatry* 30:209–213, 1989

Silva JA, Leong GB, Weinstock R: Delusions of transformation of the self. *Psychopathology* 26:181–188, 1993

Spier SA: Capgras' syndrome and the delusions of misidentification. *Psychiatric Annals* 22:279–285, 1992

Tateyama M, Asai M, Kamisada M, et al: Comparison of schizophrenic delusions between Japan and Germany. *Psychopathology* 26:151–158, 1993

▌ Six

Al-Issa I: The illusion of reality or the reality of illusion: hallucinations and culture. *British Journal of Psychiatry* 166:368–373, 1995

Allen JR: Salicylate-induced musical perceptions. *New England Journal of Medicine* 313:642–643, 1985

Asaad G, Shapiro B: Hallucinations: theoretical and clinical overview. *American Journal of Psychiatry* 143:1088–1097, 1986

Baker PB, Cook BL, Winokur G: Delusional infestation: the interface of delusions and hallucinations. *Psychiatric Clinics of North America* 18:345–361, 1995

Boudewyns PA: Posttraumatic stress disorder: conceptualization and treatment. *Progress in Behavior Modification* 30:165–189, 1996

Carter JL: Visual, somatosensory, olfactory, and gustatory hallucinations. *Psychiatric Clinics of North America* 15:347–358, 1992

Chadwick P, Birchwood M: The omnipotence of voices: a cognitive approach to auditory hallucinations. *British Journal of Psychiatry* 164:190–201, 1994

Cinbis M, Aysun S: Alice in Wonderland syndrome as an initial manifestation of Epstein-Barr virus infection. *British Journal of Ophthalmology* 76:316, 1992

de Leon J, Antelo RE, Simpson G: Delusion of parasitosis or chronic tactile hallucinosis: hypotheses about their brain physiopathology. *Comprehensive Psychiatry* 33:25–33, 1992

Dening TR, West A: The Dolittle phenomenon: hallucinatory voices from animals. *Psychopathology* 23:40–45, 1990

Fisman M: Musical hallucinations: report of two unusual cases. *Canadian Journal of Psychiatry* 36:609–611, 1991

Goodard J: Analysis of 11 cases of delusions of parasitosis reported to the Mississippi Department of Health. *Southern Medical Journal* 88:837–839, 1995

Harcourt P: Imaginary images: an examination of Atom Egoyan's films. *Film Quarterly*, Spring 1995, p 2

Hoehn-Saric R: Hallucinatory changes. *American Journal of Psychiatry* 154:293–294, 1997

Kanazawa A, Hata T: Coexistence of the Ekbom syndrome and lilliputian hallucination. *Psychopathology* 25:209–211, 1992

Lait M: Judge sentences DeHoyos to death. *Los Angeles Times*, August 28, 1993, p B6

Linn EL: Verbal auditory hallucinations: mind, self, and society. *Journal of Nervous and Mental Disease* 164:8–17, 1977

Lynch R: Lawyer claims crime itself proves DeHoyos is insane. *Los Angeles Times*, May 26, 1993, p B6

Morgan CA, Grillon C, Southwick SM, et al: Exaggerated acoustic startle reflex in Gulf War veterans with posttraumatic stress disorder. *American Journal of Psychiatry* 153:64–68, 1996

Nayani TH, David AS: The auditory hallucination: a phenomenological survey. *Psychological Medicine* 26:177–190, 1996

Post SG: Psychiatry, religious conversion, and medical ethics. *Kennedy Institute of Ethics Journal* 1:207–223, 1991

Reyes-Ortiz CA, Camacho ME, Mulligan T: Charles Bonnet syndrome in a centenarian. *Journal of the American Medical Association* 276:451–452, 1996

Rogers R, Nussbaum D, Gillis R: Command hallucinations and criminality: a clinical quandary. *Bulletin of the American Academy of Psychiatry and the Law* 16:251–258, 1988

Siegel RK: *Fire in the Brain*. New York, Dutton, 1992

Spivak B, Livnat E, Weizman A, et al: True conversive hallucinations. *Psychopathology* 24:19–24, 1991

Spivak B, Trottern SF, Mark M, et al: Acute transient stress-induced hallucinations in soldiers. *British Journal of Psychiatry* 160:412–414, 1992

Stoll AL, Oepen G: Zinc salts for the treatment of olfactory and gustatory symptoms in psychiatric patients: a case series. *Journal of Clinical Psychiatry* 55:309–311, 1994

Webster E: Cold courage: hallucinations, high winds and views like this made a new route up Everest a bittersweet test of will. *Sports Illustrated*, January 16, 1989, p 62

Weller M, Wiedemann P: Visual hallucinations: an outline of etiological and pathogenetic concepts. *International Ophthalmology* 13:193–199, 1989

▌ Seven

Ali-Gombe A, Guthrie E, McDermott N: Mass hysteria: one syndrome or two? *British Journal of Psychiatry* 168:633–635, 1996

Bannon L: Bazaar gossip: how a rumor spread about subliminal sex in Disney's "Aladdin." *Wall Street Journal*, October 24, 1995, p A1

Bartholomew RE: Redefining epidemic hysteria: an example from Sweden. *Acta Psychiatrica Scandinavica* 88:178–182, 1993

Bartholomew RE: *Mass Hysteria: A Social History of the Strange*. Durango, CO, Hollowbrook, 1995

Black DW: Iatrogenic (physician-induced) hypochondriasis: four patient examples of "chemical sensitivity." *Psychosomatics* 37:390–393, 1996

Bove RX: A textbook panic caused big bank selloff of 1990. *American Banker*, February 25, 1992, p 1

Boxer P: Occupational mass psychogenic illness. History, prevention, and management. *Journal of Occupational Medicine* 27:867–872, 1985

DeJonge J: Media blamed for clean gas hysteria. *Capital Times* (Madison, Wisconsin), September 20, 1995, p 1C

Desenclos JC, Gardner H, Horan M: Mass sociogenic illness in a youth center. *Revue d'Epidemiologie et de Santé Publique* 40:201–208, 1992

Dunn M: Taken for a ride by radio UFO tale. *Philadelphia Inquirer,* April 2, 1988, p B3

Fenton J: The disease of all diseases. *The New York Review of Books,* December 1, 1994, p 48

Gorman T: Lab suggests mystery fumes answer. *Los Angeles Times,* November 4, 1994, p A1

Göthe C-J, Molin C, Nilsson CG: The environmental somatization syndrome. *Psychosomatics* 36:1–11, 1995

Hefez A: The role of the press and the medical community in the epidemic of mysterious gas poisoning in the Jordan West Bank. *American Journal of Psychiatry* 142:833–837, 1985

Hill F: *A Delusion of Satan: The Full Story of the Salem Witch Trials.* New York, Doubleday, 1995

Lee RLM, Ackerman SE: The sociocultural dynamics of mass hysteria: a case study of social conflict in West Malaysia. *Psychiatry* 43:78–88, 1980

Mass hysteria mars the music. *Science News,* September 21, 1991, p 187

Massey EW, Brannon WL Jr, Riley TL: The "jerks": mass hysteria or epilepsy? *Southern Medical Journal* 74:607–609, 1981

Modan B, Swartz TA, Tirosh M, et al: The Arjenyattah epidemic: a mass phenomenon: spread and triggering factors. *Lancet* 2:1472–1474, 1983

Rothman AL, Weintraub MI: The sick building syndrome and mass hysteria. *Neurologic Clinics* 13:405–412, 1995

Scanlan D: Stolen children: a child-snatching hysteria sweeps the country. *Maclean's,* April 18, 1994, p 36

Shore JH: Transcultural research run amok or Arctic hysteria? *American Indian and Alaska Native Mental Health Research* 2:46–50, 1989

Showalter E: *Hystories: Hysterical Epidemics and Modern Culture.* New York, Columbia University Press, 1997

Sirois F: Epidemic hysteria. *Acta Psychiatrica Scandinavica* 252 (suppl):1–46, 1974

Small GW, Borus JF: The influence of newspaper reports of outbreaks of mass hysteria. *Psychiatric Quarterly* 58:269–278, 1987

Small GW, Nicholi AM Jr: Mass hysteria among schoolchildren: early loss as a predisposing factor. *Archives of General Psychiatry* 39:721–724, 1982

Stiehm ER: The psychological fallout from Chernobyl. *American Journal of Diseases of Children* 146:761–762, 1992

Wessely S: Mass hysteria: two syndromes? *Psychological Medicine* 17:109–120, 1987

Wilson M: Fall to grace. *St. Petersburg Times,* July 9, 1995, p 1F

▌ Final Thoughts

Ablow KR: *Anatomy of a Psychiatric Illness: Healing the Mind and the Brain*. Washington, DC, American Psychiatric Press, 1993

Andreasen NC: *Schizophrenia: From Mind to Molecule*. Washington, DC, American Psychiatric Press, 1994

Berrios G, Porter R (eds): *The History of Clinical Psychiatry: The Origin and History of Psychiatric Diseases*. New York, New York University Press, 1996

Bowden CL: Role of newer medications for bipolar disorder. *Journal of Clinical Psychopharmacology* 16 (suppl 1):48S–55S, 1996

Burns DD: *The Feeling Good Handbook: Using the New Mood Therapy in Everyday Life*. New York, W. Morrow, 1989

Engler J, Goleman D: *The Consumer's Guide to Psychotherapy*. New York, Fireside/Simon & Schuster, 1992

Galt JM: *The Treatment of Insanity*. New York, Harper, 1846

Gorman JM: *The Essential Guide to Psychiatric Drugs*. New York, St. Martin's Press, 1992

Grob G: *The Mad Among Us: A History of the Care of America's Mentally Ill*. New York, Free Press, 1994

Group for the Advancement of Psychiatry: *A Family Affair: Helping Families Cope With Mental Illness*. Washington, DC, American Psychiatric Press, 1987

Hales D, Hales RE: *Caring for the Mind: The Comprehensive Guide to Mental Health*. New York, Bantam Books, 1995

Hatfield AB: *Coping With Mental Illness in the Family: A Family Guide*, Revised Edition. Arlington, VA, National Alliance for the Mentally Ill, 1991, pp 24–25

Hatfield AB, Lefley HP: *Surviving Mental Illness: Stress, Coping, and Adaptation*. New York, Guilford Press, 1993

Inglehart JK: Managed care and mental health. *New England Journal of Medicine* 334:131–135, 1996

Kane JM: Drug therapy: schizophrenia. *New England Journal of Medicine* 334:34–41, 1996

Lesser H: Consent, competency and ECT: a philosopher's comment. *Journal of Medical Ethics* 9:144–145, 1983

Lewis S, Higgins N (eds): *Brain Imaging in Psychiatry*. Cambridge, MA, Blackwell Science Ltd, 1996

Martensen RL: Caring for the chronically mentally ill. *Journal of the American Medical Association* 273:923, 1995

Sederer LI, Rothschild AJ (eds): *Acute Care Psychiatry: Diagnosis and Treatment*. Baltimore, MD, Williams & Wilkins, 1997

Striano J: *How to Find a Good Psychotherapist: A Consumer Guide*. Santa Barbara, CA, Professional Press, 1987

John Dewey Library
Johnson State College
Johnson Vermont 05656

Styron W: *Darkness Visible: A Memoir of Madness*. New York, Random House, 1990

Swayze VW: Frontal leukotomy and related psychosurgical procedures in the era before antipsychotics (1935–1954): a historical overview. *American Journal of Psychiatry* 152:505–515, 1995

Torrey EF: *Out of the Shadows: Confronting America's Mental Illness Crisis*. New York, John Wiley, 1997

Torrey EF: *Surviving Schizophrenia: A Manual for Families, Consumers, and Providers*. New York, HarperPerennial, 1995

White BJ, Madara EJ: *The Self-Help Sourcebook: Finding and Forming Mutual Aid Self-Help Groups*, 5th Edition. Denville, NJ, Northwest Covenant Medical Center, 1995

Woolis R: *When Someone You Love Has a Mental Illness: A Handbook for Family, Friends, and Caregivers*. New York, JP Tarcher Perigee, 1992

INDEX

ACO 5453

VERMONT STATE COLLEGES

0 00 03 0584894 7

John Dewey Library
Johnson State College
Johnson, Vermont 05656